THE ART OF MIDWIFERY

THE WELLCOME INSTITUTE SERIES
IN THE HISTORY OF MEDICINE

Edited by W.F. Bynum and Roy Porter
The Wellcome Institute

THE ART OF MIDWIFERY

EARLY MODERN MIDWIVES
IN EUROPE

Edited by
Hilary Marland

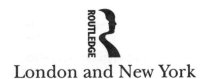

London and New York

First published 1993
by Routledge
11 New Fetter Lane, London EC4P 4EE

Simultaneously published in the USA and Canada
by Routledge
29 West 35th Street, New York, NY 10001

Typeset in 10 on 12 point Baskerville by LaserScript, Mitcham, Surrey
Printed and bound in Great Britain by
Mackays of Chatham PLC, Chatham, Kent

British Library Cataloguing in Publication Data
A catalogue record for this book is available from the British Library

Library of Congress Cataloging in Publication Data
The Art of Midwifery: Early Modern Midwives in Europe/edited by
Hilary Marland.
p. cm. – (The Wellcome Institute series in the history of medicine)
Includes bibliographical references and index.
1. Midwives – Europe – History. I. Marland, Hilary. II. Series.
[DNLM: 1. Midwifery – history – Europe. WQ 11 GA1 A7]
RG950.A69 1993
618.2′0233′094–dc20
DNLM/DLC
for Library of Congress   92-49026
CIP

ISBN 0–415–06425–2

Contents

Contents

Illustrations

Tables

Figure

Contributors

Doreen Evenden is assistant professor in the Department of History at Trent University, Peterborough, Ontario. She is author of *Popular Medicine in Seventeenth-Century England* (Bowling Green State University Popular Press, 1988). Her PhD dissertation 'Seventeenth-century London midwives: their training, licensing and social profile' (McMaster University, 1991) was awarded the Canadian Historical Association prize for the best doctoral thesis (1991) on a non-Canadian topic, and is being prepared for publication with Cambridge University Press. Professor Evenden's current research interests include early modern England, especially London, and female medical practitioners and midwives.

Nadia Maria Filippini lives and teaches in Venice. Her research concerns the history of women, in particular women's work and the history of childbearing. A founder member of the Italian Society of Women Historians (*S.I.S.*), her publications include *Noi, quelle dei campi. Identità e rappresentazione di sé delle contadine veronesi del primo novecento* (Gruppo Editoriale Forma, 1983) and, together with other scholars, *Nascere a Venezia. Dalla Serenissima alla Prima Guerra Mondiale* (Gruppo Editoriale Forma, 1985) and *Le Culture del parto* (Feltrinelli, 1985). She is editor of *Perle e impiraperle. Un lavoro di donne a Venezia tra '800 e '900* (Arsenale, 1989). She has also published extensively in major history journals, *Quaderni Storici, Società e Storia, Memoria. Rivista di Storia delle Donne, Storia e Dossier* and *Sanità, Scienza e Storia,* and is concluding her thesis for the Doctorat en Histoire (3ème cycle) at the École des Hautes Études en Sciences Sociales in Paris, where she was Maître des Conférences during the year 1988–89.

Nina Gelbart is professor of History at Occidental College in Los Angeles, California. She is the author of *Feminine and Opposition Journalism in Old Regime France: Le Journal des Dames* (University of California Press, 1987), which won the Sierra Prize, the 'Introduction' to a new translation of

Fontenelle's *Conversations on the Plurality of Worlds* (University of California Press, 1990), and of articles on Enlightenment utopias, medical journals and radical editors. Professor Gelbart is preparing a biography of the midwife Mme du Coudray, entitled *Delivering the Goods: the Midwife Mission of Mme du Coudray in 18th Century France.* Her current research focuses on the medical press and on Charlotte Corday, the 'saint/assassin' of Marat.

David Harley teaches History in Oxford. He has published several articles on early modern medicine, including a study of the midwife-witch.

Ann Giardina Hess is currently a student at Harvard Medical School. She received a BA in American Studies from Yale College in 1987. She is working towards a PhD in History from Cambridge University, England, for a thesis on local midwifery practice in village and town communities in England and New England, *c.* 1650–1750. During her tenure as a full-time PhD student and Marshall Scholar she was on leave between 1988 and 1991 to work at the Wellcome Unit for the History of Medicine in Oxford.

Helen King took her first degree in Ancient History and Social Anthropology in 1980, and completed a PhD thesis on Hippocratic gynaecology in 1985, both at University College London. Between 1983 and 1986 Dr King held a Henry Sidgwick Research Fellowship at Newnham College Cambridge and in 1986–87 a Sir James Knott Research Fellowship at the University of Newcastle. Since 1988 she has been a lecturer in History at Liverpool Institute of Higher Education. Dr King has published many articles on women in ancient myth and medicine and on the history of gynaecology, and is the author of a section on the history of hysteria from the Greeks to the seventeenth century in S. Gilman, H. King, R. Porter, G. Rousseau and E. Showalter, *Hysteria Before Freud* (University of California Press, forthcoming).

Mary Lindemann is associate professor of History at Carnegie Mellon University and author of *Patriots and Paupers: Hamburg 1712–1830* (Oxford University Press, 1990). She is currently working on a history of health and healing in northern Germany in the seventeenth and eighteenth centuries as well as preparing a volume on *Medicine and Society in Early Modern Europe* for the series 'New Approaches to European History' (Cambridge University Press, forthcoming).

Hilary Marland is author of *Medicine and Society in Wakefield and Huddersfield 1780–1870* (Cambridge University Press, 1987), and together with M.J. van Lieburg and G.J. Kloosterman of *'Mother and Child Were Saved'. The Memoirs (1693–1740) of the Frisian Midwife Catharina Schrader* (Rodopi, 1987). She jointly edited with Valerie Fildes and Lara Marks *Women and Children First.*

International Maternal and Infant Welfare 1870–1945, for the Routledge Wellcome Series in the History of Medicine (1992). She has also published on the history of dispensaries, the nineteenth-century Yorkshire medical profession, chemists and druggists, early Dutch women doctors and Dutch midwifery. Employed as research officer at the Instituut Medische Geschiedenis, Erasmus Universiteit Rotterdam, Dr Marland's interests include the history of preventive medicine in the Netherlands, women medical practitioners, and the history of Dutch midwives 1700–1945. She is holder of a Wellcome Research Fellowship for a project on the Dutch midwifery professions in the twentieth century.

Teresa Ortiz, a graduate in medicine, received a PhD in the history of medicine from the University of Granada in 1987 with a dissertation on the medical profession in twentieth-century Andalucía, *Médicos en la Andalucía del siglo veinte: distribución, especialismo y participación profesional de la mujer* (Fundación Averroes, 1987). Professor Ortiz teaches courses on the history of medicine and women in the health professions at the University of Granada. She is a member of the editorial board of *Dynamis* and of the Women's Studies Group of the University of Granada, and editor of *Feminae*, a series of volumes in women's studies (Granada University Press). With a particular interest in the health professions and women in medicine in Spain in the eighteenth to twentieth centuries, she is currently working on two projects, 'Midwives in Granada in the twentieth century' and 'Health professions in Andalucía in the eighteenth century'.

Merry E. Wiesner is an associate professor of History and director of the Centre for Women's Studies at the University of Wisconsin-Milwaukee. She is author of *Working Women in Renaissance Germany* (Rutgers University Press, 1986), *Women and Gender in Early Modern Europe, 1500–1750* (Cambridge University Press, forthcoming), and a number of articles on women and the Reformation, the relationship between work and gender, and other aspects of early modern German social history.

Acknowledgements

Although an edited volume – so much a joint effort between editor and authors – is perhaps not the most appropriate place to list acknowledgements, it is a pity to waste the opportunity. Thanks go to Bill Bynum and Roy Porter, editors of the Wellcome series, for their encouragement of the project. Gill Davies of Routledge was especially helpful in the early stages of the book, Brad Scott in the latter. I would particularly like to acknowledge the contribution of Maggie Pelling, who has been, from the first idea for the book to its final execution, a source of help, good advice and friendship. I would also like to thank the other colleagues and friends who have helped and kept me going in many different ways while this volume was being prepared: Lara Marks, Rita Schepers, Mart van Lieburg, Frank Huisman, Netty Storm, Erma Hermans and Iona Dekking (and their families), Tini Wiersma, the girls at the *Woezelhuis* and my parents. The authors have all been fantastic, co-operative, supportive and encouraging, especially in the latter stages, as I raced to complete the manuscript before the birth of my second child. But the most important people to thank of course are my husband Sebastian, victim at all times of my balancing acts, and my children Daniel and David.

Abbreviations

Chapter 1

CuRO	Cumbria Record Office
GL	Guildhall Library
GLRO	Greater London Record Office
LPL	Lambeth Palace Library

Chapter 2

BL	British Library
CCRO	Chester City Record Office
CRO	Cheshire Record Office
DM	Diocesan Miscellany
LCRS	Lancashire and Cheshire Record Society
LRO	Lancashire Record Office
PRO	Public Record Office
WRO	Wigan Record Office

Chapter 3

BRO	Buckinghamshire Record Office
CuRO	Cumbria Record Office
DRO	Dorset Record Office
FHL	Friends' House Library
HRO	Hertfordshire Record Office
PRO	Public Record Office

Chapter 4

AStB	Nuremberg Staatsarchiv, Amts- und Standbücher
BMB	Frankfurt Stadtarchiv, Burgermeisterbücher

RB	Nuremberg Staatsarchiv, Ratsbücher
RPB	Memmingen Stadtarchiv, Ratsprotokollbücher
RSP	Munich Stadtarchiv, Ratsitzungsprotokolle

Chapter 5

AGS	Archivo General de Simancas
AMM	Archivo Municipal de Málaga
LAC	Libro de Actas Capitulares

Chapter 6

BL	British Library

Chapter 7

AD	Archives Départmentales
AN	Archives Nationales
MC	Minutier Central

Chapter 8

ASV	State Archives of Venezia
ASVR	State Archives of Verona

Chapter 9

MO 1757	*Serenissimi gnädigste Verordnung, das Hemammenwesen betreffend. De Dato Braunschweig, von 18. Febr, 1757*
StadtB	Stadtarchiv Braunschweig
StAWf	Niedersächsisches Staatsarchiv-Wolfenbüttel

Chapter 10

GAD	Gemeente Archief Delft
GAR	Gemeente Archief Rotterdam
ONGD	Archief van het Oude en Nieuwe Gasthuis te Delft

Introduction

The absorption of midwifery into medical practice is a recent process, a development linked in many western countries with the diminishing role of midwives, the increased involvement of the man-midwife, the general practitioner and the obstetrician in the birthing process and, in the twentieth century, the increased hospitalization of childbirth. While it is generally recognized that the midwife has been with us since biblical times, and that midwifery is the oldest female occupation and without doubt one of the most important, the focus of historical studies has been very much on this process of decline in the midwife's place in obstetric work – on competition between the traditional midwife and her male rivals, the increase in medical intervention and, as the role of women in the birth process diminished, the shift in emphasis in childbirth from the social to the medical sphere.

This volume is concerned with midwives in the period 1400 to 1800, midwives as birth attendants, as women workers, as active members of their communities, as 'missionary' and political figures, and as defenders of their status and occupation against the invasions of male practice. It explores the period before the 'decline' and, if it challenges some of the long-held beliefs about midwives, their lives, work, social standing and place in public life, it will have achieved one of its major objectives.

The essays – covering England, Germany, Holland, France, Italy and Spain – draw on an impressive range of manuscript and printed material – church licensing records, testimonials, parish registers, baptismal rolls and records of birth registration, wills, censuses, court records, municipal ordinances, regulations and licences, midwives rolls, the archives of guilds and medical corporations, religious, political and medico-political pamphlets and obstetric literature. And, if the volume shows the vast number of possibilities in terms of source material for building up a picture of early modern midwife practice, it will have achieved a further objective.

The early modern period was neither a 'golden age' for midwives, nor was it a time when midwifery was practised by aged unskilled crones on a

1

hapless and helpless female population. The poverty of the 'ignorant midwife' theory has been further demonstrated in this volume, as has the notion that most midwives practised with only the most rudimentary knowledge and training. Yet the early modern period was, as the essays show, a period of great diversity, of variation between and within Western European countries, in terms of midwives' practices, skills and competence, their socio-economic background and education, their training and qualification to work, and their public functions and image.

The work of midwives varied greatly – what midwives were allowed by law or custom to do, and what they actually did do. Urban/rural divides were often superimposed on to national contrasts in midwives' practices. Some midwives attended births on an occasional basis, as a form of neighbourly support and female bonding, while others worked steadily at their chosen occupation for the greater part of their lives, earning a regular income. For some women attendance at a childbirth was no more than being a good friend or relation, for others it was perhaps the family's chief source of income.

The first three chapters illustrate this diversity of occupational status and practice in seventeenth- and eighteenth-century England. Doreen Evenden's essay on London midwives, drawing largely on ecclesiastical licensing records, focuses on the relationship between midwives and their clients, giving an insight into how childbearing women perceived those who delivered them (Chapter 1). The importance of 'repeat practice', sometimes stretching across generations, and the relevance of female (and male) networking and recommendations, is demonstrated, as London midwives built up a loyal clientele, often over a wide geographical area. London midwives throughout the seventeenth century attracted clients from a broad social spectrum, and well-to-do women demonstrated active support for their midwives by providing testimonials for licence applications.

In his discussion of midwifery practice in the northern English counties of Lancashire and Cheshire between 1660 and 1760, David Harley reveals great contrasts in the recognition accorded to midwives, and in their licensing and working practices and incomes (Chapter 2). Many midwives, practising on an occasional basis, found it too costly and troublesome to obtain licences; others, working more regularly at their occupation, gained esteem and co-operated closely with local medical practitioners.

The working practices of Quaker midwives in southern rural England in the late seventeenth century are explored by Ann Giardina Hess (Chapter 3). The activities and clientele of Quaker midwives are revealed through the unique system of Quaker birth registration, which listed birth witnesses, giving the opportunity to investigate the nature of neighbourly, kin and religious ties between parents and midwives. Ann Hess emphasizes the great diversity of practice, from women who attended at just a few births during the course of their lifetime, to those who worked seriously at their occupation, building up a widely distributed clientele and considerable fame across several counties. While clients often used a succession of different midwives, Ann Hess confirms the importance of networking in their selection, and demonstrates how preferences for childbirth attendants could override considerations of religious belief. There was a high level of integration of Quaker and parish women, even amongst the highest social strata, in the delivery room, as both midwives and helpers. Though Quaker midwifery practice was clearly a special case, it also provides a case study of early modern midwife practice, revealing the social exchanges between midwives and their clients.

While some midwives attended only a small number of births, in a number of countries in continental Europe a very different type of midwife was being employed during the early modern period, as a municipal employee undertaking obstetric work on a day-to-day basis, as a long-term career option, which could involve considerable investment in the costs of qualifying and obtaining a licence. The employment practices of town authorities – and the deals for the midwives as municipal employees – in Germany and the Netherlands are explored by Merry Wiesner, Mary Lindemann and Hilary Marland (Chapters 4, 9 and 10). Their conditions of work varied. Merry Wiesner, examining six towns in southern Germany between 1400 and 1800, outlines how midwives' salaries were kept to a minimum, while a stepping up of supervision by the so-called 'honourable women' and the town physicians undermined their status and independence (Chapter 4). In eighteenth-century Braunschweig, midwives were subjected to similar poor conditions of service (Chapter 9), but in the towns of Holland during the seventeenth and eighteenth centuries the picture was one of increased regulation and increased costs of qualifying to practise, but also of rising financial incentives, as the town authorities struggled to respond to a shortage of licensed midwives (Chapter 10). In France, one outstanding midwife, Mme du Coudray, whose life story is outlined by Nina Gelbart, was appointed on a very different basis, as King Louis XV's missionary and teacher, to spread obstetric knowledge and re-educate midwives throughout the French provinces, work she endured for some three decades (Chapter 7).

In all countries, there was enormous variety in the paths taken to setting up in practice as a midwife. David Harley, arguing that midwifery was a skill to be learned by experience and passed on without formal instruction, reveals the often informal and irregular routes to practice in northern England (Chapter 2). Yet in seventeenth-century London apprenticeship, often lengthy, remained important (Chapter 1), while amongst Quaker midwives the system of assisting senior midwives grounded younger women in good midwifery practice (Chapter 3). At a time when the importance of the midwife and her role as childbirth attendant was supposedly diminishing, groups of women were emerging across Europe who had undergone a sometimes extensive formal training. The town authorities and medical hierarchies of continental Europe recognized the need for trained and licensed midwives, fit and competent to practise, who were necessary for the maintenance of a healthy population. In Italy and Spain schools for midwives were established in the eighteenth century, in Holland courses set up during the seventeenth century, given by the towns' medical corporations, were extended in the eighteenth. Yet apprenticeship remained everywhere the norm and key to practice, even in countries where initiatives were being made to educate a new breed of school- or theoretically-trained midwives, and where book-learning was encouraged. Though many 'apprenticed' midwives received no recognition from the authorities, except perhaps that they constituted a danger to the health and welfare of women and the babies they delivered, they frequently enjoyed great popularity, and their skills were still in the eighteenth century often grounded in long apprenticeship with a senior midwife and years of experience.

It is the 'average' midwife, the woman who worked quietly in her community, be it village, town or metropolis, who comes to the fore in this volume. Given the enormous variety in the standing and practices of these women, can we come any closer to defining the early modern midwife? In all the countries covered, midwives shared certain characteristics – most were mature women, married or widowed, who started to practise when they had grown-up families, most were trained by some form of apprenticeship, formal or informal, most were of middling status, the wives of artisans, craftsmen, tradesmen or farmers, for whom the practice of midwifery, though not necessarily vital for the family income, was a useful addition. Several of the essays in this volume suggest that up until the eighteenth century women of considerable social and economic standing practised midwifery, although there was great variation in both directions. David Harley outlines the wide range of social backgrounds of midwives working in Lancashire and Cheshire in the second half of the seventeenth century and first half of the eighteenth – from the prosperous to the very poor who were paid for their midwifery work in lieu of poor relief. Yet many midwives, he argues, especially in the heyday of the seventeenth century, were of considerable social standing, respectable and literate (Chapter 2). These attributes of respectability and literacy were shared by many midwives across Europe during the early modern period.

The essays in this volume emphasize the need for wariness in approaching midwife history from the standpoint of a contest, in which the midwife was ultimately the loser, between female and male obstetric practitioners. The story is a much more complicated one than that of a simple decline from the seventeenth or eighteenth century onwards, of men-midwives moving into childbirth, regarded increasingly as a socially

4

acceptable and potentially lucrative field, armed with their new instruments and social charms, and eventually extending their competence to include normal deliveries. By the mid-eighteenth century, however, changes were afoot in England. While Doreen Evenden demonstrates high levels of loyalty to midwives in London during the seventeenth century, even amongst the affluent (Chapter 1), half a century later in the rural areas of the south and north of England men-midwives were carrying out more deliveries. Men-midwives officiated at Quaker births in the rural south from the 1750s onwards (Chapter 3). David Harley suggests that for a combination of reasons – exploitation by the men-midwives, boasting greater skills and education, the lack of good midwives, and changes in tastes as the social gap between clients and midwives widened – a similar process was under way in the provincial north, where male practitioners were also replacing midwives as expert witnesses (Chapter 2).

Yet, we should be wary of taking the English model as typifying what was going on in the rest of Europe. As Mary Lindemann demonstrates for the case of Braunschweig, little effort was being made to nose midwives out of obstetrics in eighteenth-century German towns (Chapter 9). In Holland, Hilary Marland argues, the stepping up of midwife regulation was geared more towards control and supervision than eliminating midwives or reducing their work-loads; on the contrary, their role as attendants in normal cases of childbirth was assured by the end of the eighteenth century (Chapter 10). Midwives themselves were concerned with issues other than the challenge of male obstetric practice – and they were not afraid to complain about their salaries and status, their duties in the community, questions of citizenship, the poor quality of training, problems between midwives and their apprentices, or annoyance about the incursions of 'quack' midwives (Chapters 4, 9 and 10). Midwives' work was just as much shaped by these issues as by the directives of the town authorities and medical hierarchies.

In Italy, as sketched by Nadia Filippini, a struggle was taking place late in the eighteenth century between the midwife and her male rivals. Yet complicated by the tussle between State and Church authorities, the latter supporting and even arguing for an extension of the midwife's obstetric and moral authority – particularly her role in performing baptisms – and by competition between the school-trained modern midwife and her traditional counterpart, who enjoyed much popular support, the conclusion of the struggle was far from clear by the turn of the nineteenth century (Chapter 8). Similarly, in Spain, as Teresa Ortiz demonstrates, the rise of a group of male practitioners who turned their attention increasingly to obstetric work and the writing of midwifery manuals – backed by Enlightenment ideals, and establishing legal and educational control over midwives by the last quarter of the eighteenth century – did not herald the immediate decline of the midwife (Chapter 5). In France, the sending out of Mme du Coudray in 1759 on her mission to re-educate the midwives of France was hardly symptomatic of a decline in the midwife's role as normal childbirth attendant; it was Mme du Coudray's niece, representing the next generation of midwives working towards the end of the eighteenth century, who was obliged to defend herself and her colleague midwives against the male obstetric practitioner (Chapter 7). In several countries, the impact of new instruments and interventions, especially the obstetric forceps, as Nadia Filippini shows for Italy, was less than we have been led to believe, while midwives themselves were not unfamiliar with the use of instruments (Chapter 8).

Many countries had their own midwife phenomena – Mme du Coudray, unsurpassed for her diligence and energy in re-educating the rural midwives of France (Chapter 7), Catharina Schrader with her great stamina and expertise in difficult childbirth (Chapter 10), the Quaker midwife Frances Kent, renowned amongst her co-religionists and Establishment aristocrats (Chapter 3), Spain's Luisa Rosado, taking on the medical authorities head on, defending her right to practise, to apply her knowledge of difficult childbirth and to administer medicines (Chapter 5), Holland's Van Putten sisters, 'female men-midwives' who crossed the boundaries between old and new, female and male spheres of practice (Chapter 10), and Italy's Teresa Ployant, author of a midwife manual, and keen to better the standards of midwife practice and to defend women's modesty from the 'horrible' interventions of men (Chapter 8).

London's 'Popish midwife', Elizabeth Cellier, is one of Europe's most famed (and infamous) early modern midwives, and Helen King shows how, embroiled in religious, political and medico-political affairs and efforts to set up a college of midwives, she straddled the boundaries between midwifery and politics in Restoration England. Her work and the pamphlets written by Cellier and the rivals who denounced her are used as sources to illustrate enduring positive and negative images of the midwife in seventeenth-century England. The shifting fortunes of Cellier and her highly public image as plotter and midwife gave contemporaries the chance to revive chiefly negative images of the midwife as drunken and lecherous bawd, even consort of the Devil, and has distorted images of the competence of seventeenth-century midwives. But as Helen King argues, we should be wary of reading too much into Cellier's pronouncements; thinking on her feet, shifting course, first advocating a male-supported college of midwives, and later criticizing male obstetric practice, may have been simple survival tactics when it was not a good time to be a Catholic midwife in London (Chapter 6).

How were midwives, famous ones apart, regarded by those they served and by the communities in which they worked? Most, even those with regular practices, had their recognition grounded on other qualities and skills than their work in delivering babies – as expert witness, public functionary, community member. In the period of the midwife's ascendancy, when childbirth, treated as a physiological process, was dominated by social norms and traditions, and was firmly rooted in female culture, the midwife straddled two spheres, helping women in the birthing process and supervising events in the delivery chamber. Ann Hess demonstrates that for Quaker midwives, their public recognition was just as likely to rest on their role as members of women's meetings, senior women in the community, and arbitrators in cases of domestic dispute and cases of sexual misdemeanour, rape, incest, infanticide or physical abuse (Chapter 3). Moral integrity and religious conformity, David Harley argues, were vital in ensuring midwives' suitability to testify in court, to question the mothers of bastard children *in extremis,* to decide on cases of ante-nuptial fornication or infanticide (Chapter 2). In Italy too, the midwife's duties went far beyond that of childbirth attendant; the Church was especially keen to preserve this role and establish authority over her administration of emergency baptisms, which brought the Church into direct conflict with the State authorities in the eighteenth century (Chapter 8).

Similar duties were expected of municipal midwives in south Germany, as explored by Merry Wiesner, who questions if and how midwives were able to bridge the gap between public and private during the early modern period. Midwives' involvement in administering emergency baptisms and reporting on illegitimate births, abortion and infanticide increased between 1400 and 1800 and yet, at the same time, became a cause of increasing anxiety on the part of town authorities concerned to reduce women's involvement in roles deemed 'public'. The duties of midwives examined in the six south German towns provide a counter-example to the notion that the trend was to reduce women's public activities and restrict them to the private domestic sphere in the early modern period. Yet it was a case of necessity. The municipal authorities, Merry Wiesner argues, were prepared to overlook the continuing public role of midwives because of midwives' perceived respectability as lower middle-class citizens and because the work they did was crucial. At the same time, the town councils were minimizing the importance of midwives' role in childbirth; their salaries were kept low, and they were placed increasingly under the control of the municipal and medical authorities (Chapter 4).

Midwives – and not just the more visible and famed ones – were subject to shifting social, economic, political and religious forces, be it the changing fortunes of Catholics in Cellier's Restoration London, the treatment meted out to Quakers, persecuted for non-payment of tithes and refusal to attend to the norms of baptism and churching, the decline in ecclesiastic licensing in England, the major shifts in du Coudray's fortunes as first war and then Revolution swept France, the economic decline of Dutch towns in the eighteenth century, and the tussles between State and Church in Italy and Spain, with the midwife caught between the forces of tradition and change, religious morality and Enlightened government. The areas of struggle which have previously been emphasized between male and female practice, interventionist versus natural childbirth and changes in social demand, were overlaid by wider forces, which could affect the work and status of midwives, even those working quietly in their village or town communities, apparently immune to such great issues and sweeping forces.

Early modern midwives were not administering angels – they were ordinary working women, wage-earners, with a sense of pride in their occupation, though, given the conditions under which childbirth often took place in this period, many midwives must have had special qualities, of patience, forbearance, physical and mental strength, and fellow-feeling. The 'art of midwifery' as practised by midwives across Europe through the early modern period was rich and diverse; the midwife remained throughout the period, the normal attendant in childbirth, and yet her role was much wider. Nor was the midwife a passive victim of events; she adapted, fought back and, though it was clear that the turn of the nineteenth century was going to mark a change, and often decline, in the practice of her art, this change was more subtle, slower to take effect and more complex than we have realized.

1

Mothers and their midwives in seventeenth-century London

Doreen Evenden

Social historians of medicine have been taken to task in recent years for their single-minded concentration on medicine and its practitioners to the exclusion of the consumer of health care services.[1] Previous studies of early modern midwifery have paid scant attention to the identities of midwives' clients and to clients' perceptions of the women who were so intimately concerned with their well-being and that of their infants.[2]

A new archivally-based study of seventeenth-century London midwives has demonstrated that midwives were better trained through an 'un-official' system of apprenticeship served under the supervision of senior midwives than has previously been assumed.[3] The period of empirical training varied, but in many cases, at the time of licensing, midwives could claim an association with one or more senior midwives which had extended from two or three years to several decades. In addition, the study has shown that London midwives were drawn from a higher social and economic stratum than has generally been accepted.[4] Many midwives were married to prosperous and influential parishioners while others were affluent widows; none of the midwives working in the twelve London parishes who were the subjects of an intensive investigation conformed to the stereotype of the ignorant, poverty-stricken crone who dabbled in deliveries to eke out a livelihood.[5] Valuable insights into the work and world of midwives can be gained, moreover, by directing our attention away from the educational or social attainments of London midwives and focusing upon their clientele, a previously undefined constituency.

Hundreds of midwives' testimonial certificates provide the best surviving evidence of the ecclesiastical licensing process in seventeenth-century London and information about the midwives' clientele. These documents were presented to church authorities by aspiring midwifery licensees residing in the metropolis of London and its environs. In addition to the ecclesiastical sources, which also include bishops' and archbishops' registers, the records of an anonymous London midwife who went about her work of child delivery in the waning years of the seventeenth and the

9

early part of the eighteenth centuries (1694–1723) supplement the more impersonal church records at several junctures. A careful examination of these records has permitted insights into the work of London midwives with regard to what we have called 'repeat business', the geographical distribution of their practices, the social standing of their clients, and the client and midwife referral 'system'. Finally, we will hear from the childbearing women themselves what they thought about their midwives.

In assessing the relationship which existed in seventeenth-century London between midwives and clients, among the most illuminating themes to emerge are those of the extent of repeat business and the nature and prevalence of personal referral from satisfied clients to prospective mothers. One might assume that midwifery services in a large cosmopolitan population centre such as London would follow a different pattern from that of the more intimate rural parish. In fact, the evidence points to the existence of long-term and intricate relationships between many London midwives and their clients, similar to what might be found in rural England.[6]

The evidence for repeat business is derived from both testimonial certificates provided by satisfied clients and the anonymous midwife's account book. Testimonial documentation in some cases specified the number of children the midwife had already delivered for the referee; for the year 1662 testimonials for all twenty-four successful candidates recorded the number of children they had delivered for each of the women testifying on their behalf. The account book provides information on the number of deliveries per client, thus giving a reasonable indication of the relationships which existed in late Stuart London between a midwife and her clients. It demonstrates that the midwife routinely carried out her work to the satisfaction of many of her clients who continued to use her services throughout their childbearing years.

Information about the number of deliveries which a prospective licensee had carried out for clients testifying on her behalf is valuable as an indication of the clientele's level of satisfaction with a midwife. The six women delivered by Debora Bromfield of St Andrew Holborn had borne a total of thirty-two children when they supported her application for a midwifery licence in 1663.[7] Elizabeth Philips of St Clement Danes had been delivered of five children by Bromfield; Susan Brownell of the parish of St Andrew Holborn of three children; Susan White of St Martin Ironmonger Lane of four children; Mary Huntley of St Salvator Southwark of seven children, and Elizabeth Boggs of St Benet Paul's Wharf had used Bromfield's services on thirteen occasions. The high degree of confidence which women placed in the skill of their midwives was exemplified by women such as Boggs or by Bridgette Richards, of St Mildred Poultry, who was brought to bed thirteen times by Elizabeth Davis of St Katherine Cree

Church and Martha Marshall, of St Martin in the Fields, who was successfully delivered by midwife Elizabeth Laywood twelve times.[8] In the year 1662 twenty-four midwives presented the sworn testimony of 142 clients; of these, eighty-six clients were delivered more than once by the same midwife, and more than 60 per cent of the deliveries by this group of midwives could be termed 'repeat business'. (For the number of women delivered more than once by the same midwife, see Table 1.1.)

Table 1.1 Frequency of contact between London midwives and clients, 1662 (based on testimonials)

No. of deliveries (same client)	Frequency (percentage)[*]
1	56 (39)
2	35 (25)
3	17 (12)
4	11 (08)
5	13 (09)
6	5 (04)
7	4 (03)
12	1 (0.7)
13	2 (01)

[*] Percentages are approximate, having been rounded off in most cases. There is no indication of whether or not any of the foregoing included multiple deliveries; calculations have assumed the delivery of a single child.

Source: GL MS 10,116/2.

The testimonial evidence sheds light on the extent of repeat business at only a single point in the ongoing relationship between a midwife and a client: the time of an application for licensing. It could be expected that the reliance of many of these women upon a particular midwife would continue, and thus that the actual extent of repeat business would exceed the figures provided above. A general pattern is discernible, confirmed by the account book of the, as yet, unidentified midwife which covers the years 1694 to 1723. During that period, this active midwife attended over 376 clients, more than one-third of whom she delivered several times. In addition to the 243 clients that Mistress X delivered on a single occasion, 433 deliveries involved clients who had previously utilized her services. That is, out of a total of 676 deliveries, 64 per cent involved a client who had used the midwife on more than one occasion. The midwife delivered eight sets of twins (counted as one delivery), and in all but one of these cases the mothers were delivered of other children by Mistress X. At least twenty-two of the clients who used the midwife's services only once did so in the last five years of her recorded practice. This would have decreased the opportunity for repeat business (see Table 1.2).

Table 1.2 Frequency of contact between Mistress X and her clients, 1694–1723 (account book)

No. of deliveries per client	Frequency (percentage)
1	243 (65)[*]
2	48 (13)
3	38 (10)
4	22 (06)
5	10 (03)
6	7 (02)
7	1 (0.2)
8	2 (0.5)
9	3 (0.8)
10	0 (00)
11	1 (0.2)
12	1 (0.2)

[*] Or 192 (58%) excluding the last five years of Mistress X's practice.
In most cases, the percentages have been rounded off. The delivery of twins was counted as one contact.

Source: Bodleian Library, Oxford, Rawlinson MS D 1141.

The majority of Mistress X's clients expressed a high level of confidence in her skills by summoning her repeatedly when they were brought to bed, and they freely recommended her services to other family members. Mrs Page, who used her services three times, told her sister about the midwife who then also became a client.[9] Mrs Duple of Blackfriars was delivered by Mistress X six times between 1703 and 1714; her sister became a client in 1704 and 1706. One of our midwife's most fecund clients, Mrs Dangerfield of Whitechapel, first used her services in July 1699. By March 1712 she had called upon the midwife nine times. Dangerfield's trust in and reliance on her midwife's skills undoubtedly influenced her own sister who became a client of Mistress X in 1713. Mrs Osten, an apothecary's wife, and her sister both placed their confidence in our midwife's abilities. All told, at least six clients referred their sisters to the midwife. Madam Blackabe, an affluent client who had been brought to bed of two sons and two daughters, referred a kinswoman who paid the midwife £4 6s., a handsome remuneration for her services.[10]

The women of the socially prominent and wealthy Barnardiston family showed a similar satisfaction with the midwife's abilities. Six Barnardiston women used her services on a regular basis. Madam Barnardiston from Leytonstone was delivered three times; Madam Barnardiston from 'The Fig Tree' twice; [11] Madam Barnardiston living in 'Cornewell' sought assistance in childbed four times, and Madam Barnardiston of Budge Row used the midwife's assistance on two occasions. Barnardiston women living on Granoch Street and Watlen Street were also delivered by the midwife. In total, fourteen small Barnardistons were brought into the world by the 'family midwife'.

Since several of the anonymous midwife's clients were themselves the daughters of women who had been brought to bed by the midwife, there is every possibility that Mistress X was attending women whom she had brought into the world, a remarkable tribute to the level of confidence and personal rapport she enjoyed. For example, Mrs Tabram of Butcher's Hall Lane was delivered by the midwife four times from 1697; 20 years later, our midwife delivered 'Ms. Tabram's daughter' who was living in Chapter House Lane.[12] Altogether at least nine daughters of former clients were brought to bed by the popular midwife. Two clients, Mrs Maret and Mrs Benet, summoned Mistress X when their serving women gave birth. Other London 'family midwives' who practised in the seventeenth century included Lucy Lodge of St Leonard Shoreditch, licensed in 1663 and supported in her application for a licence by three female members of the Samwaye family, in addition to eleven other women. Judith Tyler of Hendon, Middlesex, who was licensed in 1664, claimed four clients with the surname 'Nicoll'.[13]

London midwives did not restrict their practices to the parish in which they lived, a fact which has hitherto eluded students of seventeenth-century London midwifery, leading to the assumption that midwives carried out too few deliveries to gain the experience necessary for competence. But archival evidence shows, for example, that Bridgid Jake of St Leonard Shoreditch, who presented her testimonials for licensing in 1610, was one of the relatively few seventeenth-century midwives whose six mandatory clients all resided in her home parish.[14] Even this, of course, did not mean that Jake's practice then or in the future was restricted to her own parish. On the other hand, the abundant evidence that midwives seeking licences normally provided references from satisfied clients beyond the boundaries of their own parish demonstrates that, even at that point in their professional career, London midwives practised over a large geographical area. Rose Cumber, licensed in the same year as Jake, presented sworn testimony from women who resided in St Swithin and St Andrew Holborn although she herself resided in St Bridgid Fleet Street.[15] Elizabeth Martin of St Giles Cripplegate called on only one client from her home parish in 1626 when she applied for her licence; women from St Antholin, St Dunstan in the West, St Martin in the Fields and St Michael Pater Noster added their testimonies.[16] In 1629, Alice Carnell of St Dunstan in the West was licensed after presenting evidence from clients, none of whom resided in her parish.[17] The licensing of midwives broke down in the Civil War period but after it was reintroduced in 1661 midwives' clients were distributed much as they had been earlier in the century. Most testimonials indicated that midwives drew their clients from both their own parish and from other parishes. Some midwives found more clients close to home, in adjoining parishes, while others extended their practices far beyond parochial boundaries. In 1664 Ursula Nellham of All Hallows the Great provided testimonial support from women residing in St Dunstan in the West and the easterly parishes of St James Duke's Palace and St Botolph Aldgate, as well as from women of her own City parish which lay along the Thames.[18] While it must be borne in mind that testimonial evidence touched on only a fraction of a midwife's practice, it is still a useful indication of the geographical range of individual midwifery practices.

The account book of our unidentified London midwife, Mistress X, demonstrates a similar mobility and geographical diversity of practice. Although addresses were not recorded in every case, clients from at least thirty parishes within the city walls claimed her services. But these formed only a part of her practice: in the years covered by her records the busy and popular midwife travelled far beyond the confines of the City. To the east, she journeyed to Leytonstone, Spitalfields and Whitechapel where she attended, among others, Mrs Dangerfield in her numerous confinements; to the north, to the area of Finsbury Fields and the northern reaches of the vast ward of Cripplegate Without; to the west, she delivered women in the Strand, the Haymarket and Drury Lane. Among her clients on the South Bank was the prosperous Mrs Sims who was brought to bed five times by the peripatetic midwife. Mistress X's practice encompassed not only the City but almost all of suburban London north of the River Thames as well as Southwark. Her sprawling practice is all the more remarkable in view of the backward state of intra-metropolitan communications. At the same time as the anonymous midwife was travelling ill-lit streets to the numerous night-time confinements which she recorded, one visitor commented that the city was 'a great vast wilderness' in which few were familiar with even a quarter of its streets.[19] In the last year of recorded practice, most of Mistress X's deliveries were in the East End of London or its eastern suburbs, probably close to where the midwife resided. It can be suspected that the shrinking catchment area was a result of ill health or old age.[20] Though there is no way of determining how representative Mistress X was, it is absolutely certain that very few, if any, licensed midwives (of whom more than nine hundred have been uncovered) restricted their practice to a single parish.

There is no evidence that midwives advertised their skills by means of printed advertisements.[21] Word of mouth recommendation by satisfied clients living close to one another apparently played a key role in establishing pockets of women who used the midwife's services, and may explain some of the cases which lay at the geographical periphery of the practice of Mistress X. Mrs Rowden of Drury Lane employed her in March and less than six weeks later a client from nearby Tower Street called on her. On 29 October 1707, Mrs Nicolls of St Martin's Street was delivered; a few days later, on 7 November, Mrs Hampton of the same street called the midwife to her delivery; a month later, Mrs Wood, also of St Martin's Street, was delivered of an infant daughter by Mistress X. Mrs Field and Mrs Hobkins, both of Aldgate Street, were delivered within three days of each other. Also delivered within three days of one another were Mrs Duple's sister (referred by Mrs Duple) and her neighbour, the shoemaker's wife in Swan Yard.[22]

Testimonial evidence suggests that female clients on occasion sought a midwife on the basis of recommendations by women whose husbands were employed in the same craft or trade as that of the prospective father. For example, when Mary Taylor of St Olave Silver Street sought her licence in 1661, of the six clients who supported her application, two were butchers' wives (one from Christ Church parish and one from St Sepulchre) and two were shoemakers' wives, both from different parishes, indicating a link through their spouses' occupations.[23] The following year, Winnifred Allen of St Andrew Wardrobe enlisted the wives of three tailors from two different parishes when she applied for a licence, and Elizabeth Davis of St Katherine Cree Church supplied the names of three women (one of whom had used her services six times), all of whom were married to men employed in the exclusive goldsmith trade. Similarly, among the seven clients sworn for Elizabeth Ayre of St Giles Cripplegate in 1664, Lucy Buffington was the wife of goldsmith John Buffington of the midwife's parish, and Elizabeth Swift was the wife of Abraham Swift, a goldsmith of St Alban Wood Street; three of the remaining clients attesting to Ayre's expertise were the wives of brewers.[24] In the case of Eleanor Stanfro of the parish of St Leonard Shoreditch, where a large number of weavers made their home, parochial and occupational links converged; four of the six testimonial clients from her home parish were married to weavers.[25] Seamen's wives also apparently referred their midwives to other women whose husbands were similarly engaged. All six of Elizabeth Willis's clients, all three of Mary Salmon's, and all four of Sara Griffin's were married to seafaring men.[26]

Out of the fifty-three testimonials which gave occupational designations for clients' husbands in 1663, thirteen or almost 25 per cent demonstrated similar occupations for two or more spouses. Similarly, in the years 1696–1700, out of the forty testimonials which declared occupations, twelve, or 30 per cent, gave the same occupation for at least two of the women's husbands. Although Mistress X seldom recorded occupational information for spouses, among the few instances where she has done so, we have two examples which confirm testimonial evidence of occupational links between clients of individual midwives. In 1704 the midwife 'laid' two shoemakers' wives within five weeks of one another; similarly, in 1715, two tailors' wives were delivered less than five weeks apart, one of whom lived in the Minories and the other at a considerable distance to the west in the Strand.

The existence of other networks between women and their clients can be traced in the testimonials. Mary DesOrmeaux, wife of Daniel, a jeweller of St Giles in the Fields, was a member of the French church in the Savoy (home of the Huguenot congregation) when she applied for a midwifery licence in 1680. All five women who gave sworn testimony on her behalf were French immigrants: Catherine Faure, Marguerite Gorget and Marguerite Fournie were residents of St Giles in the Fields, while Mere Lamare and Marie Colas were from the parish of St Martin in the Fields. Catherine Bont of Stepney had been a member of the Dutch church in London for three years when she applied for a midwifery licence in 1688. Catherine was the wife of Jonas Merese, but she retained her own name after her marriage, as was the custom amongst Dutch women. Similarly, two of her clients, from Stepney and St Leonard Shoreditch, were Dutch women who gave their maiden names when they testified under oath.[27] It is apparent, and understandably so, that, whenever possible, female immigrants turned to midwives of their own nationality, who spoke the same language and shared the same cultural heritage, to assist them when they were brought to bed. Indeed, the refusal to allow midwives of their own Protestant faith to attend them was one of the precipitating factors in the flight of Huguenot women from France in the 1680s.[28] More surprising is recently uncovered evidence that ecclesiastically-licensed midwives numbered Quaker women among their clients: apparently for these women the demands of childbearing overrode, at least temporarily, religious concerns.[29]

The authors of two studies of midwifery and gynaecology in the early modern period have both concluded that women turned to male midwives because they believed that male practitioners could offer them better care.[30] If this was the case, women of the upper echelons of seventeenth-century London society could reasonably be expected to be among the first to desert the traditional midwife and seek the services of the male midwife. The evidence, however, points to a different conclusion. Wives of London gentlemen continued to use the services of midwives well into the next century, as both testimonials and the anonymous midwife's account book demonstrate.

Midwives applying for licences frequently included the name of a gentlewoman among those giving sworn testimony on their behalf. Debora Bromfield of St Andrew Holborn was exceptional with three of the five clients shown on her 1662 testimonial, delivered of a total of twelve children, married to 'gentlemen': Elizabeth Philips of St Clement Danes; Susan Brownell of St Andrew Holborn; and Susan White of St Martin Ironmonger Lane.[31] Since all three women lived in different parishes, some distance apart, the midwife was probably referred by means of a social network among women of the urban gentry. At least six midwives licensed between 1677 and 1700 included the names of two gentlewomen among those testifying on their behalf.[32] The curate of Laughton, parish of midwife Sarah Tricer, noted in 1664 that all four clients named in the testimonial were 'of the best ranck and qualitie in the parish of Laughton'.[33] Similarly, in 1669 the curate, vicar and churchwarden of Shadwell, Stepney, testified pointedly that Katherine Botts had been 'very successful in the safe delivery of many persons of very great reputation and quality in the said parish'.[34]

In rural England a midwife's practice could be expected to cover a wide spectrum of social and occupational groups. For example, the diary of the Kendal midwife lists clients whose husbands were drawn from over fifty diverse occupations. She delivered the children of professionals, including apothecaries, schoolmasters, attorneys and clergy, and members of the gentry and the aristocracy.[35] In London too midwives continued to administer to the needs of women from all classes of society. Of the seventy-five testimonials which have been preserved for the years 1663–64, fifty-three contain information on the status of clients' spouses (see Table 1.3). Out of 249 given occupations, the husbands of nine clients (4 per cent) were designated as 'gentleman'.

An indication of the continuing loyalty of gentry women to their midwives can be found in testimonial evidence at the end of the century. Of seventy-five testimonials presented to the vicar general for the City of London in the years 1690–1700, sixty-five contain occupational and status designations. Of 198 possible designations, fourteen husbands were listed as members of the gentry. Thus, 7 per cent of the women supporting the midwives' applications were from the upper level of society. The testimonials preserved in the Lambeth Palace archives were analysed separately for the purposes of comparison. Of the sixty-two testimonials which survive for the years 1669–1700, fifty included occupational information. Out of a possible 174 designations, twenty-three spouses were named as 'gentleman' (over 13 per cent). This would indicate that midwives who sought licences from the jurisdiction of the Archbishop of Canterbury, rather than the jurisdiction of the Bishop of London, not only drew their clientele from a more influential and affluent sector of society, but that this elevated group continued to use the services of the midwife.

If the occupational designations for 1663 and the 1690s from the records of the Bishop of London and the Archbishop of Canterbury are combined and averaged, we find that around 10 per cent of the designated clients giving testimonial evidence for midwives applying for licences to practise in the City of London and its environs were drawn from the gentry.

Using Gregory King's estimates for the year 1688 we might assume that the gentry made up a little more than 2 per cent of the population of England and Wales. Our figures, therefore, support the view that educated and affluent members of London society continued to look to midwives to deliver their offspring throughout the seventeenth century.[36]

Table 1.3 Occupation/status of the husbands of London midwifery clients, 1663–1700

	1663–64	*1690–1700*
Building	14	21
Clothing	54	48
Decorating/furnishing	7	2
Distribution/transport	54	33
Labouring	4	4
Land/farm workers	21	15
Leather	10	12
Merchants	5	3
Metalwork	14	7
Miscellaneous production	8	4
Miscellaneous services	8	10
Officials	1 (+2)[*]	0
Professions	9	4
Victualling	31	21
Gentleman	9	14
Total	249	198

[*] Two spouses served as churchwardens in addition to their occupations. The foregoing classifications were adapted from A.L. Beier, 'Engine of manufacture: the trades of London', in A.L. Beier and R. Finlay (eds) *London 1500–1700: The Making of the Metropolis* (London and New York, 1986), 164.

Source: GL MS 10,116/3, 13, 14.

In seeking referees, midwives quite possibly looked to respectable members of society, and the evidence from the testimonials is not necessarily representative of their practices as a whole. The practice of Mistress X, however, reflects the range of clientele listed in testimonials – indeed her accounts suggest higher levels of employment by the well-to-do. Her account book makes a clear distinction regarding the status of clients: women from the lower and middle class are designated 'Ms' or 'mistress', while women of the upper ranks of society are given the more respectful form of address 'madam'. We are, therefore, able to identify a sizeable segment of her clientele, which was largely made up of the wives of men of prestige and affluence. Although there is a very close connection between the size of the fee charged by the midwife and social designation, there are indications that occasionally the courtesy title of 'madam' was extended more for social than economic reasons. Madam Andrews of St Bartholomew Lane, for example, paid less for her deliveries, £1 14s. and £1 16s., than many a 'mistress' among the midwife's clients.

Our anonymous midwife identified no fewer than twenty of her clients as 'madam' and in addition delivered a lady. Lady Clarke paid £6 in 1720 when she was delivered of a daughter. These twenty-one women, several of whom were extremely fertile, accounted for roughly 9 per cent of the busy midwife's practice and provide some support for the argument that midwives were not deserted in favour of male practitioners by women of substance at the turn of the century. On one of the last folios of the casebook, the names of Lady Shaw, Lady Clarke, Arthur Barnardiston (a wealthy merchant), Samuel Barnardiston, John Barnardiston and Lady Barnardiston appear, indicating the elite status of a section of Mistress X's clientele.[37]

At the other end of the social scale, we find evidence that midwives remained faithful to their oath which required that they not discriminate between rich and poor women who were in need of their services. Susan Kempton's testimonial (signed by her vicar) stated that 'she is not only helpfull to the rich and those that can pay her but also to the poore'.[38] Individual parishes frequently assumed responsibility for paying for the delivery of poor women of the parish and also of vagrant women who could not be removed from the parish before they gave birth. Fees paid to the midwife by the parish ranged from the modest sum of 2s. 6d. paid by the parish of St Gregory by St Paul's in 1677 for delivering a 'poore woman that fell in labour' in the parish, to the 5s. paid in 1655 and the 10s. paid in 1684 and 1686 by the wealthy parish of St Mary Aldermanbury.[39] Mistress X delivered a female felon held 'in the stocks' at the marketplace in 1712 and was not paid for her services.[40]

If an obstetrical 'disaster' occurred which required more than the manual removal of a dead foetus, midwives were obliged to call for the help of a surgeon who owned and was permitted to use the requisite instruments such as hooks, knives and crochets.[41] Since surgeons were called upon when an operative procedure became necessary, it has been suggested that they were the group from which male midwives would logically evolve.[42] There is, however, evidence that the wives of surgeons themselves continued, throughout the seventeenth century, to turn to midwives when they were brought to bed and not to their husbands' colleagues. By the year 1662 Rebecca Jeffery of St Botolph Aldgate had delivered Susan Noxton, wife of surgeon Peter Noxton of the same parish, five times. The following year, midwife Elizabeth Dunstall of St Anne and St Agnes included the names of two surgeons' wives among the satisfied clients who supported her application for licensing. This pattern persisted throughout the century, with no evidence of change. In 1689, Catherine Goswell of St

Andrew Holborn claimed among her clientele Sara Pettit, wife of Gersham Pettit citizen and barber-surgeon of St Katherine next to the Tower. Not only did Mistress Pettit live at a considerable distance from the midwife, but there is a possibility that her husband was the resident medical attendant for St Katherine's, a hospital for almswomen, a position which afforded practical experience in treating ailing women. Even so, the Pettits chose the services of a midwife when Mistress Pettit was brought to bed. Also in 1689, Mary Garland of St Bridgid obtained sworn testimony from Susan Corpson, a surgeon's wife from St Dunstan in the West, and Mary Searle, the wife of a St Sepulchre barber-surgeon.[43] Frances Sowden of St Martin Outwich obtained sworn testimony from Alice Lovell, the wife of another St Sepulchre barber-surgeon, in the same year. As late as 1698, there is evidence in the testimonials that the wives of surgeons continued to rely on the traditional skills of a competent midwife rather than those of the surgeon. The account book of the anonymous London midwife, although containing scant reference to husbands' occupations, records that in August 1712 a Mistress Mos, who was a 'sirgung's' wife, was delivered of a son. According to Irvine Loudon, before 1730, 'the surgeon-man-midwife had . . . little or none of the extensive experience of normal midwifery which is the basis of good obstetric practice'.[44] Apparently very few surgeons were married to midwives who could have instructed them in obstetrical techniques.[45] Seventeenth-century surgeons (and their wives), aware of the shortcomings in men-midwives' knowledge and experience of normal birth processes, ensured that when their own children were born, an experienced midwife was at hand.

Finally, we may consider the role of clients in the licensing process and the significance of the testimonials as unmediated evidence of female involvement and concern for the maintenance of adequate midwifery services. As the century wore on, women's signatures, as well as their names, appeared with greater regularity and in more substantial numbers on testimonial documents presented to the courts of the Bishop of London. In the years 1661–62, out of forty-six testimonials, only one contained a statement signed in the women's own 'hands'. In it, six women, from five different parishes, appended their signatures to a statement attesting to the bearer's 'sufficient experience and ability to perform and exercise the office of a midwife'.[46] In the years 1663–64, women's voices are heard, unmediated, in five testimonials. The lengthiest list of names appeared on the documents of Isabel Ellis of St Martin in the Fields: twenty-four women were willing to vouch for the 'long experience' and competence of Mrs Ellis. In the case of Anne Gill of High Barnet, also licensed in 1664, all six women signed with their own distinctive marks. The testimonial of Mary Dowdall of Chipping Barnet contained the following statement about the woman who had been employed as a midwife 'these many years past':

wherein she hath had the blessing to be a meanes for the safe delivery
of others whose names are here subscribed and many others whome
we knowe witness our hands the 23 Day of May 1664.[47]

Similarly, the four women who signed in their own 'hands' Sara Tricer's
certificate (and who were described as 'gentlewomen' by the curate of
Laughton), noted:

> inhabitants of Laughton doo certifie that we have good tryall of the
> good skill and Gods blessings upon the endeavour of Sarah Tricer in
> the office of midwife; and have heard of the like good success to many
> more . . . we doe conceive her to be skilfull, discrete & honest . . .[48]

The 1668 testimonial of Mary Parsons of St Mary Matfellon contains the
customary sworn testimony of six clients. Eleven other women added their
names; one signed with a mark, but the other ten names appear as
signatures, presumably executed by the women themselves. In addition to
the four women who gave sworn testimony in June 1670, twenty other
women signed a 'petition' on behalf of Elizabeth Paulson of St Botolph
Aldgate stating that they had 'good experience of the great care and ability
. . . in the safe delivery of women in childbearing'.[49] Two years later fifteen
women set their marks to the certificate of Mary Burton of Rosemary Lane
in the parish of Whitechapel, confirming her suitability for the office of
midwife.[50] The testimonial of Joan Elsey of Enfield, submitted in 1689,
contained the names of ten women who had been delivered by her and
who had done very well 'under her hands'.[51] The last five years of the
century, in particular, demonstrate an increasing involvement by female
clients in the formulation of testimonial certificates. Susan Warden of New
Brentford and Elizabeth Thorowgood of Chipping Ongar presented statements containing the signatures of ten and seventeen women respectively
in the years 1697 and 1698.

The testimonial submitted in 1696 by Margery King of Chipping Ongar,
Essex, was signed by twelve women and bore witness to her

> good skill, experience and success in wifery . . . hath safely delivered
> severall women in child bed with good success, and more particularly
> some of us whose hands have subscribed to this testimoniall.[52]

The women also commented on her 'sober' life, thereby pre-empting one
of the customary concerns of the clergy who in this instance were not
represented in the testimonial.

In addition to statements by groups of women, there are examples of
individual women's voices. Ann Bell of St Martin in the Fields secured
sworn testimony from four women who appeared in the consistory court on

13 October 1677. She also obtained the following statements (all in different handwriting) from three other women:

> For I will assure you that I was safe delivered by ye help of mistris bell the midwfe of a son september ye 10 my name is Filadelfa Rogers liveing next dore to ye doge and duck in Pickadily.

> Sir my name is market Grimes I was safely delivered by *ye hands* of Mrs. Bell a midwife than is with her now that can justifie ye same.

> Ser i was safely deliverd by *ye hands* of Mrs bell the midwife the second of this present month my name is Susan Jackson.[53]

Midwife Bell's clients emphasized not only the safeness of their deliveries but their midwife's capable hands. In the previous decade, midwife Sell's testimonial certificate, written by a literate, upper-class woman, noted that no woman had ever 'failed under her hand'.[54] In the last decades of the century mothers still preferred the warm and compassionate touch of their midwives' hands of flesh and blood to the cold instruments or the 'iron hands' of the male midwives.[55]

Women were becoming more actively involved in the testimonial process of the Bishop of London's ecclesiastical courts. They were drafting petitions (either personally or with the assistance of a clerk), signing their own names (whether by mark or full signature), and continuing to appear before representatives of the vicar general to deliver evidence under oath regarding midwives' competence. One possible explanation for this trend could be that women were experiencing difficulty in obtaining the midwifery services that they needed in a city whose burgeoning population was placing increased demands on midwives.[56] Women decided perhaps to take matters into their own hands and licensing authorities acquiesced to their petitions by waiving, in some cases, the customary requirement of supportive clerical testimony.[57] The evidence clearly demonstrates the Church's perception of clients as being a (perhaps the) central feature of the testimonial system.

The clientele of seventeenth-century London midwives were drawn from a broad spectrum of society. They lived not only in their midwife's parish but, in many cases, well beyond its confines. Many of them turned time and time again to the midwife who had already proven her competence and care in previous deliveries. The gentry, as well as the poorest parish residents, continued to call on midwives throughout the century. Clients voiced their satisfaction with the services provided by these women both by maintaining a network of referral among relatives, neighbours and wives of their husbands' co-workers, and by becoming more individually (and personally) involved in the testimonial process. In all of these ways, clients not only expressed their concern for and satisfaction with their midwives, but gave their implicit stamp of approval to the traditional system in which midwives worked.[58]

Notes

1. Roy Porter has been particularly critical of this imbalance. See, for example, his introduction to R. Porter (ed.) *Patients and Practitioners: Lay Perceptions of Medicine in Pre-Industrial Society* (Cambridge, 1985) as well as the Porters' own contributions towards restoring the balance in R. Porter and D. Porter, *In Sickness and in Health: The British Experience, 1650–1850* (London, 1988); *idem, Patient's Progress: Doctors and Doctoring in Eighteenth-Century England* (Cambridge, 1989).

2. For a commentary on the authority and power invested in the midwife at the time of delivery, see A. Wilson, 'Childbirth in seventeenth- and eighteenth-century England', unpub. PhD thesis, University of Sussex, 1982, 127–8, 226; *idem,* 'The ceremony of childbirth and its interpretation', in V. Fildes (ed.) *Women as Mothers in Pre-Industrial England* (London and New York, 1990), 71–3. The testimonial evidence used in this study affords a different perspective on the perception of midwives by their clients since it was recorded sometime after the delivery, and was thus distanced from the situation which conferred unusual power on the midwife.

3. D. Evenden-Nagy, 'Seventeenth-century London midwives: their training, licensing and social profile', unpub. PhD diss., McMaster University, 1991. The sources and methodology upon which this paper is based are fully described in the foregoing thesis. The principal sources are: Testimonial certificates, Guildhall Library (hereafter GL) MS 10,116; Lambeth Palace Library (LPL) MS VX 1A/11; Vicar General's Registers, Greater London Record Office (GLRO) DLC 339–45; Anonymous midwife's account book, Bodleian Library, Oxford, Rawlinson MS D 1141. The last source was used with the kind permission of the Bodleian Library.

4. J. Donnison, *Midwives and Medical Men* (London, 1977), 9. David Harley's preliminary findings on provincial midwives support the revised view of London midwives. See D.N. Harley, 'Ignorant midwives – a persistent stereotype', *Bulletin of the Society for the Social History of Medicine*, 28 (1981), 8, 9. See also chs 2 and 3 in this volume by David Harley and Ann Giardina Hess.

5. Evenden-Nagy, 'Seventeenth-century London midwives', ch. 5: 'Midwives of twelve London parishes: a socio-economic case study'. For an example of the traditional stereotype which has persisted up until recently, see T.R. Forbes, *The Midwife and the Witch* (New York, 1966). David Harley has demolished this myth. See D. Harley, 'Historians as demonologists: the myth of the midwife-witch', *Social History of Medicine*, 3 (1990), 1–26.

6. For a rural midwife's practice, see the transcript of a Kendal midwife's diary, covering the years 1665–75, Cumbria Record Office (hereafter CuRO), MS WD/Cr. The 'diary' is a record of a midwife's practice in an area where there were one or (at most) two practising midwives and which demonstrates, not surprisingly, very extensive repeat business. For relationships between Quaker midwives and their clients, see ch. 3 in this volume by Ann Giardina Hess.

7. GL MS 10,116/3.

8. GL MS 10,116/2.

9. Bodleian Library, Oxford, Rawlinson MS D 1141, ff. 31, 32, 40, 56.

10. Bodleian Library, Oxford, Rawlinson MS D 1141, f. 15.

11. In 1726 teaman Richard Beach was located at the 'Figg Tree' in Newgate Street and in 1755 grocer George Snowball occupied the 'Figg Tree' on Salisbury Street in the Strand. A. Heal, *The Signboards of Old London Shops* (London, 1947), 164, 87. A member of the Barnardiston family of merchants may have been the owner and occupant of one of these two businesses in 1715, the year Madam Barnardiston was delivered.

12. The daughters of Mrs Abel and Mrs Chapman, both clients, were also delivered by Mistress X.

13. GL MS 10,116/3.

14. GLRO DLC/339, vol. 1, f. 102.

15. GLRO DLC/339, vol. 1, f. 133.

16. GLRO DLC/339, vol. 13, f. 172.

17. GLRO DLC/339, vol. 14, f. 68v.

18. GL MS 10,116/3.

19. J. Boulton, *Neighbourhood and Society: A London Suburb in the Seventeenth Century* (Cambridge, 1987), 231. There is no indication in the London sources of how midwives travelled to their deliveries. No doubt in many cases transportation (either by horse or carriage) or a guide would be provided by clients' families, but in others she would travel alone and on foot to the lying-in.

20. This pattern of an aging midwife restricting her practice to deliveries closer to home was also demonstrated by Vrouw Schrader, the eighteenth-century Frisian midwife. See H. Marland, M.J. van Lieburg and G.J. Kloosterman, *'Mother and Child were Saved': The Memoirs (1693–1740) of the Frisian Midwife Catharina Schrader* (Amsterdam, 1987), 11.

21. P. Crawford, 'Printed advertisements for women medical practitioners in London, 1670–1710', *Bulletin of the Society for the Social History of Medicine*, 35 (1984), 266–9. Even in the early eighteenth century advertising was restricted to special cases such as the anonymous woman purporting to be a midwife who advertised her 'cure' for an illness which could develop into a malignant 'Womb'. W.B. Ewald, *The Newsmen of Queen Anne* (Oxford, 1956), 108.

22. Although the evidence needs to be developed, I suspect that these referrals between women who delivered within a few days of one another are also an indication that at least some women limited their contact with the midwife to the actual date of delivery.

23. GL MS 10,116/1.

24. GL MS 10,116/2. All of Davis's clients were from different parishes.

25. GL MS 10,116/3.

26. GL MS 10,116/1, 2, 3, 13.

27. GL MS 10,116/11, 12. Samuel Biscope was the minister of the Dutch congregation in London and he signed the testimonial certificate.

28. A.P. Hands and I. Scouloudi, *French Protestant Refugees Relieved Through the Threadneedle Street Church, London 1681–1687* (London, 1971), Huguenot Society of London, vol. 49, 9.

29. I am grateful to Ann Giardina Hess for directing me to the sources which enabled me to establish this connection. See also ch. 3 in this volume by Ann Giardina Hess.

30. A. Wilson, 'Childbirth in seventeenth- and eighteenth-century England', 317–22; A. Eccles, *Obstetrics and Gynaecology in Tudor and Stuart England* (London, 1982), 124. The weaknesses of this argument, based mainly on the perceptions of male practitioners, have been dealt with at length in Evenden-Nagy, 'Seventeenth-century London midwives'.

31. GL MS 10,116/2.

32. This number includes only those women whose husbands were designated 'gent'. It does not include the dozens of women whose names and signatures appear on these documents, many of whom were apparently literate and probably reasonably well-to-do.

33. GL MS 10,116/3.

34. GL MS 10,116/6.

35. Transcript of a Kendal midwife's diary, CuRO, MS WD/Cr. The midwife delivered the children of at least four or five estate owners, including a squire and the two children of Sir Thomas Braithwaite. Among the less common occupations which were represented were those of a tobacco cutter and a fiddler. The clientele of the Frisian midwife Catharina Schrader was also drawn from a wide occupational spectrum, which included labourers, farmers, doctors, vicars, merchants, skippers and members of various trades associated with the sea. See Marland, Van Lieberg and Kloosterman, *'Mother and Child were Saved'*, 13.

36. Gregory King cited in D.C. Coleman, *The Economy of England 1450–1750* (Oxford, 1977), 6. King's figures are for all of England and Wales while we are dealing with London where the population would contain proportionately fewer gentry and more tradesmen, craftsmen, shopkeepers and artisans.

37. See *The Directory Containing an Alphabetical List of the Names and Places of Abode of the Directors of Companies, Persons in Public Business, Merchants etc.* (London, 1736). The midwife usually referred to Lady Clarke as 'Madam Clarke' and always referred to Lady Shaw as 'Madam Shaw'. At least one other client was the wife of a well-to-do member of London financial circles – Mrs Bodicete – whom the midwife delivered on four occasions. See *The Directory*, 8. Some sixty years earlier Thomas Barnardiston had been one of the City's parochial and civic leaders.

38. GL MS 10,116/13.

39. GL MS 1337/1, f. 16, 3556/2 (unfol.), 3556/3, ff. 33v, 47 (churchwardens' accounts). The midwife delivered 'Mr. Todds maide' in 1684 and was paid by the parish. Mr Todd would not be liable for the expense of delivering an unmarried maidservant who was probably dismissed as soon as she became the mother of a bastard, according to the accepted practice of the period.

40. There is no indication in the midwife's records whether or not the woman was temporarily released from the stocks in an unspecified London marketplace in order to give birth. For a discussion of midwives' fees, see Evenden-Nagy, 'Seventeenth-century London midwives', 224–34.

41. See Eccles, *Obstetrics and Gynaecology*, 109–18 for a discussion of the role of surgeons in the birth process which usually encompassed the death of the child, the mother or both. In 1688 midwife Elizabeth Cellier attacked the medical profession for their lack of practical experience in delivering children in a scathing, albeit humorous, pamphlet, *To Dr . . . an Answer to his Queries, concerning the Colledg of Midwives* (London, 1688). For Cellier, see also ch. 6 in this volume by Helen King.

42. Adrian Wilson has developed this argument. See Wilson, 'Childbirth in seventeenth- and eighteenth-century England', 311, 318–20.

43. GL MS 10,116/2, 3, 5, 12. The records describe the spouses of Pettit, Searle and Lovell as 'barber-surgeons'. In the light of recent research on London barber-surgeons' records, there is a possibility that these men were barbers and not surgeons. D. Evenden, 'The licensing and practice of female surgeons in early modern England', unpub. paper, meeting of British historians, Toronto, 27 Sept. 1992.

44. I. Loudon, *Medical Care and the General Practitioner 1750–1850* (Oxford, 1986), 86. Although Loudon dates the beginning of the male takeover of midwifery

at around 1730, he is sketchy about details of how the surgeons acquired their midwifery training. He suggests that treatises published by Smellie (1752) and Denman (1786) were instructive, as were Smellie's courses in London, which began in 1744. Smellie's private courses, however, were not a requirement for the practice of midwifery. Loudon, *Medical Care*, 85–94. In the late 1740s when John D'Urban, having already completed an apprenticeship in surgery, wished to become knowledgeable in midwifery, he undertook a separate course of training in London (possibly the one offered by Smellie). After successfully completing an MD degree at Edinburgh in 1753, he became physician and man-midwife at the Middlesex Hospital. British Library, Additional MS 24,123, f. 82. As late as 1788 surgeons who had completed their apprenticeship were obliged to seek out private courses in midwifery. That was the year William Savory paid 5 guineas to a male midwife in London for two courses in midwifery, given at the doctor's own residence and his 'labour house' near St Saviour's. See G.C. Peachey, *The Life of William Savory* (London, 1903), 12. The first professor of midwifery in England was appointed in 1828 at London's University College. Loudon, *Medical Care*, 92.

45.   Bloom and James list one example of a barber-surgeon married to a midwife from early in the century. J.H. Bloom and R.R. James, *Medical Practitioners in the Diocese of London, Licensed under the Act of 3 Henry VIII, C. 11* (Cambridge, 1935), 20.

46.   GL MS 10,116/1.

47.   GL MS 10,116/3.

48.   GL MS 10,116/1.

49.   GL MS 10,116/7.

50.   GL MS 10,116/7. In addition, four women gave testimony under oath, one of whom was included in the fifteen signees.

51.   GL MS 10,116/12.

52.   GL MS 10,116/14.

53.   GL MS 10,116/10 (Evenden's emphasis).

54.   GL MS 10,116/4.

55.   The eighteenth-century English midwife, Elizabeth Nihell, referred to women's preference for the midwife's 'hand of flesh, tender and safe' rather than the iron and steel forceps of the male midwife. See E. Nihell, *A Treatise on the Art of Midwifery* (London, 1760), 36. See also Joan Elsey's testimonial above.

56.   For a discussion of urban population growth which continued to the end of the seventeenth century, see R. Finlay and B. Shearer, 'Population growth and suburban expansion', in A.L. Beier and R. Finlay (eds), *London 1500–1700: The Making of the Metropolis* (London and New York, 1986), 37–57. The number of midwives who were licensed by the vicar general showed a marked decline in the 1680s with some recovery in the 1690s.

57.   Although I have not found any regulation which specifies that clerical testimony was a requirement for licensing, the evidence arising from the practice of the period indicates that it was standard practice.

58.   No examples of client dissatisfaction were found in the ecclesiastical records. For a discussion of clergy, parish officials, neighbours and medical personnel who added their support to that of clients, see Evenden-Nagy, 'Seventeenth-century London midwives', 133–51.

2

Provincial midwives in England: Lancashire and Cheshire, 1660–1760

David Harley

There was a time, when those whom Providence had blessed with Leisure, Affluence and Dignity, did not think it any Diminution of their Characters to attend the necessities of the Indigent, and alleviate the Miseries of the Diseased.

(Samuel Johnson, 1743)[1]

Despite the more positive view of midwifery that has emerged in recent years, prior to this volume little attention has been paid to the people involved in childbirth. Midwives, in particular, remain a mute group, and most of the evidence on them emanates from hostile contemporary accounts.[2] Their character and the choices made by their clients need to be reconstructed if women are not to be seen as the passive victims of the rise of the men-midwives. Propaganda and the new techniques of the surgeons were surely necessary but not sufficient causes of the change. Although the highly trained surgeons emerging from the hospitals and anatomy classes created some of the demand for their skills, changes in the supply of midwives and in the tastes of their clients also need to be considered. It is not yet clear whether men-midwives forced their way into the birthing room or simply stepped into a gap that was already beginning to open.

In early modern England, every sizeable town had at least one locally famous midwife but it is necessary to seek out more representative individuals. The Diocese of Chester offers relatively full licensing material, although mostly from the southern Archdeaconry of Chester.[3] Further information comes from wills, and the records of the poor law and coroners' courts. It is difficult to define precisely who was a midwife. For most women who practised midwifery, 'midwife' was not their main social identity.[4] Marriage bonds and parish registers rarely referred to midwives.[5] No midwives in this diocese describe themselves as such in their wills. Yet contemporaries did distinguish between a midwife and a woman like Mary Sutton of Salford who, in 1693, 'did officiate as midwife (for want of one

27

M:
skill
rather
than a
trade

att that time)'.[6] Midwifery can perhaps best be understood as a skill rather than as a trade, with few regular practitioners having it as their sole source of income and status. For the purposes of this essay, any woman described in the sources as a midwife will be considered as such.

Training, recognition and licensing

How did a provincial Englishwoman become recognized as a midwife? Not by formal apprenticeship, since only one instance is recorded in the region during this period, that of Theodoria Haddock to Dorothy Hall of Manchester in 1743, for three years at a cost of 8 guineas.[7] Even the semi-formal system of apprenticeship common in London is difficult to find in the provinces, though midwives did train friends to succeed them. In 1725, Mary Twamlow, a midwife of thirty-six years' standing, signed a testimonial for her pupil, Sarah Physwick, the wife of a Northwich shoe-maker. The elder woman was related by marriage to her pupil's husband and she left him £30 and a silver tankard in her will. Midwives often trained relatives. When Ruth Rogerson of Northwich was reported as unlicensed in 1724, she sent in a testimonial which stated that she was 'not onely a good & experienced Midwife from her own Pracktise as having laide some hundreds of ye most fashionable Women but also being instructed both by her Grandmother & Mother, Licenc'd Midwives'.[8]

Medical practitioners do not appear to have been much involved in training provincial midwives. In late Stuart London, midwives occasionally sought training in anatomy or attended the Hôtel Dieu in Paris. In the eighteenth century, a few gained access to private classes and the London hospitals but contemporaries lamented the absence of practical instruction for midwives in the provinces, where they had to rely on potentially mis-leading books for the latest knowledge.[9] Until the 1790s, when midwifery schools were created in Manchester and Liverpool, the provinces had no facilities to compare with those in London. Midwifery was a skill, like farming or child-rearing, that was passed on to succeeding generations without formal instruction.

→ Midwifery had always been regarded as a skill that could only be learned by experience. As late as 1724, John Maubray, a Bond Street lecturer on midwifery, asserted in his *Female Physician* that a midwife should have served 'as an assistant to some skilful Woman of good Business' because only practice could equip a midwife, not 'all the THEORY, that the most ingenious MAN can make himself Master of'.[10] The swelling numbers of hospital-trained surgeons denounced midwives on the same grounds of insufficient theoretical knowledge as physicians had once criticized surgeons. Sarah Stone noted that 'these young Gentlemen-Professors put on a finish'd assurance, with pretence that their Knowledge exceeds any

Woman's, because they have seen, or gone thro', a Course of Anatomy'. She was sure that more died at their hands 'than by the greatest imbecillity and ignorance of some Women-Midwives'. Henry Bracken of Lancaster, a surgeon-physician trained in Paris and Leiden who pioneered man-mid-wifery in this region, despised such men.[11] Despite their lack of formal education, midwives were generally expected by both patients and doctors to be expert in the common diseases peculiar to women and children, as the translator of a book on rickets recognized when he dedicated it to the Mayor of Oxford's wife, Mrs Mary Coombes, 'the *Oxonian* LUCINA, or *Compleat Midwife*'.[12] Everard Maynwaringe reported that, when he had attended a gentlewoman in Chester during the late 1650s, he spent time 'conferring with the Midwife'. Nathaniel Bostock MD of Whitchurch, writing to Hans Sloane in 1713, cited the gynaecological opinion of a gentlewoman's midwives. Henry Bracken thought that a midwife was better able to diagnose dropsy in a woman than was a young graduate physician.[13] Like many other women, midwives might also undertake minor surgical work, as did Elizabeth Hey, a Manchester midwife whose bill was carefully considered by the magistrates in 1702.[14]

Medical practitioners often wrote testimonials for midwives, which might suggest a close working relationship. Thomas Clayton, a former Manchester surgeon who had retired to his family estate at Little Harwood, signed four of the surviving testimonials. When John Holme, the parish priest of Blackburn, sent one of these testimonials to Chester, he described the midwife as serving 'all Persons of the best rank in this Town & Neighbourhood & desires a Lycence to Quallify her for her Practice'. When Margery Chorley of Manchester sent her testimonial, it was signed not only by two priests and forty women but also by two prominent physicians, Nathaniel Banne MD and Charles Leigh MD, FRS. In 1691, Silvester Richmond, surgeon-physician and former Mayor of Liverpool, provided a note on behalf of Ellen Fletcher, stating that she had been trained by her mother as a midwife, had practised for several years 'with great diligence and success; and I have been with her sevĩ times on that occasion; and have Observd hir to be prudent in ye manadgmᵗ of those Concerns'.[15] Actual training can perhaps be assumed only in such cases as those of the Knutsford surgeons, William Smith and John Ridge, whose wives were licensed in 1674 and 1732. Nevertheless, it is only in a single midwife's testimonial, written in 1757 for Ellen Thompson of Eccleston by the Catholic gentleman surgeon and man-midwife, Brian Hawarden of Wigan, that there is any statement of formal instruction. Formal midwife training was slow to develop in the provinces, although it was advertised in 1757 by Matthew Turner, a prominent Liverpool surgeon trained by Smellie in London, who was at pains to reassure midwives that he was not seeking 'to prejudice or undervalue them'.[16]

These testimonials, which constitute the best source of information on midwives, derive from the process of ecclesiastical licensing. The system rested on custom and power, as there was no legal authority for the penalties imposed for unlicensed practice.[17] In the Diocese of Chester, it was enforced by the courts of the Archbishop of York, at least until 1684, the triennial visitation of the Bishop, and the twice-yearly circuits of the Archdeaconry courts until about 1750.[18] Although they sometimes obtained licences as a qualification or as a precaution, midwives usually became licensed because they had been reported to a visitation as unlicensed. Apart from failing to appear and then being excommunicated for contumacy, the only other options were to deny practising or to admit the offence, be ordered to desist and pay a small fine. After Alice Massie of Great Saughall and Margaret Holland of Shotwick had been presented in June 1674, the former was licensed in the following December and their parish priest certified in February that 'Holland never practises'.[19] A midwife seeking a licence obtained signatures for a testimonial, from some combination of clergymen, parish officers, local women, midwives and medical practitioners. This would then be presented to an ecclesiastical court, a fee would be paid and the oath taken. On occasion, a midwife might be too ill to travel, so her husband or a churchwarden would appear in her stead.[20] The licence would then be sent to the midwife as soon as a clerk had written it out. Midwives were expected to present their licences at subsequent visitations but they tended to avoid doing so unless summoned as a small fee would be payable each time. In consequence, licensed midwives were often reported as unlicensed.

The initial fee was quite substantial, 18s. 8d. in the Chester courts, creating some reluctance to take out licences. Sarah Howell of Christleton did not want to be licensed as she practised among the poor without pay: 'pauperibus quibusdam opēm ferre sine mercede'. Women frequently defended themselves by asserting that they had performed the office of a midwife by chance or for no fee.[21] Parish priests interceded on behalf of women who did not regularly practise midwifery. The minister of Bromborough, supported by the women of the parish, wrote that Elizabeth Turner, cited in 1738, did not 'profess herself a Midwife' and never asked for a fee. She had no intention 'to get her self licenced, or enter further into the Profession than she has done', and she would prefer to desist rather 'than be at the trouble and charges'.[22] Churchwardens in remote parishes, such as Urswick and Aldingham, tended to report that their unnamed midwives did not intend to be licensed: 'We have one old woman who sometimes practises midwifery but her practise is so smale, yt she thinks it no advantage to her to take a Lycence.'[23]

The licensing system provoked the scorn of Henry Bracken, who complained that a Woman who can only procure the Hands of a few good natur'd Ladies, or Justices of the Peace, to recommend her to the Bishop or Ordinary, shall have a Licence to Practise, although neither those who recommended, nor the Bishop himself know any thing of the Matter.[24]

Even as Bracken wrote, medical men were replacing the clergy as signatories of the majority of Chester testimonials, which suggests a medicalization of the midwife's social role. At its best, the testimonial demonstrated social acceptance by providing evidence of satisfied clients and medical approbation as well as moral probity.

Unfortunately, the licensing system cannot indicate the duration of a midwife's practice, making it impossible to estimate the population ratio of even licensed midwives. Elizabeth Broderick of Chester, who had not appeared in the visitation records since 1725, was issued with a gate pass in 1745 so that she could pass through 'at any hour with one Servt. in order to follow her profession (being a Midwife)'. When first licensed, Alice Nabb of Bury had been a midwife for thirty years and Elizabeth Scholefield of Atherton had practised for twenty years but neither had ever appeared in any visitation records.[25]

Social and economic status

What sort of women became midwives in late Stuart and early Hanoverian England? The belief that they were 'ignorant, unskilled, poverty-stricken and avoided', as Forbes has put it, has been abandoned by students of English midwifery in recent years because it owes more to medical disdain than historical accuracy.[26] Nevertheless, it remains difficult to assess the social and educational status of midwives because precise information is scarce and of dubious representativeness. Little information has yet emerged on the social status of midwives prior to the Restoration in 1660. The few who appear in published sources seem to have been literate and respectable, such as the widow of a clergyman who attended a Catholic mother near Preston, as related in the pamphlet account of a monstrous birth, published in 1646.[27] Most of the women who applied for licences during the 1662 visitation of the Archbishop of York appear to have been reasonably prosperous. Dorothy Walker was the wife of a busy Manchester master clothworker. Mary Steele of Nantwich was the widow of a yeoman who had left her lands and the use of his personal estate for life. Maude Rowe of Witton inherited half of her husband's yeoman estate in 1670. Anne Penlington of Acton was in possession of goods worth over £250 when she died in 1672. Margaret Strettell, a Mobberley spinster, left £78 worth of goods, livestock and money owed to her on her death in 1674. Mistress Jane Pennington, a yeoman's wife near Wigan, inherited goods worth over £160 from her husband in 1691.[28]

One member of the 1662–63 cohort is well known only by chance, because of the cutaneous horns that grew on her head. Her biography suggests that this respectability of the midwives is not a product of the bias inherent in record linkage. Mary Davies of Saughall in the parish of Shotwick, near Chester, was summoned by the York visitation in 1662, so she obtained a Chester licence which she produced at the Archbishop's court in August 1663. She was also summoned for initially failing to produce her licence at the Bishop's visitation of 1665. Her horns became valued curios and at least two portraits of her were painted in 1668. She travelled to London and exhibited herself near Charing Cross in 1676, at which time she was 76, a tenant farmer paying £16 per annum to the Crown. 'She was Wife to one Master Henry Davies, who dyed Thirty five Years pass'd; and since she hath lived a Religious Widow, all along of a spotless and unblameable Life and Conversation, of singular use to her Neighbours, for she is a professed Mid-wife.'[29]

Such respectable midwives appear to have been particularly concentrated in the major towns during the late seventeenth century. In 1704, an ecclesiastical lawyer proudly noted in his diary that his wife had been delivered by the Mayoress of Chester, 'Domina Anderton praetoris uxor obstetrix'.[30] Late seventeenth-century Liverpool was served by notably prominent midwives. The first recorded midwife, Margery Heald, was licensed in the 1662–63 visitation. When she died in 1669, her personal estate totalled over £800, a sum that it would have been difficult to accumulate from the profits of midwifery. Her successor, Jane Hunt, was only the widow of an innkeeper but, as the town's wealth and population rapidly increased, later midwives were more substantial members of the community. Hannah Brancker was the daughter of a former Oxford academic interested in chemistry and mathematics who taught in Macclesfield until his death in 1676. She was licensed in 1679 and practised in Macclesfield for several years but she did not marry until 1699, when she was living in Liverpool with her brothers, a goldsmith and an apothecary. Her husband was a writing master and mathematician, William Moss. Katharine Warbrick, licensed in 1684, was the pious wife of a very wealthy merchant who founded a charity for sailors' widows. Ellen Fletcher, licensed in 1691, was the daughter of Jane Hunt and the wife of a wealthy mariner who left her his Little Eccleston estate.[31] Such women cannot be found practising midwifery in the genteel Liverpool of the mid-eighteenth century.

It is possible to trace midwives in many of the parishes of Lancashire and Cheshire who possessed adequate financial resources apart from what they could earn from midwifery, although few matched Alice Kay, a Bury nonconformist and founder of a medical family, only known to have practised midwifery because she witnessed a bastardy deposition in 1704. Despite her late husband having disposed of most of the family property, she left a personal estate of over £1,300.[32] Most midwives in villages and small towns were less fortunate but they were usually the wives or widows of tradesmen, yeomen farmers or professional men. Personal possessions in the region of £50 to £200 were common until about 1730.

Even in the heyday of midwifery there were, of course, some midwives whom their contemporaries described as poor, women who practised because they needed the income. Dorothy Rowland of Holt, Iscoed, was excused licensing in 1662 because she was old and poor.[33] Martha Leigh of Ormskirk, formerly of Manchester, had been licensed as a midwife in 1674. In 1704, she petitioned the Lancashire Quarter Sessions for an increase in the poor relief paid to her and her daughter because she was too old to practise.[34] Elizabeth Fletcher, a Wrenbury widow, was described as 'one of ye poor of the Town' when she was cited as unlicensed in 1722. A clergyman gave her a testimonial, which was also signed by the curate, the churchwardens and twenty-six women, and she continued to practise for at least twenty-five years.[35] More remarkable perhaps, as indicating the decline of midwifery, is the case of Mary West, a Blackburn spinster, who was first recorded as a midwife in 1747. In 1752, she was examined as a pauper, at which time she was 33 years old and lived with her mother and step-father, tenant farmers who provided her with food and clothing in return for her work about the house. She had learned midwifery eight years previously, 'allways applying ye money she acquired by it to her own Use'.[36] Midwifery declined so steeply that in 1774 it was possible for a Catholic midwife to go bankrupt at Great Crosby, in the Catholic heartland.[37]

Payments to midwives varied widely, in part because wealthier families gave substantial tips. After a birth among even minor gentry, the female relatives would give graces of at least a shilling or half a crown. The godfather and even absent male relatives might give rather more at the baptism. Arthur Jessop wrote in 1668 to his daughter, Anne Hilton of Hilton Park, 'If out of ye mony in y^r hands yo^u would giue something as from me to yor Midwife & Nurses employed when litle Jess was borne I think it might doe well and I should take it well giuen.'[38] Gentry families also paid fees higher than those paid by other clients, since the midwife would be expected to spend several days in the house. Ann Aspinwall of Wigan had a riding practice among the Catholic gentry. For the birth of Nicholas Blundell's eldest child, she stayed 18 days and was paid 7 guineas. When she travelled to Northumberland to attend a Lancashire-born Catholic woman, she was paid £2 7s.[39]

A yeoman family would usually pay half a crown to the midwife, as did Richard Latham of Scarisbrick in the late 1720s when his first three children were delivered by Elizabeth Gill or Elizabeth Ditchfield of Ormskirk.

Thereafter, he employed a neighbour on five occasions, for fees of 1s. to 3s.[40] Overseers of the poor usually paid midwives between half a crown and 5s., although this might include two visits or services other than midwifery. The bill submitted by Mary Peers for delivering a vagrant's bastard near Warrington in 1745 included three items: midwifery, washing linen, and laying out the dead child in its coffin.[41] The midwife's fee was a small part of the total costs of childbirth, but, in some parts of Lancashire, frugal overseers managed to pay midwives 2s. or less.[42]

Such indications as can be gathered from signatures and surviving letters suggest that many midwives before the decline were highly literate, even though their skills were practical rather than learned from books. Most books in a household would belong to the husband, so it is difficult to assess what midwives were reading. Only one midwife can be identified as owning a midwifery manual, Anne Crompton of Breightmet, who also left several nonconformist devotional works when she died in 1681, but other licensed midwives can be identified as possessing small collections of books. The largest collection found is that of Margery Chorley, who left a bookcase and forty books.[43] Samples of bastardy depositions suggest that fewer of the mainly unlicensed midwives who delivered village bastards were fully literate, perhaps only 20 per cent in Cheshire. Some parts of Lancashire, especially those areas with strong religious traditions, did rather better. Of the thirty-two bastardy depositions witnessed by sixteen midwives in Bury between 1700 and 1760, only five were witnessed by midwives unable to sign their names.[44]

Only experienced midwives obtained licences, so it is difficult to know at what age most midwives commenced practice. Mary West seems to have been exceptionally young when she began practising at the age of 21. William Sermon justified the advanced age of midwives on the grounds that 'a woman that beareth Children is over-much troubled, so the more unfit to labour in so great a task'.[45] Licensed midwives were usually widows or women whose children were old enough to look after themselves, but this may simply indicate that they came to the notice of the court when they were devoting more time to midwifery, whether because they had more need or more opportunity. There were a few young licensed midwives, such as Hannah Brancker. She practised in Macclesfield and Liverpool for several years before marrying in 1699. She was widowed in 1708 and her younger children died in childhood. She had resumed practice by the time the eldest was 10. Since her late husband was far from poor, it seems unlikely that her resumption of practice was brought about by financial need.[46] The marital status of midwives is often unclear, but other examples of unmarried licensed midwives can be found, such as Margaret Strettell and Hannah Sutton, a Knutsford spinster recommended by Thomas White of Manchester in 1760.[47]

Midwives, religion and morals

In all their functions, the integrity of the midwives was paramount. They were central figures in women's culture, acting as advisors and conciliators as well as organizing the rituals surrounding childbirth, but at times they also had to represent the more respectable section of the town or village. The oath and licence laid a wide range of duties on licensed midwives, most of which were also recognized by their unlicensed colleagues.[48] Discretion and modesty were primary qualifications for a midwife. Esther Fogg of Salford was 'a Gentlewoman of modest & sober behavior' and Elizabeth Walker of Ashton-under-Lyne was 'a Gentlewoman of a sober & an honest Conversation', according to the clergymen who gave them testimonials.[49] Such qualities were also highly regarded by a midwife's neighbours, who trusted her not to upset patients or reveal their secrets. When Anne Knutsford, the wife of a prosperous Nantwich grocer, engaged in a costly and protracted series of slander suits to recover her good name and her 1662 midwifery licence, her skills were not in dispute between the two factions, led by the wives of the minister and the doctor. Mrs Knutsford had to defend herself against accusations of cursing, swearing, slander, neglecting the poor and revealing the secrets of women. She successfully rebutted the charges although she did admit attending women in emergencies while inhibited from practice by the court.[50] For the pious, profane speech on the part of a midwife was an abomination. Widow Maurice of Whitchurch, 'in ordinary Conversation, lifting up her two Hands towards Heaven, and stretching out her Fingers to the full length, used to swear by these Ten Bloody Bones'. God's punishment led to her son and grandson being born with additional thumbs which she herself had to hack off.[51]

Religious conformity was also one of the key characteristics of the ideal licensed midwife, but midwives were not expected to obtain certificates confirming that they had taken the sacrament.[52] Presbyterian midwives probably experienced few difficulties as long as they were occasional conformists, although religious scruples may have been behind the persistent failure to appear of such women as Elizabeth Pickering of Warrington, 'an experienced Midwife but not licensed', or the refusal of a licensed midwife, Sarah Faulkner of Middlewich, 'to bring ye Children to be baptizd in time of Divine Service'.[53] Since licensed midwives were expected to bring children to the parish church for Anglican baptism, it was important for Quakers and Catholics to have access to sympathetic midwives, although these were not necessarily co-religionists.[54] Elizabeth Gill of Ormskirk dined with the Blundells, after delivering a baby which was baptized by Mrs Blundell, and Hannah Moss of Liverpool lodged with the Blundells after attending Catholic families in the neighbourhood.[55] Catholic midwives were probably not resented by their Protestant colleagues, as long as they practised only among their fellow Catholics. In 1738, however, the

Protestant midwives of Wigan complained that 'two papish stroulers' had come to town and the wife was persuading women, 'by her fair speeches', to let her act as midwife. 'And some few dayes after the birth of the said children shee takes them away to a papish preist And getts them baptizd.' They were expelled from Wigan.[56] Such motives probably lay behind the last ecclesiastical case against a midwife, brought in Preston in 1776 'against Elizabeth Sharrock otherwise Cowper for that she being a Roman Catholic and having no License practises Midwifery in this Parish and other places in the Diocese of Chester'.[57]

Before the passing of the Toleration Act in 1689, Quaker midwives were sometimes vigorously pursued. The Quaker community of Stockport possessed three midwives in the late seventeenth century, Ann Shield, her daughter-in-law Constance, and Elizabeth Owen. Ann Shield came to the notice of the Archbishop's court in 1662–63 as a midwife but she and Constance were usually noticed for failing to attend the parish church or for keeping their shop open during divine service. The two women ran a draper's shop which sold imported silks and taffeta, Scots and English cloth, and a range of medicines and groceries such as treacle, strong waters and tobacco. Constance was assisting Ann in midwifery by 1674, when they were both reported to the courts of the Archdeacon and the Bishop. Presumably Constance, whose eldest child was then 15, was preparing to take over from Ann, who died in 1675. She continued to be presented for not appearing until 1686, but she was untroubled thereafter until her death in 1703, either as a result of the Toleration Act or because she ceased to practise after her only surviving daughter's wedding, handing over her practice to Elizabeth Owen, the widow of a Quaker weaver.[58] In the Quaker heartland of north Lancashire, persecution was rather more sporadic. The two Quaker midwives of Hawkshead, Dorothy Beck and Dorothy Satter-thwaite, were intermittently cited by the churchwardens for unlicensed practice during the period 1680–1700. Although the Quaker midwives of Westmorland and North Lancashire do not appear to have had their own meeting, unlike the Quaker midwives of Barbados, the Women's Meetings exercised close supervision of their activities. The two Hawkshead midwives also acted as poor relief agents for their Women's Meeting.[59]

Parish and county officials might call upon midwives to act as expert witnesses in a variety of circumstances. Like any other medical practitioner, they might have to make a statement that a witness was unable to attend a trial.[60] The most frequent role of midwives in legal proceedings was their responsibility under the poor law to question mothers of bastard children during labour as to the identity of the putative father and then provide a deposition at the petty sessions which could form the basis for a maintenance order.[61] It was in the interest of the parish officers and all the ratepaying households that the father should be identified, so the midwife was acting as the representative of the respectable parishioners. In cases where pregnancy was denied by the expectant mother, a midwife might be called in well before the birth.[62]

The statement to the midwife *in extremis* generally took precedence over depositions taken before the birth. When Hannah Jones of Nantwich, 'a common whore', falsely named a local miller in 1721, the magistrates refused to allow her to retract her sworn statement so the midwife's evidence was crucial. The mother admitted 'in her greatest extremity' that her original statement 'was in prejudice to and to be revenged on Mr. Cook's wife with whom she had a Quarrel'.[63] The midwife's opinion remained crucial even when the mother attempted to mislead her or named more than one man as the father.[64] If the midwife arrived too late to deliver the child, she still might find the mother *in extremis,* so she could still question her and report the dying words.[65] This role of midwives gradually disappeared in the eighteenth century as courts gave priority to the pre-birth statement and as printed forms, which called only for the mother's statement, replaced handwritten depositions made after the birth.[66]

Midwives who failed to ensure the filiation of bastards might well fall foul of the ecclesiastical authorities since participation in the legal process was regarded as one of their principal duties. Ann Witter of Tarporley, who had previously denied practising midwifery, was later implicated as the midwife when her widowed daughter was presented for failing to name the father of her bastard.[67] Alice Hodgson of Dent failed to question a mother in 1714 and Jane King of Moor was cited by the curate of Daresbury in 1727 'for practiceing the Mistery of Midwifery without a License from the Ordinary and thereby makeing great gain to her Self and does not Cause the Naugty Women to filiate their Children'.[68]

Thanks to their respectability, midwives were credible witnesses on behalf of married couples accused of ante-nuptial fornication. Some midwives would merely add their signatures to statements that birth was premature, citing the lack of hair and nails. Sometimes the midwife herself would write, invoking community support for her expertise:

> This is to satisfy this Honourable Court that I Mary Cheetham Midwife do fully believe that Elizabeth Daughter of Aaron Hilton was born before it's full time, Likewise severall other women att that time p'sent do believe the same as Witness my hand, Mary Cheetham.[69]

Rape was a capital crime in which the midwife's evidence could be essential for the securing of a conviction. Since she would often know all the people involved and be called upon to examine the alleged victim by interested parties, it was vital that her moral probity be above suspicion. Adam Martindale vividly recalled the behaviour of the jury of matrons when his young daughter had been a witness in a rape case:

A midwife, being one of them, was much his friend, and talked hard for him; but when it came to swearing, she joyned with the rest, and tooke her oath, as all of them did, that (to the utmost of her judgement) the child was carnally known by some man.[70]

The deliberations of juries of matrons are generally lost to history but midwives were also called in for preliminary investigations.[71] When two apprentices were accused of raping the daughter of a Chester barber-surgeon in 1685, a midwife was called by the father of one of the accused to examine the child. She later deposed that she 'could not *p*ceive or Finde any probabillity or signe or tocken in the least of any Rape'.[72] A Warrington midwife called in by the mother of an 11-year-old girl in 1738 stated 'that she did this day Examine the private parts of the said Judith Henshaw and saith that some man hath lately Ravished or attempted to Ravish her the sd Judith, for that she had several marks of violence upon those parts'. The hesitancy of this evidence led to the man being accused and convicted of the non-capital offence of attempted rape.[73]

The other capital crime that required the evidence of midwives was infanticide. Although the Infanticide Act of 1624 had shifted the onus of proof on to a defendant, once she had been identified as having secretly borne a child that had subsequently been found dead, in practice it was even more difficult to obtain a conviction than in cases of rape, because of the problem of providing convincing evidence that the child had been born alive.[74] A respected midwife could exonerate an accused mother simply by testifying that the child was stillborn or premature. Mary Trygorne, the wife of a Chester saddler, signed a deposition in 1678 that she could not have saved a bastard child born dead even if she had been present at its birth as she estimated it to have been about 3 months premature.[75]

The usual procedure when an infant's body had been discovered was for some respectable women of the neighbourhood, usually led by the midwife, to interrogate the most likely suspect, attempting to draw milk from her breasts if a confession was not forthcoming. The greatest asset of midwives in such investigations was probably their personal authority. In 1696, the midwife who was questioning a Clayton-le-Dale spinster 'said unto her can you looke me in ye face and say you have not borne a Child'.[76] By the time the coroner arrived, the identity of the mother had often been established. The midwife might also be required to consider the cause of death. In 1739, Anne Elliott had to inspect a child buried secretly in Leyland churchyard. She declared that it 'was come to its full Growth but cannot say whether the said Child was born alive'.[77] The main handicap of midwives as witnesses was not a lack of competence but the very reticence imposed on them by the oath and social expectation. When Chorley midwives gave evidence before a knight and a baronet in petty sessions in

1684, they stated that 'the sd Mrs Ellin Ainsworth hath borne a Child but how lately they can none of them sweare and that they drew ye Brests of ye sd Mrs Ellin Ainsworth and found Milk therein; and likewise that there were other signes on her of haveing a Child but they cannot with modesty express it'.[78]

The rise of the man-midwife

Surgeons had always been required to operate on parturient women in emergencies but after the 1720s they began increasingly to move into the field of normal deliveries. The practice of man-midwifery could, on occasion, be highly profitable. In an infanticide case, a Cartmel apothecary was reported to have delivered a child in 1733, 'for wch trouble he recd five Guineas & was pmisd five Guineas more & sd he would not live but by such Businesse'.[79] Even for delivering a poor law patient, a man-midwife could expect to be paid a guinea, as were William Oddie, a Clitheroe gentleman surgeon-apothecary, in 1750 and Richard Guest, a Pennington apothecary, in 1757. A wealthy pupil of Boerhaave, Edward Pemberton of Warrington, was paid 2 guineas for attending 'a poor Woman in labour in Cronton' in 1760, as was an unnamed man-midwife in Bickerstaffe in 1750. Atherton employed men-midwives occasionally from 1737 and normally paid a guinea, although they managed to find a surgeon for 16s. in 1741.[80] Yet no man could comfortably maintain himself through obstetrics alone. There was not enough demand and it was too time-consuming and exhausting. In an overcrowded profession, man-midwifery was a route to more lucrative kinds of family practice.[81]

Before 1750, few surgeons seem to have distinguished man-midwifery from their surgical practice, although licences for man-midwifery were issued to Peter Key of Dunham in 1691 and Jonathan Hall of Nantwich in 1731.[82] Thomas White, the Manchester surgeon-physician who had been apprenticed to a London apothecary and became an extra-licentiate of the Royal College of Physicians in 1733, was credited with developing the methods that ensured the fame of his son Charles, but he does not appear as a man-midwife in contemporary records.[83] Of the leading surgeon-physicians in this region, only Henry Bracken sought to publicize his intrusion into midwifery. Country practitioners were voraciously reading the new obstetrics texts but were slow to recognize changing patterns of practice.[84] Unfortunately, this makes it impossible to estimate the availability of men-midwives since often only a stray reference indicates that a surgeon-apothecary regularly offered midwifery attendance.[85]

This was beginning to change during the 1750s. As the system of licensing midwives fell into disuse, along with other aspects of the ecclesiastical court system, there was a little flurry of men-midwives who sought licences to justify their expanding practice. Among others, Ralph Holt of Liverpool presented a testimonial signed in 1755 by his former master, Henry Bracken, who testified to his pupil's abilities 'in the buisnesses I do profess (that is to say) as a Surgeon, Physician, and man Midwife'. John Wareing of Liverpool, who had been apprenticed to James Bromfield in 1730, presented a testimonial signed by his former master and another surgeon in 1757. In 1762, some twenty years after his apprenticeship to an Ormskirk apothecary, Miles Barton of Hoole, a gentleman surgeon-apothecary, took out a man-midwifery licence.[86]

The transition to using surgeons as the practitioners of first resort was far from straightforward. Just as there was a reluctance to commit a sick relative to the hands of surgeons before all physical means had been exhausted, so too in difficult births relatives tended to procrastinate before calling in a male practitioner, partly because of the association with death. Henry Bracken complained that during sixteen years he had only been called as the practitioner of first resort some four or five times. In 1744, a letter from Chester about a woman's death in childbed revealed that 'she was in ye Agonyes of death before a Man-midwife reacht her'.[87] This reluctance was probably increased by the reputation of the men-midwives for immodest behaviour. In the case of Henry Bracken, this appears to have been deserved. He was named as the guilty man in a 1734 fornication case and even his admiring biographer had to admit that he was 'addicted to unlawful commerce with the sex'.[88]

The surgeons also started to be called as expert witnesses by the coroners in cases of infanticide, because of their increasing post-mortem experience. There was, however, no guarantee that the surgeon would be called at the trial. Henry Bracken complained that he had not been called to give evidence in an infanticide trial, despite having viewed the body, and he blamed the woman's acquittal on this. Yet when Bracken was Mayor of Lancaster and sat as coroner *ex officio* in 1748, the only expert witness he called in a case of infanticide was Mrs Sarah Haresnape.[89] Initially, midwives were still closely involved even when surgeons were called, as in a 1741 case before Sir Henry Hoghton of Walton-le-Dale. A surgeon pronounced on the causes of death but it was a midwife who drew milk from the breasts of the suspect, the traditional means of identifying the guilty woman, and pronounced on the likelihood of her still having milk five years after the birth of her last child.[90] Fairly soon, however, surgeons supplanted midwives in court as autopsies became more routine in infanticide cases. In February 1755, a surgeon of New Church in the Forest of Rossendale opened an infant corpse and found its breast bone broken and, in the same month, a Liverpool surgeon examined a body found in a midden, but their evidence was no more decisive than that which a midwife could have given. Ralph Holt of Liverpool examined a dead child's body in 1761 'but cannot really tell whether it was born alive or not but it seems to have come to a proper time of Birth or nigh it tho he cannot be Exact as to that'.[91] The supplanting of midwives in one of their most prominent public functions seems to have been brought about by the coroners' growing familiarity with surgeons as witnesses rather than by any superiority of their evidence.

It has been suggested that the use of the forceps broke the association of the surgeon with certain death, for either mother or child.[92] Yet not all men-midwives were enthusiastic users of tools and it remains unclear why the midwives eschewed their use in the eighteenth century. They had formerly employed them on occasion. A Liverpool woman owned 'a midwife's stoole and instruments' when she died in 1669 and one of the most horrific tools, the griffon's foot, was described in a 1688 book sponsored by Chester medical practitioners as 'an Instrument used by Midwives and Chyrurgions, that follow the Occupation of Midwifery'. A Shropshire midwife of the same period is known to have employed hooks to deliver a stillbirth.[93] Nevertheless, it is clear that midwives increasingly left the emergency use of such tools to their male colleagues. William Sermon, discussing stillbirths in 1671, did not describe the use of crochets, hooks and tongs because 'such remedies are most commonly made use of by men'.[94] Thus the use of tools became the exclusive preserve of surgeons just as the use of the forceps was about to become widespread and instruction in their use became the monopoly of the London men-midwives. Among Catholics, the spread of man-midwifery may have been further encouraged by the use of a less arcane tool, the syringe. Baptism *in utero* by a Catholic man-midwife is recorded in Staffordshire as early as 1733.[95]

Although he complained that midwifery was dominated by 'a Pack of young Boys, and old superannuated Washer-women', George Counsell claimed that a local examination system for both men and women who wished to practise midwifery would be feasible because, in 1752, there was 'scarce any City, or very large Town, in which a Practitioner in Midwifery of some Eminence does not now reside'.[96] Indeed, some towns were overstocked with men-midwives, as William Holbrooke complained of Manchester as early as 1737, contrasting it with Leicester. As a result, man-midwifery was a fertile source for the professional disputes that bedevilled mid-eighteenth-century English medicine, a vicious one breaking out between Ralph Holt and John Wareing of Liverpool in 1757.[97]

In response to the incursions of the surgeons, some enterprising midwives actually advertised the very services that in London had given rise to accusations of conniving at infanticide, made by moralists from Dekker to Defoe. In 1752, Mary Welch of Chester offered secret birth for a select clientele, safe from the prying eyes of parish officers.[98] Despite the rise of the men-midwives, some respectable midwives continued to practise successfully, such as the Wiltshire midwife who delivered over ten thousand women or the Derbyshire woman said to have practised for over eighty years.[99] In some towns, well established dynasties of midwives were able to resist the general trend.

Conclusion

As in Italy, it may be that the decline of traditional licensing was partly responsible for the devaluing of midwives' skills.[100] In England, this was caused by the decline of the ecclesiastical court system as a whole, independent of any medical interests. Perhaps midwives would have been better served by the imposition of the kind of state licensing attempted in more bureaucratic countries.[101] Women were not politically impotent in England during the eighteenth century, despite not having the vote, and the introduction of such a system would have been more likely had it not been for articulate women's desertion of the practice of midwifery and the employment of midwives.

The precise causes of midwifery's decline remain obscure, now that the simple story of the midwives' ignorance has to be rejected. Further research into English midwifery is clearly needed, to reveal the situation before the Civil War and at the end of the eighteenth century, to identify the precise social location of midwives within specific communities of different sorts and in different regions, and to shed further light on the cultural changes involved in women's choices. Even in the late eighteenth century, there clearly were a few educated women who continued to practise in some parts of the country, especially London, and the social distribution of their clients is still unknown.

It is possible to sketch the outlines. In the seventeenth century, midwives were often women of considerable social status, both central figures in local women's culture and representatives of the respectable part of the local population. Some were able to move as equals among the more affluent of their clientele, by virtue of both their skills and their social standing. The midwives' position, as brokers or intermediaries amid the network of women and parish notables represented by their testimonials, suggests that they should not simply be seen as offering a trade in a metaphorical 'medical marketplace'.[102]

In the mid-eighteenth century, the gentry withdrew behind their park walls while prosperous merchants and professionals cultivated the decorum of assemblies, societies and committees. Increasing aspirations to 'respectability' meant that affluent and educated townswomen were no longer recruited to the art of midwifery. Gentry families, becoming distant from their tenants and no longer finding suitable urban midwives, were obliged to rely on the surgeon's visit. The ever-widening gap between genteel and popular cultures made the village midwife, whatever her technical skills, an unsuitable person to take into a gentry household. The women's space of the elaborate lying-in ritual, governed by the midwife and excluding the husband, had no place in the companionate home of the Enlightenment. As ever, males defined the meaning of childbirth but it may be that they increasingly controlled the event too, husbands choosing a man-midwife from among their acquaintances.[103]

As a corrective to older views that saw women as passive victims of change, the interpretation presented here has laid more stress on changes in women's tastes than on the creation of new demands by male practitioners, responding to the oversupply of medical services, but these are not mutually exclusive explanations. The men-midwives, boasting greater skills and education than their female rivals, were able to exploit the lack of good midwives, driving home their advantage through the publication of propaganda. Men-midwives, even if they were Tories in politics like Bracken and the Whites, represented metropolitan modernity and scientific progress, a fashionable posture that few midwives could hope to emulate. The apparent willingness of polite society to be persuaded by this strategy suggests a shift in attitudes towards the value of science and the acquisition of knowledge. By the end of the century, it is possible that in some parts of England about half of all deliveries were attended by men.[104] The change to man-midwifery meant that, although the best available skills were available to all, they were most used by the rich and the poor, the latter in the insanitary conditions of lying-in hospitals. Such changes may have been consequences rather than intentional results but the shift to man-midwifery, with the associated change to the lithotomy position for childbirth, helped to inculcate concepts of the natural passivity of women and encouraged the infantilization of parturient women that was to reach its apogee in twentieth-century maternity hospitals.[105]

Notes

1. [S. Johnson and R. James], *A General Account of the Work* [proposal for the *Medical Dictionary*] (London, 1743).

2. For discussions of the midwifery literature, see J. Donnison, *Midwives and Medical Men* (London, 1977); J. B. Donegan, *Women and Men Midwives* (Westport, CT, 1978); A. Wilson, 'The ceremony of childbirth and its interpretation', in V. Fildes (ed.) *Women as Mothers in Pre-Industrial England* (London and New York, 1990), 68–107. On mute groups, see E. Ardener, 'Belief and the problem of women', in S. Ardener (ed.) *Perceiving Women* (London, 1975), 1–17.

3. I.M. Green, *The Re-establishment of the Church of England, 1660–1663* (Oxford, 1978), 117–42; W.F. Irvine, 'Church discipline after the Restoration', *Transactions of the Historic Society of Lancashire and Cheshire*, 64 (1912), 43–71; 'List of clergymen, &c., in the Diocese of Chester, 1691, recorded at the first visitation of Nicholas Stratford, Bishop of Chester', ed. J. Brownbill, *Chetham Miscellanies*, new series, vol. 3 (Chetham Society, 2nd series, 73, 1915).

4. See ch. 3 in this volume by Ann Giardina Hess, cf. chs 9 and 10 in this

volume by Mary Lindemann and Hilary Marland for Germany and Holland.

5. In this diocese, only two marriage bonds and one parish register entry have been discovered that refer to women as midwives.

6. Lancashire Record Office (hereafter LRO): QSP 751/12; cf. Cheshire Record Office (CRO): QJF 129/3/24.

7. Public Record Office (hereafter PRO): IR 1/50/214 for a Staffordshire example from 1738, costing £40 for a 5-year apprenticeship cf. IR 1/15/169.

8. CRO: WS 1727, Mary Twamlow of Northwich; EDV 1/106, f. 56; Diocesan Miscellany (hereafter DM). When this collection of testimonials was consulted, it consisted of three unnumbered bundles.

9. Guildhall Library, MS 25,598, file 8, testimonial of Elizabeth Beranger, 9 Sept. 1674; W. Clarke, *The Province of Midwives in the Practice of their Art* (London, 1751), 2–4; Middlesex Hospital: Quarterly General Court, 4 Aug. 1763; Weekly Board, 31 May and 11 Oct. 1763, 17 Sept. 1764, 15 Oct. 1765, 17 April 1770. I am grateful to Susan Lawrence for this reference.

10. J. Maubray, *The Female Physician* (London, 1724), 176–7.

11. S. Stone, *A Complete Practice of Midwifery* (London, 1737), xi–xii; H. Bracken, *The Midwife's Companion* (London, 1737), 36, 65, 149, 163, 171–2. For Bracken's career, see W.C., 'Some account of Henry Bracken, MD late of Lancaster', *European Magazine*, 45 (1804), 26–30, 100–4, 176–81.

12. J. Mayow, *RHACHITIDOLOGIA*, trans. W. Sury (Oxford, 1685). I am grateful to Barbara Simon for this reference.

13. E. Maynwaringe, *Morbus Polyrhizos & Polymorphaeus: A Treatise of the Scurvy*, 3rd edn (London, 1669), 31; British Library (hereafter BL): Sloane MS 4043, ff. 155–6. Bracken's pamphlet is quoted in D.N. Harley, 'Honour and property: the structure of professional disputes in eighteenth-century medicine', in A. Cunningham and R. French (eds) *The Medical Enlightenment of the Eighteenth Century* (Cambridge, 1990), 163.

14. LRO: QSP 881/24; 889/3; 909/13.

15. CRO: DM; EDC 6/1/7; EDC 5/1691/30.

16. *Marriage Licences granted within the Archdeaconry of Chester*, vol. 6, 1667–80 (Lancashire and Cheshire Record Society (hereafter LCRS), vol. 69, 1914), 142; *Liverpool Chronicle*, 6 May 1757, quoted in the *Lancet*, 27 March 1897, 905; CRO: DM.

17. H. Rolle, *Un Abridgment des Plusieurs Cases et Resolutions del Common Ley* (London, 1668), pt 2, 286; J. Godolphin, *Repertorium Canonicum* (London, 1680), 126; R. Burn, *Ecclesiastical Law* (London, 1763), vol. 2, 47–9. See also ch. 1 in this volume by Doreen Evenden.

18. Most studies of the church courts deal with the period before 1640, but J. Addy, *Sin and Society in the Seventeenth Century* (London, 1989) uses later material from the Diocese of Chester. The York visitation records are kept at the Borthwick Institute, York (York V.); the Chester records are at the Cheshire Record Office (EDV); the Archdeaconry of Richmond records are held mainly at the Lancashire Record Office (ARR).

19. CRO: EDV 1/44, f. 64; *Chester Marriage Licenses*, vol. 6, 151.

20. CRO: EDV 1/34, f. 24; 1/64, f. 32; EDC 5/1691/30.

21. CRO: DM; EDV 1/111, f. 8; 1/45, f. 18; EDC 6/1/13; 5/1667/13.

22. CRO: EDV 1/126, f. 51/5, loose letter.

23. LRO: ARR 17/1/10, 17/41; CRO: EDV 1/35, f. 103v; 1/56, f. 100; 1/61, f. 36. See ch. 8 in this volume by Nadia Filippini for Church involvement in midwife licensing in eighteenth-century Italy.

24. Bracken, *Midwife's Companion*, sig. A6.

25. Chester City Record Office (hereafter CCRO): CR 74; CRO: EDV 2/21, f. 20v; DM.

26. T.R. Forbes, 'Midwifery and witchcraft', *Journal of the History of Medicine*, 17 (1962), 264; cf. D. Harley, 'Historians as demonologists: the myth of the mid-wife-witch', *Social History of Medicine*, 3 (1990), 1–26. Margaret Pelling's work on Norwich suggests that it is possible to find out a great deal about midwives before the Civil War. M. Pelling and C. Webster, 'Medical practitioners', in C. Webster (ed.) *Health, Medicine and Mortality in the Sixteenth Century* (Cambridge, 1979), 165–235.

27. *Five Wonders Seene in England* (London, 1646), 2–5.

28. York V. 1662–63/Exh.Bk., f. 33; York V. 1662–63/CB2, ff. 38v, 44v, 66v, 75v, 143v; LRO: WCW 1679 supra, Randle Walker of Manchester; WCW 1691 supra, Andrew Pennington of Orrell; CRO: WS 1661, Thomas Steele of Leighton; WS 1670, William Rowe of Hartford; WS 1672, Anne Penlington of Acton; WS 1674, Margaret Strettell of Mobberley.

29. York V. 1662–63/CB2, f. 25v; *Marriage Licences granted within the Archdeaconry of Chester*, vol. 5, 1661–67 (LCRS, vol. 65, 1912), 46; CRO: EDV 1/34, f. 21; R.T. Gunther, *Early Science in Oxford* (Oxford, 1926), vol. 3, pt 2, 372–3; BL: Sloane MS 4042, ff. 41, 51, 229; A. Macgregor, 'Mary Davis's horn: a vanished curiosity', *The Ashmolean*, 3 (Oct.–Dec. 1983), 10–11; *A Brief Narrative of a Strange and Wonderful Old Woman that hath A Pair of Horns Growing upon her Head* (London, 1676), 4–6.

30. *The Diary of Henry Prescott, LL.B., Deputy Registrar of Chester Diocese*, ed. J. Addy, vol. 1 (LCRS, vol. 127, 1987), 15.

31. York V. 1662–63/CB2, f. 135v; 'List of clergymen, &c.'; *Dictionary of National Biography*, entry for Thomas Brancker; CRO: WS 1676, Thomas Brancker of Macclesfield; LRO: WCW 1669 supra, Margery Heald of Liverpool; WCW 1669 supra, William Hunt of Liverpool; WCW 1708 supra, William Moss of Liverpool; WCW 1706 supra, Richard Warbrick of Liverpool; WCW 1728 supra, Katherine Warbrick of Liverpool; WCW 1703 supra, William Fletcher of Liverpool.

32. LRO: CBB 32; WCW 1697 supra, Richard Kay of Baldingstone; WCW 1711 supra, Alice Kay of Cross Hall, Walmersley.

33. York V. 1662–63/CB2, f. 11v; cf. CRO: EDV 1/34, f. 10v.

34. *Chester Marriage Licenses*, vol. 6, 145; LRO: QSP 909/2, 3.

35. CRO: EDV 1/102; DM; EDV 2/33, f. 13r.

36. CRO: EDV 2/33, f. 29r; LRO: PR 1560/2/8, 9.

37. LRO: QJB 41/27.

38. *The Household Account Book of Sarah Fell of Swarthmore Hall*, ed. N. Penny (Cambridge, 1920), 241, 335, 439; Donnison, *Midwives and Medical Men*, 10; LRO: DDHu 47/34.

39. *The Great Diurnall of Nicholas Blundell of Little Crosby, Lancashire*, 3 vols (LCRS, vols 110, 112, 114, 1968–72), vol. 1, 1702–11, 66–9; *Selections from the Disbursements Book (1691–1709) of Sir Thomas Haggerston, Bart.*, ed. A.M.C. Foster (Surtees Society, vol. 180, 1969), 50.

40. *The Account Book of Richard Latham, 1724–1767*, ed. L. Weatherill (Oxford, 1990), 9, 12, 16, 20, 24, 29, 36, 48.

41. LRO: QSP 1549/19–22.

42. LRO: PR 3168/7/9; Wigan Record Office (hereafter WRO): TR Ath/C1/1/97, 100, 169, 170, 176, 177, 184, 204, 564, 606.

43. LRO: WCW 1681 infra, Anne Crompton of Breightmet; WCW 1708 infra, Jane Runnigar of Manchester; WCW 1729 supra, Margery Chorley of Manchester; CRO: WS 1674, Margaret Stretell of Mobberley; WS 1685, Ann Hagar of Duddon.

44. LRO: CBB 32. Out of a hundred depositions, only two of the mothers

could sign. For literacy amongst Quaker midwives, see ch. 3 in this volume by Ann Giardina Hess.

45. W. Sermon, *The Ladies Companion, or the English Midwife* (London, 1671), 4.

46. 'List of clergymen, &c.'; LRO: WCW 1708 supra, William Moss of Liverpool.

47. CRO: DM. For the age and marital status of Quaker midwives, see ch. 3 in this volume by Ann Giardina Hess.

48. For a discussion of the position of midwives within women's culture, see Wilson, 'The ceremony of childbirth'. For the duties peculiar to midwives, see *The Book of Oaths* (London, 1649), 284–90; *The Book of Oaths* (London, 1689), 229–31; Donnison, *Midwives and Medical Men*, 229–31.

49. CRO: DM.

50. York V. 1662–63/CB2, f. 44v; CRO: EDC 5/1663/16, 54; 5/1664/6, 57, 68; 5/1667/2, 62; 1668/10; WS 1690, will of Thomas Knutsford.

51. W. Turner, *A Complete History of the Most Remarkable Providences* (London, 1697), pt 1, ch. 105, 17.

52. Alice Stamp, a Manchester innkeeper's wife who got a certificate in 1673, appears to be the only Lancashire example. LRO: QSJ/8/1/56.

53. A. Mountfield, *Early Warrington Nonconformity* (Warrington, 1922), 51; CRO: EDV 1/38, f. 87v; 1/54, f. 85v; 1/87, f. 7; EDC 6/1/1.

54. See ch. 3 in this volume by Ann Giardina Hess.

55. *Blundell's Diurnall*, vol. 1, 1702–11 (LCRS, vol. 110, 1968), 84, 281; vol. 2, 1712–19 (LCRS, vol. 112, 1970), 17. One of Mrs Moss's brothers, the goldsmith Benjamin Brancker, was a friend of Nicholas Blundell.

56. WRO: CL/Wi, Roll 156/Mich.1738.

57. LRO: ARR 15/128, f. 2v.

58. York V. 1662–63/CB2, f. 83v; York V. 1669–70/CB, 112; York V. 1684–85, f. 333; CRO: EDV 1/37, f. 34v; 1/38, f. 45v; 1/39, f. 31; 1/40, f. 70; 1/44, f. 52v; 2/7, f. 12v; 1/44, f. 52v; 1/52, f. 48v; 1/64, f. 30; EDC 1/14/2, 1/14/3, 12/1/1; will of Ann Sheilds, WS 1675; will of Elizabeth Owen, WI 1695.

59. LRO: ARR 15/29, f. 6v; 15/33, f. 3; 15/34, f. 4; 17/33; *Account Book of Sarah Fell*, 307, 363, 375, 397–8; 'At a meeting of the midwives in Barbadoes', *Journal of the Friends Historical Society*, 37 (1940), 22–4. See also ch. 3 in this volume by Ann Giardina Hess.

60. PRO: PL 28/40/2: affidavit of Joyce, wife of Charles Brooks of Halsall, 26/8/1737.

61. For a discussion of the origins of this system and some early cases, see P.C. Hoffer and N.E.H. Hull, *Murdering Mothers: Infanticide in England and New England, 1558–1803* (New York, 1984), 13–7.

62. CRO: EDC 6/1/9, statements on behalf of Robert Pont, 25/10/1728.

63. CRO: EDC 6/1/6; QJF 149/3/49, 78; QJB 3/7; Nantwich Parish Register, baptism on 29/8/1721.

64. CRO: EDC 5 (1704) no. 7.

65. LRO: QSP 697/10, bastardy deposition re Grace Pollard.

66. The change occurs around 1750. WRO: TR Ath/C7/1. The printed forms used in Bury from 1722 required witnesses. LRO: CBB 32.

67. CRO: EDV 1/34, f. 13; 2/6, f. 4v; 1/45, f. 5; 1/51, f. 8.

68. LRO: ARR/15/84, f. 6v; CRO: EDV 1/109, f. 30v.

69. CRO: EDC 6/1/12, letter re Abraham and Mary Barlow, signed by Mary Farmer of Manchester, 4/5/1729; EDC 6/1/7, undated letter re Silence and Thomas Hardman, written in 1724 by Elizabeth Walker of Radcliffe; EDC 6/1/8, letter on behalf of Aaron Hilton, 3/11/1725.

70.   *The Life of Adam Martindale*, ed. R. Parkinson (Chetham Society, vol. 4, 1845), 206–7.

71.   T.R. Forbes, 'A jury of matrons', *Medical History*, 32 (1988), 23–33.

72.   CCRO: QSF/83/181–4, 219, 268.

73.   PRO: PL 27/2, depositions re Judith Henshaw, 9/8/1738; PL 25/103.

74.   21 James I, c. 27 (1624); Hoffer and Hull, *Murdering Mothers*; T.R. Forbes, *Surgeons at the Bailey: English Forensic Medicine to 1878* (New Haven, 1985), 96–108; R.W. Malcolmson, 'Infanticide in the eighteenth century', in J.S. Cockburn (ed.) *Crime in England, 1550–1800* (London, 1977), 187–209.

75.   CCRO: QCO/I/14/7.

76.   PRO: PL 27/2, depositions re Elizabeth Boulton, 16/6/1696, 23/6/1696.

77.   PRO: PL 27/2, inquest on bastard of Margery Thornley, 15/11/1739.

78.   PRO: PL 27/1, depositions re bastard of Ellin Ainsworth, 28–29/4/1684. For the moral functions of midwives in early modern Germany, see ch. 4 in this volume by Merry Wiesner.

79.   PRO: PL 28/13, 5; PL 27/2, depositions re child of Margaret Lickbarrow, 12/5/1736–28/6/1736.

80.   LRO: PR 2995/1/22, 2995/1/9 (9); Warrington Library: MS 1115; LRO: PR 607; PR 418; WRO: TR Ath/Cl/1/118, 121, 126, 281, 370.

81.   I. Loudon, *Medical Care and the General Practitioner 1750–1850* (Oxford, 1986), 94–9. See chs 5, 8, 9 and 10 in this volume for the relationships between men-midwives and midwives in Spain, Italy, Germany and Holland.

82.   *Marriage Licences granted within the Archdeaconry of Chester*, vol. 8, 1691–1700 (LCRS, vol. 77, 1924), 1; CRO: DM.

83.   PRO: IR 1/1/179; CRO: EDV 2/21, f. 10r; W. Munk, *The Roll of the Royal College of Physicians* (London, 1878), vol. 2, 129; J.G. Adami, *Charles White of Manchester (1728–1813) and the Arrest of Puerperal Fever* (Liverpool and New York, 1923), 23, n. 2.

84.   BL: Sloane MS 4040, f. 84; *A Catalogue of Books in Various Languages contained in the Library collected by Richard Shepherd, Esq., M.B.* (Preston, 1839), 106–7.

85.   For example, the registering of an apprentice by William Barrow of Lancaster in 1754. Lancaster City Library: MS 208, p. 179, but not PRO: IR 1/52/25; the will of Thomas Frith of Middlewich: CRO: WS 1765; an advertisement for an apprentice in the *Manchester Mercury*, 25 March 1766, by James Ward of Stockport, but a druggist in his will. CRO: WS 1775.

86.   CRO: DM; PRO: IR 1/16/165, 1/49/269; LRO: WCW 1758 supra, will of Henry Barton; W.R. Hunter, 'William Hill and the Ormskirk medicine', *Medical History*, 12 (1968), 294–7.

87.   Bracken, *Midwife's Companion*, 64–5; LRO: DDX/207/1/25.

88.   R. Porter, 'A touch of danger: the man-midwife as sexual predator', in G.S. Rousseau and R. Porter (eds) *Sexual Underworlds of the Enlightenment* (Manchester, 1987), 206–32; W.C., 'Some account of Henry Bracken', 102; LRO: ARR/15/105A, f. 24.

89.   Bracken, *Midwife's Companion*, 38; PRO: PL 26/290, inquest on bastard of Mary Parker, 22/8/1748; PL 28/2, p. 73. No guilty verdicts were returned in the twenty-two infanticide cases at Lancaster assizes, 1730–60.

90.   PRO: PL 27/2, inquest on infant found in millstream, 6–9/2/1741.

91.   PRO: PL 27/3, inquest on bastard of Mary Mather, 26/2/1755; inquest on bastard of Ann Kenion, 14/2/1755; PL 27/2, inquest on the bastard of Martha Woods, 17/7/1761.

92.   For a discussion of this, see A. Wilson, 'William Hunter and the varieties of man-midwifery', in W.F. Bynum and R. Porter (eds) *William Hunter and the*

Eighteenth-Century Medical World (Cambridge, 1985), 343–69.

93. LRO: WCW 1669 supra, Margery Heald of Liverpool; R. Holme, *The Academy of Armoury* (Chester, 1688), vol. 2, 421; R. Gough, *The History of Myddle*, ed. P. Razzell (Firle, 1979), 99.

94. Sermon, *Ladies Companion*, 4.

95. *Roman Catholic Registers, 1720–1830* (Staffordshire Parish Register Society, vol. 53, 1959), 34. For the use of instruments by midwives in Italy and Holland, see chs 8 and 10 in this volume by Nadia Filippini and Hilary Marland.

96. G. Counsell, *The Art of Midwifery: or, the Midwife's Sure Guide* (London, 1752), x–xv.

97. *Notes and Queries*, 2nd series, 10 (25 Aug. 1860), 144; J. Nichols, *History and Antiquities of the County of Leicester* (London, 1800), vol. 3, pt 1, 161n; Harley, 'Honour and property'; *Lancet*, 10 April 1897, 1047. For a detailed examination of the problems that could beset an early man-midwife, see D.N. Harley, 'Ethics and dispute behaviour in the career of Henry Bracken of Lancaster, surgeon, physician and manmidwife', in R. Baker, D. Porter and R. Porter (eds) *The Codification of Medical Morality in the Eighteenth and Nineteenth Centuries* (Dordrecht, 1993), 47–71.

98. [Thomas Dekker], *Lanthorne and Candle-light* (London, 1608), sig. K4v; [Daniel Defoe], *Augusta Triumphans* (London, 1728), 9; *Adams's Weekly Courant*, 14 July 1752.

99. *Adams's Weekly Courant*, 9 June 1767; *Newcastle Chronicle*, 23 Jan. 1790.

100. N.M. Filippini, 'Levatrici e ostetricanti a Venezia tra sette e ottocento', *Quaderni Storici*, 58 (1985), 149–80. See also ch. 8 in this volume by Nadia Filippini.

101. R.A. Dorwat, 'The Royal College of Medicine and public health in Brandenburg-Prussia, 1685–1780', *Medical History*, 2 (1958), 13–23; R.L. Petrelli, 'The regulation of French midwifery during the *ancien régime*', *Journal of the History of Medicine*, 26 (1971), 276–92.

102. For an analysis of the limitations of current economic interpretations of eighteenth-century medicine, see D.N. Harley, 'Restricted markets and complex demand in early modern English medicine', forthcoming in a collection of essays on consumption edited by A. Offer.

103. H. Callaway, 'The most essentially female function of all: giving birth', in S. Ardener (ed.) *Defining Females: The Nature of Women in Society* (London, 1978), 163–85. The classic portrayal of the relationship between husband and man-midwife is, of course, Laurence Sterne's *Tristram Shandy* (York and London, 1759–67), which satirizes a famous York physician.

104. I am grateful to Irvine Loudon for this information. For an example of the proportion of births that a single man-midwife could deliver, see J. Lane, 'A provincial surgeon and his obstetric practice: Thomas W. Jones of Henley-in-Arden, 1764–1846', *Medical History*, 31 (1987), 345.

105. A. McLaren, *Reproductive Rituals: The Perception of Fertility in England from the Sixteenth Century to the Nineteenth Century* (London, 1984), 13–29; R.E. Davis-Floyd, 'The technological model of birth', *Journal of American Folklore*, 100 (1987), 479–95; S. Kitzinger, 'The social context of birth: some comparisons between childbirth in Jamaica and Britain', in C. P. MacCormack (ed.) *Ethnography of Fertility and Birth* (London, 1982), 181–203.

3

Midwifery practice among the Quakers in southern rural England in the late seventeenth century

Ann Giardina Hess

In the autumn of 1677 the Quaker matron Margaret Treadway paid a visit to Elizabeth Crouch at the Quaker girl's home in the Buckinghamshire parish of Prestwood. She was there to warn Elizabeth of the impropriety of her continued residence at her widowed father's house. According to the men delegates to the Upperside monthly meeting of south Buckinghamshire, 'Elizabeth stood charged by some of her Neighbours of the World with having behaved herself very immodestly with her father'. Judging the matter 'more proper and comely for women to examine than for men', they had referred it to the newly formed Upperside women's business meeting attended by fifty-three Quaker matrons from south Buckinghamshire and the neighbouring villages of Hertfordshire. Margaret Treadway was one of the three women entrusted to investigate the charges against the miscreant girl who, she reported, was 'hard and insensitive to the truth'. Her evaluation was vindicated when, at the winter's end, Elizabeth Crouch committed a second offence of being married by a priest.[1]

Margaret Treadway was a woman well chosen for the delicate task of investigating the case of incest. She was a long-standing member of the Upperside community, and both her husband and her son-in-law were men delegates.[2] She dealt frequently with the more routine matters of the women's administration, such as investigating the 'clearnes' of marriage intentions and reproving Quaker girls for dancing, keeping 'evil company', and marrying non-Quaker men 'of the World'.[3] Margaret Treadway also officiated at local Quaker births as a midwife. According to the Buckinghamshire quarterly meeting birth register she attended childbirths in the Upperside community for over twenty years.

The fact that the men delegates consulted with Margaret Treadway before taking punitive action against the wayward girl was not a disciplinary procedure unique to Quaker society. Seventeenth-century midwives were commonly consulted by male authorities for their expert opinion in cases of sexual misdemeanours. In the English quarter sessions courts, midwives certified in countless cases of bastardy after questioning the mother during labour about the identity of the baby's father. In the quarterly courts of Puritan New England, midwives were also involved in prosecuting cases of ante-nuptial fornication, examining infants born before nine months of wedlock for signs of prematurity. Midwives were also called upon to testify in more serious offences which involved unsanctioned household relations, such as rape, infanticide, physical abuse and even witchcraft.[4] Like Margaret Treadway, many of the matrons so consulted by the authorities were women who had waited until their children were grown and their domestic duties lessened before taking up midwifery and its associated social obligations.

Margaret Treadway's story reflects another feature common to early modern midwifery practice, in that many women donned the role of midwife on an occasional basis only, being content to offer their skills to a neighbour or relative, or to assist a more experienced midwife, as the situation demanded. In 1672 Margaret Treadway travelled to Hitchin to attend her daughter, Sarah Dell.[5] However, when Sarah had her second baby in 1674, she did not choose her mother as midwife, even though the birth took place in Upton, Margaret Treadway's home village. Instead Sarah went to the considerable expense of employing Frances Kent, a Quakeress from the Berkshire town of Reading 20 miles away.[6] In 1690 Margaret Treadway was invited together with several other women to assist a Chesham midwife deliver the baby of a Quaker merchant's wife at Chalfont St Peter.[7] Two years later, Margaret Treadway was employed[8] as officiating midwife by the same family. Her last recorded attendance at a childbirth took place in 1694, when she presided at the delivery of a blacksmith's wife at Farnham Royal.[9] Like other English women whose names are documented as 'midwife' in seventeenth-century Quaker birth registers, court depositions and churchwardens' presentments, Margaret Treadway probably was not primarily identified as such. It is feasible that the Upperside people knew her as a yeoman's wife, a grandmother and as a delegate to the women's meeting.

The woman designated as 'midwife' by the Quaker clerk might have been a helpful woman who had presided at a neighbour's childbirth or a fee-collecting practitioner active in the towns and villages of several neighbouring counties. Seventeenth-century midwives could be affluent or needy, literate or illiterate, rural or urban, young or old.[10] However, all midwives were influenced by the events of the life cycle. Like other women, Quakeresses combined the responsibilities of childbearing, family life and religious duty with the activities of a midwife in a variety of ways, and their stories have a broad application to the study of early modern midwifery practice. Although the Quaker records do not provide details on reimbursement (fee-for-service versus charitable neighbourly assistance), the detailed birth registers kept by the Quakers specify more routine information often absent from other sources such as court depositions and

Anglican licensing records. They reveal the identity of the parents who 'employed' midwives, the names of the women who assisted them, and the dates and places of the births which the midwife attended.

The nonconformist system of birth registration developed in contrast to the parochial system whereby the clerk simply entered the date of the baby's christening and the name of the baby's father into a yearly register.[11] William Penn, a famous member of the Upperside monthly meeting, recorded the Quakers' procedure for registering births in his book, *A Brief Account of the Rise and Progress of the People Call'd Quakers* (1694), by noting that,

> For Births, the Parents Name their own Children; which is usually some Days after they are born, in the Presence of the Midwife, if she can be there, and those that were at the Birth, who afterwards sign a Certificate for that Purpose prepared, of the Birth and Name of the Child or Children.[12]

Unlike Anglican baptisms, which usually occurred during the mother's lying-in,[13] Quaker registration required the active participation of the mother who, together with her husband, presented the new-born for naming at the local meeting a few weeks to a few months after the birth. Typically, the midwife and four or five women who had been present at the birth attended. One copy of the signed certificate was returned to the parents. The other was retained by the clerk of the monthly meeting who entered the details into a general register and then forwarded it to the clerk of the quarterly meeting, where it was similarly registered.[14] The births of stillborns and infants who died in the first few weeks of life most often went unrecorded.

Quaker birth registration was by no means a tightly regulated affair, and there are some problems attached to using registers and certificates. Original birth certificates seldom survive for rural meetings outside of London and Norwich prior to 1700, and not all meetings even recorded information on birth witnesses. The ones that did were at best sporadic in their reporting habits. The Buckinghamshire Quakers were particularly efficient in recording information on witnesses, and yet only 15 per cent of the 526 births entered by the quarterly meeting clerk between 1652 and 1702 included the names of midwives.[15] Thus, information about the 'case-loads' of rural Quaker midwives is typically limited to a few births, and the volume of their practices can only be guessed at. Other dissenting churches, such as the Presbyterians, Independents and Baptists, also documented information on birth witnesses. However, these other non-conformist birth registers generally survive only from the mid-eighteenth century onwards and for London. Quakers maintained their own system of registration from the beginnings of the movement in the 1650s until the administration of vital statistics became incorporated with the British public civil registry in the early nineteenth century.[16] As such, the lists of birth witnesses are a unique source for a case study investigating the nature of the neighbourly, kin and religious ties which midwives shared with parents. In addition, they provide an insight into contemporary employment practices.

Quaker midwifery is also clearly a special case, with respect to the effect of religion on childbirth practices, neighbourly bonding and employment opportunities. The Quakers were officially under siege by ecclesiastical and State authorities until the Toleration Act of 1689, and Quaker midwives were not immune to the religious persecution of their sect. They were jailed for their beliefs and their families were stripped of their household goods for refusing to pay church tithes. After the Restoration, midwives' names appeared on episcopal returns listing the hosts and hostesses of local conventicles.[17] Even some local churchwardens were at daggers drawn with Quaker midwives and harassed them by repeated presentments for unlicensed practice and refusal to attend church.[18] Midwives were not the only Quaker female practitioners to be persecuted. During the tumultuous years of the Civil War, the governors of hospital boards, including that of St Thomas's, discharged Quaker sisters from their posts.[19] Both at the level of the parish neighbourhood and at that of the urban charitable institution, administrators were active in weeding out this dangerous sort of woman.

From the 1670s onwards the social integration of Quakers into village life was becoming increasingly apparent. Parishioners protected their Quaker neighbours from persecution by the Church and State authorities by paying their tithes and by concealing the whereabouts of their conventicles. In some parishes, Quakers were even invited to fill parochial posts, acting as constables, vestrymen and overseers of the poor.[20] As to churchwardens, the vast majority did not bother to report the unlicensed activities of local Quakeresses. Perhaps nowhere was neighbourly bonding and community religious integration more evident than amongst women. As we shall see, the mutual willingness of Quaker women and their parish neighbours to exchange help during childbirth was apparent from the settling of the first Quaker communities in the mid-seventeenth century.

Religious integration at childbirth in the Buckinghamshire quarterly meeting, 1652–1718

The Upperside monthly meeting, of which Margaret Treadway was a member, was held in the Chiltern hills of south Buckinghamshire and the bordering parishes of Hertfordshire. Like many Quaker meetings, this one was drawn largely from the rural population – yeomen, husbandmen, small craftsmen and traders[21] – although it also had amongst its members several gentry families including the Penns and Peningtons. The less prosperous Lowerside monthly meeting was located in the mixed farming region of the north Buckinghamshire Vale of Aylesbury. Altogether, thirty-one midwives were registered as witnessing the births of seventy-two Quaker mothers in the Buckinghamshire quarterly and monthly meetings between 1652 and 1702.[22] Twenty-three (74 per cent) of the midwives are thought to have been Quakers. Of these, nine have been positively identified in the Quaker vital statistics. Fourteen shared the surname of a local Quaker family or had some other strong association with the Society, such as having their will witnessed by a local Friend. However, six (19 per cent) of the midwives were definitely selected from outside the Society of Friends. The names of the remaining four women cannot be traced definitively in either the Quaker or parochial registers.[23]

Not only did Quakers apparently use non-Quaker 'parish midwives',[24] they commonly engaged the help of non-Quaker neighbours to assist the midwife. Seventy-five (32 per cent) of the 235 witnesses attending births with the thirty-one midwives possessed surnames not traceable to Quaker records in Buckinghamshire or any of the surrounding counties. In several instances the Buckinghamshire clerks were explicit in their designation of witnesses as 'neighbours', the customary distinction used for non-Quaker friends and kin who attended their births, marriages and burials. Some of the women who helped out at these births were perhaps maidservants from more distant counties such as Yorkshire and Lancashire. Notwithstanding this possibility, it appears that it was common for a Quaker mother to invite non-Quaker friends and kin to her confinement. These women were asked to help out at childbirths, and were given the honorary role of acting as witnesses to the baby's birth certificate. Non-Quaker women helped at Quaker childbirths in Buckinghamshire as early as 1654, the year in which the first list of witnesses survives. By 1669, if not earlier, parish midwives had begun to officiate at Quaker births.

Inviting non-Quaker women into their homes for a birth involved the attendant risk that one of their parish friends would attempt to baptize the infant. Yet the desire to have a skilful and familiar midwife and to have good neighbours present at the birth could overcome religious differences. Quaker women were no doubt ostracized to some degree from the rest of the female parish community because of their peculiar religious beliefs, namely their rejection of baptism and churching rituals. Although Catholics performed such rites in the privacy of their own homes and chapels, and Puritan women practised modified forms of churching rituals devoid of the purification rites,[25] Anglican, Catholic and Puritan women shared a belief in the efficacy of such religious rituals as the christening of the infant and formal thanksgiving by the safely delivered mother. Baptism and churching were central events in parish life which provided a chance

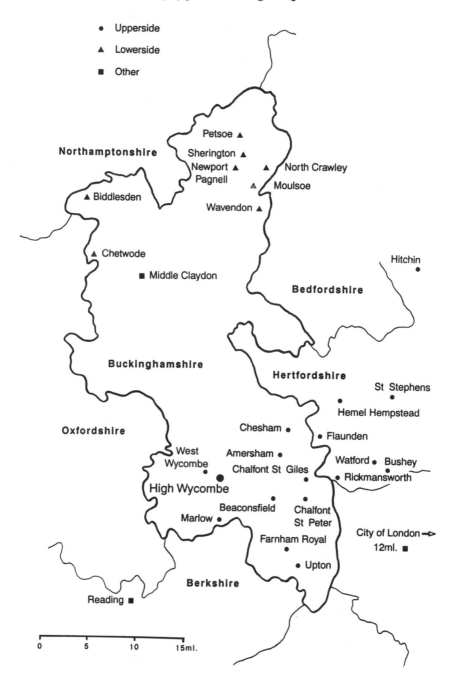

Figure 3.1 Location of Quaker childbirths attended by thirty-one midwives active in the Upperside and Lowerside monthly meetings of Buckinghamshire, 1652–1718

for women to get together, and they were an occasion for neighbourly bonding both in rural and urban communities.[26] The village midwife who attended a Quaker birth was deprived of her honorary role in presenting the infant at the baptismal font and of leading the mother and gossips in the churching procession. At a Quaker birth, tips from godparents were also forgone. The six midwives who attended the Buckinghamshire Quaker births thus gave up these important social rights as midwives in order to lend their services to their Quaker friends. may not have been that important

Religious integration at childbirths was not confined to small villages, such as those dotting the Chiltern hills and the Vale of Aylesbury, where women were undoubtedly constrained by virtue of geography and population distribution in their choice of help. Quakers of the Buckinghamshire market town of High Wycombe also employed non-Quaker women. The Buckinghamshire scene was apparently not unusual. A diary kept between 1665 and 1675 by an unknown, but non-Quaker, midwife from Kendal offers evidence that this custom was practised in north-western towns where Quaker populations proliferated. On two occasions, the Kendal midwife recorded her employment by a Quaker family. Of the fifty-six births she attended in 1670, on 24 February, at one o'clock in the morning she delivered the baby daughter of George Taylor, 'Quaker'. The Taylors again employed the experienced midwife when their son George was born in 1674.[27]

Such religious integration was also common in the city. Evidence based on my work on London Quaker birth certificates and Doreen Evenden's work on the City's licensing records shows that twenty (12 per cent) of the 168 midwives who signed Quaker birth certificates in London between 1676 and 1718 were in possession of an Anglican church court licence.[28] Some of the licentiates were quite well established, having been licensed more than 10 or 20 years before being engaged by Quaker families.[29] Although these women were obliged by oath to see to it that the baby they delivered had a proper Anglican baptism, the London licentiates were obviously willing to overlook that duty, be it through a sense of neighbourly obligation or financial incentive.

Like their London counterparts, Quakers in the Buckinghamshire quarterly meeting employed ecclesiastical licentiates. Licensed by the St Albans archdeacon's court in 1682,[30] Mrs Elizabeth Finch of Watford delivered over thirty Quaker babies in Watford and the neighbouring parishes of St Stephens, Rickmansworth and Bushey between 1689 and 1712. Mrs Finch was a member of an established and wealthy family of churchgoers and vestrymen in Watford with well-educated women members.[31] Mrs Finch was herself a literate woman and signed her name to Quaker birth certificates in a neat and legible hand as 'Elizabeth Finch medwife'. She was a widow who lived a comfortable existence, surrounded by a large family. At her death, the affluent midwife distributed £200 in cash gifts to her son, three married daughters, and her sixteen grand-children, also leaving them such household items as silver, curtain valances, tablecloths and needlework.[32]

Mrs Finch was popular amongst Upperside Quakers as well as amongst those from the neighbouring Hertfordshire meetings. Among the fourteen Quaker families who employed Elizabeth Finch as their midwife, the heads of household included a surgeon-apothecary, a grocer, a maltster, a shoe-maker, two husbandmen and a labourer. The Quaker surgeon-apothecary, William Wells, employed her for the births of all his seven children to his three wives.[33] The Quakers also employed other members of the Finch family. Several months before her death in 1712, Elizabeth Finch's kins-woman, Mary Finch, took over some of her Quaker clients.[34] The last recorded Quaker delivery that Elizabeth attended occurred on 9 August 1712. Four days later she made out her will[35] and was buried in the parish churchyard on 27 August.[36] The Quakers noted the decease of this venerable midwife on the baby's birth certificate.[37]

Although popular with local Quakers, Elizabeth Finch was only one of at least twelve midwives who practised in the same four parishes. Nine of the others were employed by Quaker families, and two more had been presented for unlicensed practice by the St Albans archdeacon's court.[38] An additional eleven women were registered as midwives amongst Quaker families in the neighbouring parishes of Chalfont St Peter, Chalfont St Giles, Hemel Hempstead, Flaunden and St Albans.[39] In sum, at least twenty-four midwives were active within 5 miles of Elizabeth Finch's Quaker clientele, and at least four of them were Quaker women. As with other informally qualified early modern practitioners,[40] midwives proliferated even in rural areas.

When choosing from outside the Society, the Quakers selected women who were known by local parishioners for their skill, not women from the fringe of the village or town community. In the heartland of the Upperside monthly meeting, in parishes such as Amersham, Chalfont St Peter and Rickmansworth, Quaker families frequently engaged the services of such women. In 1699 the Quaker husbandman James Weedon and his wife Elizabeth employed the elderly parish widow, Bridget Allday, at their home in Rickmansworth. Two years after delivering the Weedons' baby, the parish clerk entered her name in the church burial register, identifying her by occupation: 'The Widdo Allden Ahanshent [an ancient?] midwife was Buryed.'[41] Mrs Jane Ives, whose career in Rickmansworth resembled that of Bridget Allday, was employed by three Quaker families in the parish and locality between 1692 and 1705. Mrs Ives attended births in Quaker families until the end of her life. In 1705 she signed a Quaker birth certificate,[42] and upon her death the following year her name was entered in the church burial register: 'Mrs. Ives a midwife buried.'[43]

Leading members of the Society were included amongst those engaging non-Quaker women. Mrs Ives was employed on at least two occasions, in 1693 and 1695, by John Bellers, a successful merchant and well-known philanthropist and social reformer.[44] Had he and his wife Frances objected to relying on the services of a parish woman like Mrs Ives, they could have employed any of three Quaker midwives who were active within 5 miles of the Bellers' estate at Chalfont St Peter, or could have afforded to have a Quaker midwife come from London, where they had a winter home. Indeed, on previous occasions, the Bellers had used other midwives. In 1690 they had employed the Chesham widow, Anne Wilkinson, and two years later invited the Upton Quakeress Margaret Treadway to officiate.

The Bellers' habit of switching midwives reflected a common practice; it was not unusual for a Quaker family to use two or three different women in the course of a mother's childbearing years. Families alternated between Quaker and parish women, between local and non-local women, between literate and illiterate women and, later in the eighteenth century, between men and women practitioners. This last practice was especially evident amongst Quaker families in the rural south from the 1750s, when men first started officiating at Quaker childbirths in Buckinghamshire and the surrounding counties. By the 1790s, surgeons and men-midwives, London based and those working in small towns and villages, were attending over 85 per cent of the registered Quaker births in the Buckinghamshire quarterly meeting. The number of births attended by women practitioners dwindled thereafter. On the occasions in which a midwife and a surgeon appeared together at a birth, both signing the certificate, only the occupation of the male practitioner was specified. The last woman to sign a Buckinghamshire quarterly meeting birth certificate did so in 1829. By the time the register ended in 1837, the only women practitioners who were being identified were the surgeons' nurses.[45] The Quakers' habit of engaging the services of a variety of obstetric practitioners was symptomatic of the way in which early modern villagers and townspeople actively selected from and bargained with a myriad of surgeons, healers and lay practitioners.[46]

Quaker midwives and their Buckinghamshire quarterly meeting practices

As we have seen, nearly one out of every five midwives who was active amongst Upperside and Lowerside Quakers in the second half of the seventeenth century was herself not a member of the Society. Yet the majority of Quaker childbirths were probably attended by Quaker midwives – women who came from the local Buckinghamshire and Hertfordshire villages, and those who travelled in from the City of London and surrounding market towns. These women came with a varied set of recommendations for their expertise and skill.

Women like Sarah Harris of High Wycombe took up midwifery with important social connections to back their reputations in the Quaker community. Medicine and religion were predominant influences in Sarah's home life from an early age. She was the daughter of John Raunce, a 'practiser of physick'.[47] Among her father's clients were the most important leaders of the Upperside Quaker movement, including Thomas Ellwood who went to Raunce for a cure for lung trouble contracted in London.[48] The Harris home was a gathering place for prayer meetings, and both Sarah's parents were religious leaders. Her father was a delegate of the men's meeting and a teacher at conventicles, who was on more than one occasion committed to prison for his Quakerism.[49] Sarah's mother, Frances Raunce, was one of the 'first publishers of Truth' who preached at Quaker meetings in Oxfordshire.[50] Sarah's husband Charles Harris[51] was another dynamic figure in the Upperside community. With his father-in-law, John Raunce, he led a separatist movement of Upperside Quakers in objection to the founding of the women's business meeting there in 1677.[52]

Although Sarah's husband and father rejected her participation in the business meeting, they sanctioned her activities as a midwife. Sarah waited until her own children were grown before taking up midwifery. She had at least five babies in the 1670s, two of whom died as children. In 1699, when her youngest had reached the age of 22,[53] Sarah officiated at the childbed of Ruth Costard, an Amersham mealman's wife.[54] In addition to attending births in outlying villages, Sarah was employed within the market town of High Wycombe itself. There her clientele included the wives of two maltsters and a chapman, whose babies she delivered on five occasions between 1699 and 1704. She, like Elizabeth Finch, signed the babies' birth certificates in a self-assured and educated hand, as 'Sarah Harris, midwife'.[55]

Not all Quaker midwives had such auspicious social backgrounds as Sarah Harris and Margaret Treadway, two women who were sure to have known each other from their attendance at the same Upperside prayer gatherings and weddings.[56] Other Upperside midwives had humbler backgrounds. Sarah Body of the village of Chalfont St Giles[57] was the wife of a husbandman and practised midwifery in the Upperside region for at least ten years. At the time she was first recorded as officiating at a birth, Sarah had two adult daughters, the younger of whom was 19 years old.[58] She would have been at least a middle-aged woman, in any case old enough to be a delegate to the women's business meeting. However, Sarah Body was never distinguished in this way. Nor was her husband a delegate to the men's meeting.

Despite her family's anonymity amongst the Quaker leadership, Sarah

Body was respected for her midwifery skills, not only by Upperside Quakers but also by Londoners. Two of the Quakeresses whom Sarah attended were affluent city women who returned to the countryside for their confinements. One was Elizabeth Heywood, the wife of a London drysalter, who came to Amersham to have her baby in 1686. The Quaker gentlewoman Mary Penington was one of seven women present at Elizabeth Heywood's travail. Mary Penington must have been impressed with Sarah's skills. Two years later, Sarah Body was asked back to Amersham when Mary Penington's sister-in-law, Mary Wharley, the wife of a London woollen draper, was staying at the Peningtons' house during her confinement. In addition to being employed by London Quakeresses, Sarah Body was invited to local childbirths. She officiated at the birth of a member of a Quaker yeoman's family in the nearby parish of Rickmansworth in 1696. Five months later, she delivered the baby of a Quaker labourer in her own village of Chalfont St Giles.[59]

Sarah Body's London patron, Mary Wharley, had returned to her family home to have her first baby in 1688, although her next two children were born at her city home.[60] Mary Wharley again travelled to Chalfont St Giles for the births of her last three babies in 1698, 1700 and 1702. She did not rely upon her sister-in-law's recommendation or use Sarah Body as a midwife for these later country births. Instead Mary Wharley brought her own midwife, Margaret Wigan, with her from London.[61]

Margaret Wigan, the wife of a Quaker saddler, lived at St Anne Aldersgate in the City of London about 600 yards away from the Wharleys' home in St Lothbury's, where she began her midwifery training as a young mother. In 1689, when Margaret had four children, aged between 5 and 9,[62] she assisted the midwife Alice Boulton at the birth of a Quaker goldsmith's wife at Allhallows Lombard Street, about 250 yards from her own home. Nine years later, in 1698, she attended a birth with the midwife Elizabeth Gabird on Milk Street in the parish of Mary Magdalene, half a mile from her home in St Anne's.[63] In the same year she assisted Elizabeth Gabird and, when her youngest child was 14 years old, Margaret Wigan began to officiate at births on her own. She practised as a midwife mostly in the City of London, but also in parishes outside the City walls, until 1718, during which time she delivered at least thirty-one Quaker babies. The Quaker fathers included a cheesemonger, a clockmaker, a clothworker, an ironmonger, a silkthrower, a tobacconist, a tallow chandler, a winecooper and two glovers. Margaret Wigan, like the midwives she had assisted, was also a literate woman who signed her name, 'Margaret Wigan midwife'.[64] She spent at least five years practising midwifery as a widow.[65]

Privileged city Quakeresses like Mary Wharley could afford to travel back to the country with their city midwives. Affluent countrywomen likewise procured the services of reputable, urban women like Margaret Wigan. Mary Wharley's half-sister, Gulielma Maria Penn, the wife of William Penn, employed two different townswomen to travel to her childbirths in the village of Rickmansworth on at least three occasions. In 1672 Guli's first baby was delivered by Frances Kent, the Quaker midwife from Reading.[66] When she became pregnant again in 1674, Guli decided to employ Elizabeth Kemble, a Quakeress from Bromley in Middlesex, a village located about 8 miles outside the City walls. Although they lived in London, Elizabeth Kemble and her husband had ties with both the Reading and Upperside monthly meetings. Elizabeth had grown up in Reading, and her first child had been born there. Her marriage had taken place at an Upperside monthly meeting, and her husband witnessed Upperside marriages at Rickmansworth on at least two occasions.[67] The Kembles' wide social network must have facilitated Elizabeth's entry into midwifery. Indeed when Elizabeth Kemble was first employed by Guli Penn, she was still only a young mother with three small children.

In order to attend Guli Penn's confinement in February 1674, the young Elizabeth Kemble travelled 30 miles along winter roads to the Penns' home in Rickmansworth. Unfortunately, the twins she delivered died soon after their births. Despite their disappointment, one which would have been tragically common to seventeenth-century mothers and their midwives, the Penns employed Elizabeth Kemble again in 1676. This time Guli was staying at her husband's family home in Walthamstow, Essex, so Elizabeth Kemble did not have to travel far from Bromley. Elizabeth was helped by several distinguished women, among them Guli's mother-in-law, Lady Penn, the mistress of the house. Four other women, including Guli's mother, the gentlewoman Mary Penington, travelled from the Upperside area to help Elizabeth Kemble deliver the baby at Walthamstow. Happily, the child survived.[68]

Based on her financial means, a Quaker mother might employ a reputable urban midwife or choose a respectable rural one, who came recommended by friends and kinswomen. Other Quakers did not look beyond the sphere of their own relatives and neighbours. The less affluent Lowerside Quakers were especially provincial in their employment practices. Whereas the Upperside Quakers occasionally employed women from London and market towns outside Buckinghamshire, Lowerside Quakers did not go even so far as to employ Quaker midwives from the constituent Upperside meeting.

When her own daughters and daughter-in-law began to have babies, the Lowerside Quakeress Mary King, the wife of Henry King of Moulsoe,[69] was always on hand to officiate at the births. Mary was midwife to her own daughter, Mary Steele, as well as to her daughter-in-law, Ann King. She delivered at least four of her grandchildren between 1656 and 1664.[70] On only one recorded occasion did Mary King attend an 'outside' childbirth. In 1661 she travelled a few miles across to North Crawley to offer assistance to the Quakeress Elizabeth Ireland to deliver Susanna Mouse's twins.[71]

Although both Elizabeth Ireland and Mary King were named as midwives for the Mouse birth, Elizabeth Ireland was the primary midwife in North Crawley. She had delivered babies there on at least nine other occasions between 1663 and 1670.[72] Alice Hasker of Northampton was another Lowerside Quakeress who was recorded as officiating only at the births of other family members.[73] Alice Hasker was still married and her youngest child had reached the age of 15 when she was first documented as officiating at a delivery of a kinswoman in the neighbouring Lowerside parish of Biddlesden.[74]

A third Lowerside Quaker midwife, Elizabeth Glidwell of Newport Pagnell, started practising midwifery during difficult early married years. Her husband William was repeatedly imprisoned between 1656 and 1666 for refusing to pay tithes and for attending conventicles, leaving Elizabeth harassed by the authorities and with six young children in her care.[75] A year and a half after the birth of her second baby, and while 4 months pregnant with her third child, Elizabeth acted as midwife to Susanna Newman, a Quaker woman who lived in North Crawley, a few miles away. A few months after the birth of her third baby, in November 1654, Elizabeth attended a North Crawley kinswoman, Hannah Glidwell. During the period of her husband's imprisonment in London, she officiated at five more births in North Crawley. While the family's goods were being taken away by the exchequer of tithes and while she had four hungry little mouths to feed, midwifery earnings could have contributed to her family's support. Notably, Elizabeth Glidwell's last recorded attendance at a delivery was in February 1659, the year that her husband was first released from prison.[76] From then on the Quakeress Elizabeth Ireland (the midwife who delivered Susanna Mouse's twins with Mary King in 1661) was employed by all the North Crawley mothers who had previously employed Elizabeth Glidwell as their midwife.[77]

Despite minor harassment by the authorities who fined William for attending conventicles,[78] life settled down for the Glidwells in the course of the next ten years, during which time there is no record of Elizabeth having acted as a midwife. During this time, she raised her five surviving children, kept her home at Newport Pagnell, and participated in the Society of the Lowerside meeting where she and her husband attended Quaker prayer meetings and marriages.[79] Tragedy struck again, in 1677, when an illness appears to have swept through the family, resulting in the deaths within five days of two of Elizabeth's adult children.[80] Two years after her children's deaths, Elizabeth buried her husband.[81] As a widow, Elizabeth continued actively to participate in the Quaker community of Newport Pagnell by hosting local conventicles in her home.[82] Yet, even in her final separation from her husband in widowhood, there is no evidence that she returned to midwifery practice.

The employment of Quaker midwives by 'people of the world'

While village women were willing to show up at the births of their Quaker neighbours, they may have been less amicably disposed to having a Quaker woman act as their own midwife. Quite simply a Quakeress fell short in terms of the social niceties required. She could not participate in the baptism, churching or the gossips' party. Her disapproval of laced linens and frivolous gossip would have been unpleasant for the mother and the other women during the long hours of waiting during delivery. There was also a danger that the Quaker midwife might use the opportunity to attempt to convert the parturient mother and her helpers.

However, benefits were to be gained by employing a Quakeress, who was guaranteed to be honest and plain in her dealings and who would refuse to accept tips from the godparents. She was unlikely to be a gossipy woman who spread tales from the home of her employer. The Quaker midwife was also likely to be educated, possibly well read in contemporary midwife manuals. Twenty-two (67 per cent) of the thirty-one midwives who autographed birth certificates in the Upperside meeting between 1702 and 1752 were not only able to write their names but many also signed as 'midwife'. Using signatures as an indicator of literacy, these Buckinghamshire midwives were more than twice as likely to be able to read and write as their non-Quaker female neighbours.[83] The Quakers also had some reputation for medical skill. The roots of Quaker ascendancy in medicine and pharmacy during the eighteenth century[84] were presumably also to be found in the occupational respectability of seventeenth-century Quakers as apothecaries, surgeons and midwives.

Quaker birth registers are not forthcoming on the subject of whether Quaker midwives attended the births of the 'people of the World'. Fortunately, however, Friends were keen on communicating about such matters of social policy. In 1677 an epistle was issued by the national men's meeting at Dublin which sent instructions to local Irish women on how to conduct themselves at non-Quaker childbirths. The Dublin letter requested that the local meetings, presumably the women members, supervise the activities of midwives, as well as nurses and

> looke into & consider whether there be amongst you any women who profess truth [that] take upon them [the] office of a midwife, nurse or nurse-keepers who have occasion to be employed by [the] world whether they keep truth cleare & keep up their testimonys for [the] Lord in faithfullness & whether any such be present at their sprinkling of children & at their gossips, feasts, & receive their offerings money, w[hi]ch at such times is usually given, if any be

found to practice such things, they are to be reproved and admonished . . .[85]

Quaker midwives took the initiative in discussing matters concerning the attendance of Friends at non-Quaker births. In the same year that the instructions were issued at Dublin, the Quaker midwives of the West Indian colony of Barbados formed their own meeting, where they formulated a protocol for attending the births of 'people of the World'.[86] Such organization of midwives was likely to have occurred amongst Quaker midwives in England as well. Quaker women were used to practising their administrative skills. In their local business meetings they were responsible for disciplining Quaker girls and approving Quaker marriages. In central meetings they distributed poor relief and medical care, placed out Quaker maidservants, and issued policy epistles on matters of female dress and etiquette.

The Barbados midwives met on at least five occasions between 1677 and 1679. At their first meeting in January 1677 the midwives committed to paper some basic rules of their profession, such as that of receiving moderate payment and performing charitable work amongst the poor. As to the custom of lying-in parties, the midwives bore testimony 'against the World and their ways, who as soon as the Woman is delivered, do run into eating and drinking & foolish talking & jesting to the grieving of God's spirit, instead of returning praise to God'. Instead of joining in such frivolities, the Quaker midwife was to 'exhort the Woman to return praise to God for her deliverance'. It was further agreed

> that if we should be in any place & they should bring us laced linen to put upon the Child, that then we call for plain & if they have none, that then we put on the head cloaths & blanket, & what is necessary to keep it warm & bear a testimony against all superfluous ribbands & lace in Gods behalf, unto w[hi]ch we did all consent.[87]

At the second meeting in November the Barbados midwives took up only one matter, and that was of sending for other midwives when confronted by a difficult labour. They determined that if a Quaker midwife found herself in need of help that she should not 'go to the World for help but take advice one of another'. At a third meeting in January, they expressed their concern with the administration of the meeting itself. In order to ensure that the meetings were run on orderly lines, they enjoined against the 'disorderly manner of speaking, more than one at a time' (a provision which echoed the ordinances of surgeons' guilds and many other trade and craft companies). At a fourth meeting in February, the midwives returned to what had been discussed at the November meeting. They decided that 'if near the Meeting', the midwife should repair to the meeting for advice in the case of a complicated childbirth. As to delivering Negro slave women, the Barbados midwives sanctioned payment by the master or mistress but mandated against taking money from poor slaves. At the last meeting in April, the women again returned to the point which had vexed them at the meetings of November and January – the issue of receiving help from non-Quaker women. They decreed that if she found herself at a non-Quaker childbirth, the Quaker midwife could receive assistance from non-Quaker women. If the mother insisted on having a non-Quaker midwife co-officiate at the birth, the Quaker midwife was to decline her help.[88]

The Quakeress midwife, Frances Kent of Reading

Judging from the notes of the Dublin men's meeting and the Barbados midwives' meeting, Quaker women officiated at the childbirths of non-Quaker people and did so in these places as early as 1677. In Buckinghamshire, collateral evidence survives from as early as 1667. In this year, Sir Edmund Verney of the north Buckinghamshire village of Middle Claydon invited Frances Kent of Reading to be his wife Mary's midwife. Mary Verney was a sick woman, and her husband had contracted for the services of local 'women doctors' and engaged the help of several aristocratic lady friends in London to try to cure Mary of her fits of depression and violent raging, with secret powders and sleeping pills.[89] When Mary became pregnant in 1666, Edmund was anxious to find a skilled midwife to attend his wife. He heard about the fame of the Quakeress Frances Kent of Reading and wrote to his father, who was in France, to ask for advice about employing a Quaker.

Edmund corresponded extensively with his father, Sir Ralph Verney, about the arrangements for Mary's childbirth and lying-in. The two men wrote fourteen letters between November 1666 and February 1667 and were in communication up until a week before the birth. The letters are a poignant testimony of the interest and care taken by fathers and husbands in matters of childbirth. The two men made arrangements for the employment of a midwife, a monthly nurse and a wet-nurse, and decided who amongst the female relatives would be asked to come to Middle Claydon to help out at the birth. Ralph advised his son on the minutiae of the arrangements for Mary's lying-in. He instructed Edmund on how to turn old linens into makeshift bed clothes, where to find a good cradle, and how often to light the fires in Mary's room.[90]

Edmund was preoccupied with the dilemma of whether or not to employ the skilled Quakeress, Frances Kent, and eight of the men's letters discussed the matter. The first one was written (in French) by Edmund to Sir Ralph on 8 December 1666.

I went to visit my cousin Dormer at Lee, and I asked her about good midwives, and she spoke to me about several, among others of one, who she told me was the best reputed by all the doctors of Oxford as the best in England, her name is 'Mamoiselle' Kent, she is a Quaker and she lives in the town of Reading in Berkshire, and I was advised to assure myself of her as soon as possible, for fear of not being able to have her, but I dont know how to do it, because I dont know if she will please my wife, who will not hear of anything of that sort, even though she is very pregnant.

Sir Ralph warned his son about the considerable dangers of employing a Quaker when he wrote back (in English) on 13 December 1666.

if you, & your Wife resolve uppon the Quaker for Midwife, I pray never lett her bee alone with her, for those persons are apt to instill theire ill principles into the mindes of weake persons, & you well know, if your Wife get any thing in her Head, all the reason in the World will not perswade her out of it. I know not this Quaker but I am sure they are a dangerous sort of people, & those that couler theire designes with a shew of Religion, are ever most dangerous, God direct you for the best.

Edmund acquiesced that it was unwise to have a Quaker woman, but still pressed his father to consult Sir Thomas Lee's wife, a Buckinghamshire lady who knew Frances Kent as both she and her mother had employed her. In a letter dated 24 December 1666, Edmund had encouraging news for his father.

Last Wednesday I went to visit my cousin Woodward expressly to ask her about a wet-nurse . . . and speaking also with her by chance about a midwife we spoke of that 'Demoiselle' Kent that Quaker of Reading, and she praised her highly as being very skillful in her art, and 'Damoiselle' Woodward said the same, who was not long ago in an area where this Quaker exercised her office and she said she had never seen such a learned and adroit midwife, and that anyone would think themselves happy if they could have her, and that one gave her ordinarily £20, £10, and at the least £5 for her pains, and that this woman would take nothing from the godfathers or godmothers, and that she never meddled in speaking of her religion to her patients, and that if the Queen had continued pregnant she would have been her midwife, and that if she promised to come she is perfectly faithful to her word; these are great eulogies such that I am inclined to have her, but yet I wish to know first what 'Madame' Lee of Hartwell says of it.

The two men stalled the decision until a month before Mary's lying-in, at which time Edmund again urged that Mrs Hartwell or Lady Lee be consulted about the Quakeress. Ralph Verney was able to respond on 10 January that Lady Lee had given good testimonial for Frances Kent's skills, but he also reported that 'unlesse she is bespoke 2 or 3 moneths before hand, tis a Thousand to one shee cannot be had'. Five days later, Edmund Verney sent one of his servants to Reading to ask the well-known 'bien nomee' midwife to come to Middle Claydon to attend his wife.[91]

Frances Kent was the wife of a Quaker clothier and a prominent member of the Quaker Reading community, where she was a delegate to the women's business meeting.[92] On two occasions she was jailed at Newgate for attending Reading conventicles, once only three years before she was employed by the Verney family.[93] She was an accomplished midwife while still only a young mother. When she was invited to attend the Verney birth at Middle Claydon she had two daughters who were only about 10 years old.[94] In addition to being employed by Buckinghamshire aristocrats, Frances Kent was also employed by the county's affluent Quakers, women like Guli Penn, who employed her at Rickmansworth in 1672, and Sarah Dell, the wife of a wealthy yeoman and the daughter of the midwife Margaret Treadway, who employed her at Upton in 1674.[95] In 1684 Frances Kent went to London to attend Sarah Meade when Sarah was pregnant with her first baby at the age of 42. Frances Kent may well have been recommended to Sarah Meade by Guli Penn. Guli was a good friend and correspondent of Sarah's mother, Margaret Fox of Swarthmore Hall, Lancashire.[96] After the birth of her son, Sarah Meade wrote to her mother to tell her of the talented midwife. Sarah described her six-hour travail, the good health of her 'sweet babe', her plans to nurse, along with other chatty details of the weather and of visitors. In a postscript Sarah added:

> Frances Kent stayed with me a week after I was laid. She is a fine woman; it was the Lord sent her to me. It was the Lord's mercy to me that I had her, who is a very skilful and tender woman for that imployment.[97]

Sarah Meade was a discriminating employer. While still unmarried and living with her mother at Swarthmore Hall, she had had the opportunity to help supervise midwifery practices. At a gathering of the women's business meeting at Swarthmore in February 1675, Sarah was the clerk who penned the minute which directed the midwife Mabell Brittaine to desist from practice.[98]

The year after she delivered Sarah Meade's baby at London, on 27 August 1685, Frances Kent died at Reading. Despite her fame as a midwife, the inscription at her death in the Quaker burial register was simple and made no mention of her vocational calling: 'Frances Kent wife of John Kent Sr clothier was taken out of this life [the] 27th day of [the] 6th month and was buried the first day of [the] 7th month 1685.'[99] Her reputation lived on through her female descendant, Sarah Kent, who practised as a midwife in the Witney monthly meeting of Oxfordshire, where she delivered at least six Quaker babies between 1715 and 1725.[100]

Conclusions

Many features of Quaker midwifery practice and childbirth were shared by non-Quakers. Quaker families often engaged the services of several different women and, as such, their employment practices reflect what was a defining feature of the early modern person's consumption of medical care. Neighbourly and personal ties could take precedence over considerations of religious affiliation when Quakers chose non-Quaker women who practised in the parishes in which they resided or nearby ones as their midwives. There was a mutual willingness on the part of some non-Quakers to employ Quaker midwives, despite their reservations about the dangers of Quaker beliefs and practices. Some features of Quakerism were repellent to prospective employers, while others, such as honesty and medical skill, were attractive. According to Quaker writings, employment by 'people of the World' was common as early as 1677.

Yet, despite a significant degree of integration, most Quaker births in the seventeenth century were probably attended by Quaker midwives. Nine midwives practised amongst Buckinghamshire quarterly meeting families and Quaker families from London and Hertfordshire between 1652 and 1718 – Margaret Treadway, Sarah Harris, Sarah Body, Margaret Wigan, Elizabeth Kemble, Alice Hasker, Elizabeth Glidwell and Frances Kent. They acted as midwives for a variety of shared reasons, including social duty, vocational interest, neighbourly obligation and financial need. Their stories illustrate typical ways in which the demands of women's household duties were combined with midwifery. According to records of their first appearances in the birth registers, six of the nine midwives started practising midwifery when their youngest children had reached their teens, though some women, like Margaret Wigan of London, must have begun to assist other midwives while they still had young children at home. Three of the nine midwives were young mothers when they began officiating at births on their own. Frances Kent of Reading and Elizabeth Kemble of London were both urban midwives who built their reputation outside of their own home county while young women with toddlers at home. Elizabeth Glidwell was probably forced to take up midwifery when her husband was thrown into jail. Her story suggests how women turned to midwifery – as to other forms of paid female work – on a temporary basis in order to support their families. More specifically, it shows how Quaker women could be thrust into the role of breadwinners owing to religious persecution.

What is known of the occupations of the husbands and fathers of the nine women, which included agrarian callings, crafts and trades, and medical occupations, indicates that they, like most other Quakers, were of solid middling status. What evidence survives also suggests that these midwives, like many Quaker women, were literate. While the social status of this small group of Buckinghamshire Quaker midwives fits with the social profile of the Quaker population as a whole, it contrasts sharply with the social diversity of Anglican licentiates on whom most of studies of local English midwifery practice have focused.[101] Although many of the women who took out an Anglican church court licence were of middling status, they varied from urban gentlewomen, who paid high fees to have a licence as a social cachet, to poor, illiterate, country widows who were charitably given a licence to practise midwifery in lieu of receiving poor relief.[102]

Some midwives took an active role in the administrative affairs of their religious community, but, as few rural women's meeting books survive, it is difficult to determine how common it was for midwives to serve as delegates. Of the midwives active in the Upperside area, two of the nine attended their women's business meeting, and one hosted a Quaker conventicle in her home. More evidence survives from London but does not support a connection between midwifery and administrative leadership. Of the 168 midwives who autographed London birth certificates between 1676 and 1718, only two were in attendance among the seventy-five delegates of the central London women's box meeting held between 1681 and 1717. None was among the twenty-four participants at the Barking women's monthly meeting in 1699.[103] The delegation of authority amongst Quakeresses in urban areas may well have been different to that in rural settings. Rural midwifery indeed attracted women who wished to perform the work as an expression of their social status. It is notable, however, that none of the most affluent and prominent of Buckinghamshire Quakeresses, such as the gentlewomen of the Penn or Penington families, acted as midwives in the Buckinghamshire quarterly meeting region. The messiness of childbirth and long hours of waiting in the birthing room were not perhaps deemed as befitting women of the highest social rank.

In certain respects the world of the Quaker midwife was a small, familiar one. Six of the midwives stayed within a 10-mile range to deliver babies and not infrequently these midwives shared the same clientele. Yet the Quaker midwife's employment was not solely dictated by the bounds of geography, and she did not find her nucleus of support within the bounds of the parish church. Although some of her employment might indeed have been found in the neighbourhood, it was also very much shaped by networks of religious affiliation, for example by the monthly meeting which encompassed scattered populations of Quakers residing in several ecclesiastical parishes.

All nine of the Quaker midwives travelled outside the parishes in which they resided in order to attend Quaker births, and three of them came from urban centres outside Buckinghamshire – one from Reading and two from London. Quaker midwives probably travelled further and more frequently than other midwives. Travel was a normal feature of life for Quaker women. Even women with young children travelled across the country to attend meetings and the geographic mobility of women was actively encouraged by the women's business meeting which provided travelling expenses. The active correspondence of women – through personal letters and official epistles – encouraged this type of long-distance and literate networking amongst women, who also wrote and exchanged information about their midwives.

Finally, although not all midwives were delegates to the local women's business meetings, the organization of Quaker midwifery differed from that of other seventeenth-century English female medical work because Quaker women had formal methods of supervising midwives and of regulating their childbirth practices. In the villages and towns of England, parish matrons had local control over the standards of midwifery practice, though only in an informal capacity, as senior midwives, employers and gossips. There were no guilds or companies for women medical practitioners. However, the Quaker women's business meeting provided a unique forum in which the supervisory role of local matrons was made explicit. The delegates of the women's monthly business meeting reprimanded individual midwives and supervised proper childbirth practices. On their own, midwives developed procedural forms for consulting each other as colleagues. They organized themselves into meetings in which they discussed religious policies and issued written mandates, such as that to deliver amongst the poor and to send for the help of other midwives during a complicated labour. The latter two mandates were common to Anglican licensing oaths as well as to civic ordinances drawn up in Germany, France and America during the course of the seventeenth and eighteenth centuries. However, in all other cases, these oaths and ordinances were issued by ecclesiastical officials and city fathers.[104] Quaker midwives had the opportunity to publish their own rules and regulations, in a grassroots occupational organization peopled exclusively by women midwives.

A woman's Quakerism no doubt affected the way she practised midwifery – it influenced her scope of employment, the way she swaddled a baby and her occupational relations with other midwives. Religion profoundly influenced childbirth practices and the social aspects of medical practice, but at the same time a study of Quaker birth registers also reveals the commonalities shared by any woman undertaking the practice of midwifery in seventeenth-century English society. The minutiae of evidence on childbirth in the Society's registers offers valuable information on training, employment and the geographic distribution of clientele. This study has focused on a rural community during the seventeenth century and early part of the eighteenth. However, detailed information in the registers holds the key to birthing rooms of rural and urban homes well into the nineteenth century, when the configuration of practitioners surrounding the parturient mother was changing from parish neighbours, local Quakeresses and imported city midwives to male surgeons and their nurses. Quaker midwifery is at once a special case and a case study of early modern midwifery practice. The Society's records are a unique source for documenting the social exchanges of rural and urban women and the activities of midwives at the level of the village household.

Acknowledgements

I would like to thank Margaret Pelling, Hilary Marland and David Harley for commenting on earlier versions of this article. I am also grateful for the help given by the archivists at the Buckinghamshire County Record Office, the Hertfordshire County Record Office, the Friends' House Library and Claydon House. I would also like to acknowledge the Marshall Aid Commemoration Commission and the Wellcome Trust for funding my research.

Notes

1. Buckinghamshire Record Office (Aylesbury) (hereafter BRO), NQ/2/3/1, Upperside Monthly Meeting, Women's Meeting Minute Book 1677–78 to 1736–37 (minutes 2/11/1677); B.S. Snell (ed.) *Minute Book of the Monthly Meeting of the Society of Friends for the Upperside of Buckinghamshire 1669–1690*, Buckinghamshire Archaeological Society, vol. 1 (High Wycombe, 1937), v–vi, 55–65.
2. Snell (ed.) *Minute Book*, 8, 12.
3. BRO, NQ/2/3/1 (minutes 3/5/1678, 2/8/1678, 1/11/1678, 5/1/1678–79, 2/11/1692, 7/9/1693).
4. For the role of the midwife as expert witness in England and Germany, see chs 2 and 4 in this volume by David Harley and Merry Wiesner.
5. Public Record Office (hereafter PRO), RG/6/1367 (Dell: 28/8/1672). Although the clerk failed to designate a midwife out of the four women witnesses present at her grandchild's birth, Margaret Treadway's name was listed first, in the usual place of the midwife.
6. PRO, RG/6/1367 (Dell: 15/12/1674).
7. PRO, RG/6/1367 (Bellers: 28/6/1690).
8. The term 'employed' will be used rather loosely, as not all midwives received cash payment or goods for their services. The Quaker records give no information on the reimbursement of midwives.
9. PRO, RG/6/1367, Quaker Register, Buckinghamshire Quarterly Meeting, Births 1654–1775 (Bellers: 18/8/1692; Pearce: 8/6/1694).

10. See chs 1 and 2 in this volume by Doreen Evenden and David Harley.

11. The only initiative of documenting midwives in Anglican childbirths occurred in London in 1747. J.S. Burn, *History of Parish Registers in England* (London, 1829), 71–2.

12. W. Penn, *A Brief Account of the Rise and Progress of the People, Call'd Quakers* (London, 1694), 870.

13. E.A. Wrigley and R.S. Schofield, *Population History of England 1541–1871* (London, 1981), 96–7; S.J. Wright, 'Family life and society in sixteenth and early seventeenth century Salisbury', unpub. PhD thesis, University of Leicester, 1982, 152; A. Wilson, 'The ceremony of childbirth and its interpretation', in V. Fildes (ed.) *Women as Mothers in Pre-Industrial England* (London and New York, 1990), 80.

14. *Works of George Fox*, vol. 7 (Philadelphia, 1831), 331, 347 (Epistle, 1669); J. Willsford, *A Brief Exhortation to All Who Profess the Truth* (Philadelphia, 1691), 5; A.R. Barclay (ed.) *Letters of Early Friends* (London, 1841), 279, 283–4, 307 (Letters: 1657, 1659, 1662); Dorset Record Office (Dorchester) (hereafter DRO), NQ1 Al8, 'Propositions by way of advise' from the Cerne General Meeting to Friends in Dorset, 1659.

15. PRO, RG/6/1367.

16. PRO, RG/4–RG/8, Non-Parochial Registers and Records.

17. G.L. Turner (ed.) *Original Records of Early Nonconformity Under Persecution and Indulgence*, vol. 1 (London, 1911), 82, 840.

18. A. Giardina Hess, 'Social aspects of local midwifery practice in latter seventeenth-century England and New England', unpub. PhD thesis, University of Cambridge, forthcoming; M.J. Galgano, 'Out of the mainstream: Catholic and Quaker women in the Restoration Northwest', in R.S. Dunn and M.M. Dunn (eds) *The World of William Penn* (Philadelphia, 1986), 126; A. Wilson, 'Childbirth in seventeenth- and eighteenth-century England', unpub. PhD thesis, University of Sussex, 1982, 113.

19. F. G. Parsons, *History of St Thomas's Hospital*, vol. 2 (London, 1932–36), 85; J. Besse, *Collection of the Sufferings of the People Called Quakers*, vol. 1 (London, 1753), 366.

20. T.A. Davies, 'The Quakers in Essex 1655–1725', unpub. DPhil thesis, University of Oxford, 1986, 292–3, 300.

21. Most recent scholars have taken issue with Vann's thesis that Quakerism, in the early years, attracted members of the 'middle to upper bourgeois' and that the social base of Quakerism narrowed and declined over time. R.T. Vann, 'Quakerism and the social structure in the Interregnum', *Past and Present*, 43 (1969), 71–91; *idem, Social Development of English Quakerism 1655–1755* (Cambridge, MA, 1969); A. Cole, 'The social origins of the early Friends', *Journal of the Friends Historical Society*, 48 (1957), 99–118; J.J. Hurwich, 'The social origins of the early Quakers', *Past and Present*, 48 (1970), 156–62; B. Reay, 'The social origins of early Quakerism', *Journal of Interdisciplinary History*, 11 (1980), 55–72; Davies, 'The Quakers in Essex 1655–1725', 50–61; W. Stevenson, 'The economic and social status of Protestant sectarians in Huntingdonshire, Cambridgeshire and Bedfordshire 1650–1725', unpub. PhD thesis, University of Cambridge, 1990, 3–25, 61–2, 80–1, 116, 174–6, 247, 263–4, 265–75, 272–6, 348.

22. PRO, RG/6/922, Quaker Birth Notes, Buckinghamshire, 1702–1807; RG/6/1304, Quaker Register, Leighton Monthly Meeting, Wavendon, Buckinghamshire, 1665–1776; RG/6/1305, Quaker Register, Leighton Monthly Meeting, Sherington, Buckinghamshire, 1645–1774; RG/6/1367, Quaker Register, Buckinghamshire Quarterly Meeting, Births 1654–1775; RG/6/1406, Quaker Register, Upperside Monthly Meeting, Buckinghamshire, Births

1656–1775; RG/6/1599, Quaker Register, Leighton Monthly Meeting, Biddlesden, Buckinghamshire, 1675–1778.

23. Giardina Hess, 'Social aspects of local midwifery practice'. Although records for the parishes in which the babies were born were examined for evidence of the relevant midwives, it was beyond the scope of this study to examine all of the local Anglican parish records in the county and neighbouring areas. It is possible that some or all of the four midwives were Anglicans from a different parish.

24. I will use the expression 'parish midwife' to refer to any woman who was not a Quaker herself but who attended Quaker childbirths in the parish in which Quakers resided. This does not necessarily imply that the midwife only delivered in that parish, or that only one midwife served the parish.

25. Wilson, 'The ceremony of childbirth', 88–93. For a discussion of Puritan objections to ceremonies associated with childbirth and popular participation in or evasion of these rites, see K. Thomas, *Religion and the Decline of Magic* (New York, 1982), 41, 43, 63, 65, 68–9, 87, 190, 197.

26. Boulton shows that during the 1620s over 90 per cent of childbearing women of the Boroughside district of London participated in the churching ceremony. J. Boulton, *Neighbourhood and Society: A London Suburb in the Seventeenth Century* (Cambridge, 1987), 276–8.

27. Cumbria Record Office (Kendal) (hereafter CuRO), MS WD/Cr, Kendal midwife's diary 1665–75 (Taylor, 24 Feb. 1670, 26 March 1674).

28. Friends' House Library (London) (hereafter FHL), Digested Copies of Births, Marriages, and Burials for London and Middlesex, 1644–1837. It is unlikely that these twenty women were Quakers who had somehow obtained an Anglican licence. None of them is registered in the extant Quaker records of births, marriages or burials. Local informal integration was well in advance of formal ecclesiastical procedures.

29. PRO, RG/6/1626–28, Quaker Birth Notes, London and Middlesex, 1676–1701; D. Evenden-Nagy, 'Seventeenth-century London midwives: their training, licensing and social profile', unpub. PhD diss., McMaster University, 1991, Appendix G, 402–23.

30. Hertfordshire Record Office (Hertford) (hereafter HRO), ASA 17/2, Archdeaconry Court of St Albans, Churchwardens' Presentments, 1680–89, ff. 21, 24.

31. HRO, D/EFn (Finch family papers, 1597–nineteenth century), F9, Faculty for pew in Watford parish church; HRO, ASA 17/2, ff. 21, 24; HRO, D/EFn, F1, Will of Elizabeth Finch, 1675.

32. HRO, 149 AW5, Will of Elizabeth Finch, 1712.

33. PRO, RG/6/1367 (Weedon: 3/7/1694, 2/12/1695–96, 3/11/1697–98, 6/7/1699; Wells: 29/10/1695, 27/11/1696–97, 30/3/1698, 14/9/1699; Woods: 6/9/1696, 19/11/1698–99; Parker: 9/9/1700); RG/6/919 (Smith: 13/10/1689, 15/7/1691, 7/7/1707, 4/2/1710, 9/6/1712; Wise: 25/6/1702, 2/5/1703, 14/7/1705; Pritty: 7/5/1703, 7/9/1704, 22/12/1705–6; Neale: 24/3/1704; Skidmore: 14/11/1707, 12/6/1710); RG/6/1248, Quaker Register, St Albans Monthly Meeting, Watford, Hertfordshire, 1702–75 (Parker: 20/4/1703; Wells: 15/10/1703, 9/6/1705); RG/6/1406 (Parker: 17/12/1701; Wells: 16/9/1702).

34. PRO, RG/6/919, Quaker Birth Notes, Bedfordshire and Hertfordshire, 1700–94 (Parker: 1/12/1711). Mary Finch was employed as a midwife by the Quaker husbandman, Thomas Parker and his wife Sarah of St Steven's parish. The Parkers had previously employed Elizabeth Finch on three occasions: PRO, RG/6/1367 (Parker: 9/9/1700); PRO, RG/6/1406 (Parker: 17/12/1701); PRO, RG/6/1248, Quaker Register, St Albans Monthly Meeting, Watford, Hertfordshire,

1702–75 (Parker: 20/4/1703).

35. HRO, 149 AW5, Will of Elizabeth Finch, 1712.

36. HRO, D/P117 1/4.

37. PRO, RG/6/919 (Smith: 9/8/1712).

38. HRO, ASA 17/2 (presentments: 5/5/1685, 20/4/1686); PRO, RG/6/919 (Rickmansworth: Ann Hall, 1712–27; Ellen Woods, 1706–10; St Steven's: Jane Edmonds, 1705–10; Mary Finch, 1712–13; Mary Switch, 1711–12). Another local midwife who was not a Quaker, but who was employed by local Quaker families was Elizabeth Boro, who attended the wife of a Quaker husbandman at Watford in 1701. PRO, RG/6/1406 (Pritty: 22/11/1701).

39. PRO, RG/6/919 (Margaret Bullingham, 1703–10; Elizabeth Crawley, 1709–14; Sarah Gladman, 1703; Hannah Haydon, 170?–17; Margaret Marston, 1708–10; Ann Martin, 1704; Sarah Seers, 1709–11). Giardina Hess, 'Social aspects of local midwifery practice' (Hannah Alford, 1701–8; Margaret Treadway, 1672–94; Margaret Wigan, 1698–1702; Anne Wilkinson, 1690–96).

40. M. Pelling and C. Webster, 'Medical practitioners', in C. Webster (ed.) *Health, Medicine and Mortality in the Sixteenth Century* (Cambridge, 1979), 231–5.

41. PRO, RG/6/1406 (Weedon: 14/1/1698–99); HRO, D/P85 1/1–2, Rickmansworth Parish Burials, 1698–1730.

42. PRO, RG/6/1248 (Greenhill: 1705).

43. HRO, D/P85 1/1–2, Rickmansworth Parish Registers, 1653–1716, 1704–1722–23 (Allden: 13/5/1701; Ives: 22/11/1706).

44. RG/6/1406 (Bellers: 20/10/1693); RG/6/1367 (Bellers: 5/9/1695).

45. Giardina Hess, 'Social aspects of local midwifery practice'. See esp. Quaker sections 4 and 5.

46. M. Pelling, 'Medical practice in early modern England: trade or profession?', in W. Prest (ed.) *The Professions in Early Modern England* (London, 1987), 100–1, 106–9.

47. Turner (ed.) *Original Records*, vol. 1, 843.

48. Snell (ed.) *Minute Book*, xvii.

49. Besse, *Sufferings*, vol. 1, 77, 80; Snell (ed.) *Minute Book*, 8, 46, 69. Sarah was on hand at other Quaker gatherings in High Wycombe, and in 1671 witnessed a Quaker marriage there. PRO, RG/6/1024, Quaker Register, Buckinghamshire Quarterly Meeting, Marriages, 1658–1769, f. 9.

50. Vann, *Social Development of English Quakerism*, 14.

51. PRO, RG/6/1024, f. 10v. Among the witnesses of Sarah's marriage to Charles was Rebecca Zachary, wife of a Quaker physician from Rickmansworth.

52. Snell (ed.) *Minute Book*, xvi–xix. By 1688, her father and husband had set up their own meeting at High Wycombe.

53. PRO, RG/6/1367 (Harris: 2/10/1674, 20/2/1676, 11/8/1677); RG/6/1401, Quaker Register, Buckinghamshire Quarterly Meeting, Burials, 1656–1711 (Harris: ?/4/1685, 20/2/1676, 11/8/1677). Sarah's 8-year-old daughter Ruth and her son John died in the summer of 1685.

54. Ruth Costard had used the parish midwife, Jane Ives, 7 years previously. PRO, RG/6/1367 (Costard: 13/10/1692); PRO, RG/6/1406 (Costard: 15/8/1699).

55. PRO, RG/6/1367 (Steevens: 12/4/1701); PRO, RG/6/922 (Albright: 29/11/1702; Wilson: 2/8/1702, 14/3/1704; Steevens: 13/6/1704).

56. PRO, RG/6/1024, ff. 16v, 19.

57. FHL, Digested Copies of Births and Burials, Buckinghamshire, 1645–1837.

58. FHL, Digested Copies of Births, Buckinghamshire; PRO, RG/6/1024, ff. 12v, 31v, 22.

59. PRO, RG/6/1367 (Heywood: 17/4/1686; Wharley: 17/2/1688; Bowry: 15/6/1696; Heywood: 24/11/1696–97).

60. FHL, Digested Copies of Births, London and Middlesex (Wharley: 23/9/1693, 26/10/1696).

61. PRO, RG/6/1367 (Wharley: 22/2/1697–98, 29/8/1700); RG/6/1406 (Wharley: 31/6/1702).

62. FHL, Digested Copies of Births and Burials, London and Middlesex. Her daughter Elizabeth Wigan had been buried on 30/8/1679, aged 2.

63. PRO, RG/6/1626 (Boulton: 29/11/1689; Collen: 19/4/1698).

64. PRO, RG/6/1367, 1406, 1626, 1627.

65. FHL, Digested Copies of Marriages, London and Middlesex (Hannah Wigan and James Spelling: 22/8/1713). William Wigan was dead by the time his daughters married.

66. PRO, RG/6/1367 (Penn: 23/11/1672).

67. PRO, RG/6/1024, ff. 5v, 21, 21v; RG/6/1255, f. 30v; FHL, Digested Copies of Births, London and Middlesex.

68. PRO, RG/6/1367 (Penn: 28/12/1673–74, 25/11/1675–76); L.V. Hodgkin, *Gulielma: Wife of William Penn* (London, 1947), 157–8.

69. Mary King's husband was imprisoned under the terms of the Conventicle Act and died at Moulsoe in 1676. Besse, *Sufferings*, vol. 1, 77. Mary died only 7 months after her husband and was buried at Sherington with him. FHL, Digested Copies of Burials, Buckinghamshire (King: 2/12/1676–77, 13/7/1676).

70. PRO, RG/6/1367 (King: 8/2/1656; Steele: 22/8/1660, 8/11/1662–63, 25/8/1664).

71. PRO, RG/6/1367 (Mouse: 25/5/1661).

72. PRO, RG/6/1367 (Marks: 23/1/1661, 3/5/1666, 10/9/1668; Mouse: 26/5/1661, 24/8/1663; Glidwell: 17/8/1664, 25/12/1666–67, 23/2–1667, 31/8/1670; Newman: 24/8/1664).

73. PRO, RG/6/1599 (Ashby: 3/3/1698, 1/8/1699).

74. Alice married Thomas Hasker, a fellow member of the Northampton monthly meeting in 1671. The couple initially settled in the parish of Bugbrook, where Alice gave birth to four baby girls and where one of Thomas's relatives died at the hands of the persecuting authorities. Eventually, the Haskers moved to Northampton where the birth of their last daughter, Alice, took place in 1683. Thomas Hasker died in gaol, having been imprisoned for non-payment of tithes. He was buried on 1 July 1684. FHL, Digested Copies of Births, Marriages, and Burials for Northamptonshire. Thomas Hasker married Alice Ashby on 6/2/1671. Ann Hasker was born on 19/11/1671, Sarah 5/1/1673, Elizabeth 1/5/1677, Jane 10/3/1680, Alice 16/3/1683; Besse, *Sufferings*, vol. 2, 547.

75. The couple had at least six babies between 1650 and 1664. FHL, Digested Copies of Births, Buckinghamshire; FHL (no ref.); *Great Book of Sufferings 1650–1725*, vol. 1, f. 95; Besse, *Sufferings*, vol. 1, 75–7.

76. PRO, RG/6/1367 (Newman: 18/1/1654; Glidwell: 4/9/1654, 18/2/1657; Mouse: 9/2/1656, 18/8/1656, 20/9/1658; Marks: 28/12/1658–59).

77. PRO, RG/6/1367 (Newman: 24/8/1664; Glidwell: 17/8/1664, 25/12/1666–67, 23/2/1667, 31/8/1670; Mouse: 26/5/1661, 24/8/1663; Marks: 23/1/1661, 3/5/1666, 10/9/1668).

78. Besse, *Sufferings*, vol. 1, 81.

79. PRO, RG/6/1024, ff. 5v, 6v, 7v, 9, 12, 13.

80. PRO, RG/6/1401 (Hannah Glidwell: 3/5/1677; John Glidwell: 8/5/1677).

81. FHL, Digested copies of Burials, Buckinghamshire (Glidwell: 28/2/1679).

82. Snell (ed.) *Minute Book*, v.

83. Giardina Hess, 'Social aspects of local midwifery practice'.

84. D.H. Pratt, *English Quakers and the First Industrial Revolution* (London, 1985), 129; A. Raistrick, *Quakers in Science and Industry* (London, 1950), 277–315.

85. Swanbrook House, Dublin, 1/2 YMA1, National Men's Meeting at Dublin, 1671–88, 47 (Epistle 12/9/1677).

86. 'At a meeting of the midwives in Barbadoes', *Journal of the Friends Historical Society*, 37 (1940), 22–4.

87. Ibid., 22.

88. Ibid., 22–3.

89. H. Verney, *Verneys of Claydon* (London, 1968), 153–7, 169–72.

90. Middle Claydon, Buckinghamshire, Claydon House, Verney Letters (Nov. 1666 – Feb. 1667: Correspondence of Sir Edmund Verney and Sir Ralph Verney). Translations courtesy of the archivist at Claydon House.

91. Ibid.

92. PRO, RG/6/1255, Quaker Register, Reading and Warboro Monthly Meeting, Reading, Berkshire, 1650–1730, ff. 10, 13, 14, 18, 20, 26v, 28, 30v, 31v, 33, 35, 42, 44, 47.

93. Besse, *Sufferings*, vol. 1, 14, 19; N. Penney (ed.) *Extracts from State Papers Relating to Friends 1654–1672* (London, 1913), 344.

94. PRO, RG/6/1255, ff. 30v, 31.

95. PRO, RG/6/1367 (Penn: 23/11/1672; Dell: 15/12/1674–75).

96. Hodgkin, *Gulielma: Wife of William Penn*, 87.

97. 'Sarah Meade to her mother' [1684], *Journal of the Friends Historical Society*, 30 (1933), 42.

98. Mabell Brittaine was a member of the women's business meeting and the mother of five children, when she came under fire from the Swarthmore women delegates for her bad practice.

From A Womens Meettinge at Swarthmore the 10:th day of the 12:th mo:th 1675

Where as Wee have beene Informed, that Mabell Brittaine hath Exercised the place of A Midd wife; And [that] certaine Women have beene Longe in travell, and have beene delivered of dead Children under her hands: And some doth suppose, [that] it was for want of Judgment & skill in her. Therefore in tendernesse & Love to [the] Lord, who is the Author & giver of life, & to his truth w[hi]ch wee are made per takers of; And in Love & tendernesse to Women & Children (Haveinge had many things under Examination, & thereupon doe finde her defective, in some Cases:) Itt is our Judgement & Testimony (And wee doe warne her) That shee doe not meddle in [the] Imployment here after; (where there is any difficulty) without the helpe & Assistance of another Middwife; And if any doe sufferr therron makeing use of her, for [the] futer they must take it upon themselves: For Wee have given this forth, for the cleareinge of the truth, and our selves; haveing A Godly Care upon us, and desires, for the Good of all. And As for all words & Discourses that hath beene past, touchinge this Concerne; Lett them not bee mentioned any more.

CuRO, BDFC/F/2/5, Swarthmore Monthly Meeting, Women's Meeting Minute Book, 1671–1700 (minute: 10/12/1675).

99. RG/6/1255, f. 54v. Her husband, John Kent Sr, died two years after her on 24/4/1687.

100. RG/6/1378, Quaker Register, Reading and Warboro Monthly Meeting, Witney, Oxfordshire, 1656–1776 (Clark: 3/4/1715, 28/9/1716, 17/5/1718, 28/5/1721; Wiggins: 19/3/1722; Flexney: 24/12/1725).

101. See chs 1 and 2 in this volume by Doreen Evenden and David Harley.

102. An apt social comparison to the Buckinghamshire Quaker community can be drawn with the Puritan New England town, another society defined by its middling-class bias and radical Protestantism. In Essex County, Massachusetts, twelve midwives testified in cases of fornication, infanticide, rape and abuse at the quarterly courts between 1657 and 1686. Nine were residents of small fishing or farming communities and three more practised in and around Salem. Their husbands and fathers variously combined the activities of craftsmen and tradesmen (weaver, carpenter, cooper), retailers (tavern keeper, butcher) and entrepreneurs (mill proprietor, merchant), as well as fishermen and farmers. One of the Essex midwives was a recipient of poor relief, but only as an elderly widow, long after she had testified as a midwife. By the time each of these midwives testified, at least nine of them had adult children and none was known to have a child who was younger than 7 years old. This was with the exception of a Salem woman who acted as a midwife during her childbearing years. Like Frances Kent and Elizabeth Kemble, this young midwife came from a large population centre, in this case a port town. Another similarity between the Essex and Buckinghamshire midwives was that none was a member of the highest 'governing' classes, though the Essex midwives were often women from the top quarter ranks of the town in terms of wealth and social status. Seven were the wives of selectmen, grand jurymen or high-ranking officers in the town's militia and one other was married to a wealthy merchant. However, the wives of magistrates did not appear at the court to testify as midwives. See Giardina Hess, 'Social aspects of local midwifery practice'.

103. FHL, London Box Meeting Accounts, 1681–1750, 1672–84, 1713–25; FHL, Barking Monthly Meeting Women's Meeting Minute Book, 1675–1721.

104. For a comparison with municipal ordinances in Germany and Holland, see chs 4, 9 and 10 in this volume.

4

The midwives of south Germany and the public/private dichotomy

How did this affected their status & role?

Merry E. Wiesner

As the essays in this volume demonstrate, the history of midwifery may be placed within a number of different frameworks – medical practice, women's work, relations between women, women's place in the community. In earlier studies, I chose to analyse midwifery within the context of women's work, viewing it as women's most important occupation and the one which offered them the greatest opportunity for independence.[1] In this article, I would like to examine it from a slightly different perspective by exploring how midwifery fits in with what many historians perceive as a growing split during the period 1400 to 1700 between a male public and female private realm. As we shall see, at least in the south German towns that are the focus of this study, midwives continued to be public officials with a municipal salary throughout this period, though their primary responsibility was taking care of women within a private household setting. They thus appear to have maintained a position that bridged the gap between public and private, but changes in their status and role need to be explored more carefully to see if or how this 'new division between personal and public life' affected them.[2]

The growing split between the public and the private (or, as it is sometimes termed, 'domestic') spheres and the simultaneous privatization of women have been traced in a number of realms of life. Joan Kelly-Gadol, in her classic 'Did women have a Renaissance?' points to the decreasing political role of upper-class Italian women and their increasing dependence on their husbands and families.[3] Christiane Klapisch-Zuber documents the increasing importance of the patrilineal lineage, noting that the public functions of the family were carried out largely by men, and that women were often not considered true members of a lineage, but simply 'borrowed' for their child-producing capacities.[4] Mary Elizabeth Perry notes that any attempt by women in Seville to assert a public role, even through religious activities, was seen as a sign of disorder by male authorities,[5] a phenomenon that Natalie Davis has described more generally as the equation of all female power with disorderliness.[6] Heide Wunder finds that by the late seventeenth century, bourgeois women could no longer frequent streets and public squares without being held suspect.[7] Women who did assert a public role by publishing their writings or speaking out on religious matters often justified their actions by commenting that their private responsibilities – to their children, their families, younger women friends or to God – required them to act.[8]

Recent examinations of the ways in which the lines between public and domestic were drawn also indicate that by the nineteenth century, the association of men with public and women with domestic was so firm that women doing exactly the same occupation in exactly the same place as men were not considered workers (and thus eligible for publicly-funded pensions), but simply housewives who happened to work.[9] Public and private had thus become codes for male and female. Several cultural anthropologists have speculated as to whether this is a transhistorical, transcultural phenomenon – that is, whether what men do is simply defined as 'public' in most societies and what women do as 'private' – but medieval scholars have noted that public and private were not sharply distinguished throughout much of the Middle Ages, nor associated with a single gender.[10] Ancient historians and political philosophers have pointed out that the public/private, male/female association was extremely strong in ancient Athens, so that what we are seeing in the early modern period is a reassertion of divisions, and not a totally new phenomenon.[11] This does not make it any less important, however, and actually results in a more interesting question: why, at certain historical periods, is the association of men with the public sphere and women with the private stronger than at others?

This question takes us far beyond the scope of the present study, for it is one of the basic questions underlying much current analysis of the actual and symbolic links between gender and power.[12] Because midwives appear to have straddled the line between public and private, however, we can use their situation as a means of testing the limits of the public/private division. Like female monarchs, whose existence inspired countless sermons and pamphlets, midwives could pose a challenge to theoretical ideas of proper gender divisions.[13] Examining their situation thus might enable us to observe, on a very different class level from female monarchs, the possible contradictions between theoretical gender divisions and actual social practice, and the ways in which these were resolved.

I shall be limiting my focus to seven south German cities – Nuremberg, Frankfurt, Stuttgart, Memmingen, Augsburg, Munich and Strasbourg – largely because this is where I have conducted intensive archival research, but also because these cities offer good test cases. Midwives became sworn city officials very early in several of these cities – 1417 in Nuremberg, 1456 in Frankfurt, 1480 in Munich, 1489 in Stuttgart – and continued to serve in this capacity until at least the end of the eighteenth century. The city councils in all of them took great care to license, regulate and oversee the midwives, frequently issuing and changing ordinances.[14] These ordinances provide us with an excellent picture of how male authorities fit midwives into their theoretical understanding of gender divisions. Some records regarding the actual practice of midwifery have also survived in these cities, enabling us to see how authorities handled cases which did not fit with their theories. Unfortunately, no diaries or case books of midwives working in these cities have as yet been discovered, and so we can only assess the midwives' attitudes toward their own role obliquely, through the lens of official records.

Though these cities differed in size, governmental structure, economic base and, after the Reformation, religion, their governments all implemented restrictions on women's ability to act independently in economic and legal matters during the early modern period, so that in fields other than midwifery, the public sphere was becoming increasingly male.[15] Masculinity was also becoming a more important component of symbols and representations of public political power and of the right to work in the public arena.[16] For a number of reasons, then, these cities are good places to observe the way in which midwifery fitted in with or challenged new gender divisions. To test this, I will focus on a number of somewhat distinct issues: midwives' salaries and fees; the structure of municipal midwifery systems; licensing procedures and ordinances; emergency baptisms; illegitimate births, abortion and infanticide.

Midwives' salaries and fees

Midwives supported themselves both from fees paid directly by their clients and from salaries paid by the city treasury, and changes in the latter suggest that city officials grew increasingly uncomfortable with the midwives' public role. In records of the salaries paid to city officials, midwives were generally listed right after surgeons and apothecaries, but their salaries were much less – 2 to 8 gulden a year, compared to 10 to 25 gulden for city barber-surgeons – and the salary differential increased throughout the sixteenth and seventeenth centuries.[17] Midwives' salaries were more closely comparable with those of employees of city hospitals, though the latter received room and board in addition to their salaries, so they were actually better compensated than midwives. This meant that though midwives were technically independent, they could not live on their salaries alone. Those who did not have a husband who also worked or a significant income from private clients were forced to ask the city council for assistance. They generally asked directly for a salary increase, but city councils instead granted them 'special' gifts of wood, grain or relief from taxes.[18] This eased the financial plight of the midwives, but allowed the council to avoid validating their rights to a salary more in line with that of male medical practitioners; such grants were viewed rather as a sign of generosity and largesse – 'of our good will and not their rights', in the words of the Memmingen city council.[19] Thus midwives were regarded as part of the urban medical establishment, but clearly the lowest ranking part entitled to the smallest salary for their public services. When midwives were granted additional payments or gifts for special services, such as caring for pregnant women during times of the plague or caring for women in the city hospital, these were also lower than the additional payments made to male medical practitioners for similar services.

One might suppose that the salary differential between midwives and barber-surgeons resulted from the judgment that a barber-surgeon's strictly medical services were more valuable than a midwife's, but municipally-approved fee schedules indicate that this was not the case. Fees for all medical services were often set specifically according to social class or expressed as an allowable range rather than a single price, but in all cases midwives' fees for their private clients were set at a level comparable with those of a barber-surgeon – the cost of a simple birth was similar to that of a circumcision, and of a more difficult birth, such as breech presentation or the delivery of twins, comparable to the fees for setting a bone or removing tonsils.[20] It was midwives' public salaries, and not their private fees, that city authorities kept unusually low, thus minimizing the importance of the midwives' public duties.

Municipal midwifery systems

Changes in the way in which municipal systems of midwifery were structured give further evidence of the attempts of the male authorities to control the midwives' public role. Initially midwives were responsible directly to the city council in these seven cities, and appeared at council meetings with their concerns, such as requests for higher salaries or complaints about women acting as midwives without a licence.[21] Apparently the appearance of such women of the lower social orders before the city fathers was unwelcome, and during the late fifteenth or sixteenth century most city councils began to appoint other women, usually members of upper-class families, to oversee the midwives. Known by various names – 'honourable women' (*Ehrbare Frauen*), 'sworn women' (*geschworene Frauen*), 'women assigned to the midwives' (*zugeordnete* or *verordnete Frauen*), 'wise women' (*Weise Frauen*) – in every city their function was the same. They examined those wishing to become midwives, assigned midwives to indigent mothers and assessed whether these mothers needed food or clothing, disciplined midwives who they believed were not living up to their oath. In most cities they could revoke a midwife's licence for what they considered a serious infraction.[22]

The 'honourable women' were not to deliver children themselves, but were to give pregnant women 'help, advice and assistance' whenever they judged this necessary.[23] They, and not the midwives, were to make an annual report to the city council noting any problems, obviating the need for the midwives to appear themselves. It is clear that the councils did not see these 'honourable women' as taking over the midwives' medical functions, but as serving as their voice in the public sphere and keeping this aspect of city life under the control of members of patrician families.[24]

Thus the first step by city councils to limit midwives' independence was motivated by class interests, interests which were strong enough to cause them to appoint as overseers women who had no formal medical training. This parallels developments in other medical institutions, for at the same time city councils often appointed patrician overseers for the municipal hospitals and pesthouses. These steps did not keep lower-class individuals out of council meetings, however, for both male hospital workers and midwives continued to appear, in the midwives' case now with complaints about the 'honourable women' – they were providing more assistance in deliveries than the midwives appreciated, or were even delivering babies on their own, though this was termed as simply providing emergency assistance to friends.[25] The midwives demanded that if the 'honourable women' wanted to deliver babies, they should take the formal examination and apply for a licence like anyone else, something that would have been incongruous with their status as members of the city's elite.

The concern with class status which led to the original appointment of the 'honourable women' in some cases also worked against their effectiveness. In 1549 in Nuremberg, for example, the midwives requested that the council appoint a different type of group if it wanted supervision of their work, for the 'honourable women' were now apparently refusing to assist the city's poor and were unresponsive to the midwives' requests.[26] The midwives requested that this new group be chosen from the wives and widows of craftsmen rather than patricians – in other words, women more like themselves. The city council agreed, particularly as it had been having difficulty finding enough patrician women willing to serve as 'honourable women' during this period of more rigid social stratification, a problem which had also emerged in Memmingen.[27] Unlike the 'honourable women', the '*geschworene Weiber*' in Nuremberg were paid for their services, with their salaries being roughly equivalent to those paid to midwives.

Licensing procedures and ordinances

At the same time as many city councils were placing midwives under the jurisdiction of women without medical training, they were also calling for improvements in midwives' education. Never realizing that this was rather ironic, the councils increased the irony by giving the city's university-trained physicians the right to decide who could receive a midwife licence, at a time when university medical training included very little even remotely connected with pregnancy and delivery.

Midwives received their training through apprenticeship which generally lasted at least a year, during which they accompanied an experienced midwife on all her deliveries. Until the late fifteenth century, those who chose simply to practise privately apparently determined for themselves when they were ready to practise on their own, while those who wished to become sworn city midwives were examined by the city council. The council may have been assisted in this by city physicians, but this is not clear from the records. Beginning in the late fifteenth or sixteenth century, the 'honourable women' took over this examination, assisted in Frankfurt, Strasbourg, Memmingen and many other German cities by several of the city's doctors. City councils decided that not only those midwives who received municipal salaries, but also those who simply practised privately, should be examined and swear an oath of office.

The questions in such an examination reveal the level of knowledge which city councils hoped every new midwife would have. First came questions about her training and experience. With whom had she studied and for how long? Had she had children herself? How many births had she seen or taken part in? Then came questions about the content of her training. What food, drink and baths will help a woman have an easy birth? How does she know if a woman is pregnant and does not simply have some other kind of swelling? How does she know whether the foetus is healthy or sick, alive or dead? What is the normal position for birth, and how is this to be brought about in the case of abnormal presentation? What should be done with the umbilical cord and afterbirth, especially to make sure that the latter has emerged? How are the new mother and infant to be best taken care of, and what advice should she give the new mother?[28] The doctors judged the prospective midwife's answers about the medical aspects of delivery and pre- and post-natal care while the 'honourable women' assessed her morality and character. Though the questions appear sensible, it is important to remember that the physicians holding the examination had received all their training through the reading of classical medical texts and perhaps observing a single autopsy on a female cadaver; they were thus testing the skills of women who may have observed or assisted in as many as a hundred deliveries, while they had never even witnessed the birth of a live child.

Giving university-trained physicians the right to approve midwives' licences was in line with the growing professionalization of medicine. Physicians persuaded cities to pass laws against empirics – now dubbed 'charlatans' (*Pfuscher* or *Zuckermacher*) – and to keep barber-surgeons restricted to a narrow range of activities.[29] Because women could not attend

universities, professionalization automatically excluded them from officially practising medicine, an exclusion which was also intentional, as the
laws often used the phrase 'women and other untrained persons' in describing those who were now forbidden to practise. Individual women were
occasionally allowed to practise medicine by city councils despite a lack of
formal training, but they were usually forbidden to charge for their services
and had to limit themselves to treating women and children. Like the
special payments to midwives, such permission did not give these women a
formal right to practise, and could be revoked by the city council at any
time if it was felt that their services were no longer needed.

Though city councils granted university-trained physicians a role in the
licensing procedure as early as 1500, it was not until the late seventeenth
century that the ordinances suggest that midwives should turn to physicians or other male practitioners for advice or assistance in anything other
than caesarean sections.[30] This indicates that the councils recognized that
the involvement of a physician would probably not improve the process of
delivery, and that their decision to grant physicians a licensing role was
motivated, as with their appointment of 'honourable women', more by
considerations of status than of public health. In this instance gender was
also an issue, for, though councils could not exclude women from the
practice of midwifery as they could female practitioners from other areas
of medicine, they could place them under the control of male authorities
and so convince themselves that the women were not practising independently. In reality, of course, the women were, for it was not until the
mid-eighteenth century that a man was recorded as practising midwifery in
these cities, and not until the early eighteenth century did midwives receive
any part of their training from university-educated physicians.[31]

The presence of both 'honourable women' and physicians at the midwives' examinations demonstrates that considerations of class and gender
often outweighed strictly medical concerns when cities established their
systems of midwifery. These same considerations emerge again when we
examine the regulations and ordinances which cities expected their
midwives to follow, particularly those which were related to midwives'
responsibilities beyond delivering babies and caring for new mothers.

Most cities in southern Germany first promulgated midwife ordinances
in the late fifteenth or sixteenth centuries. The first ordinance in all of
Germany was that of Regensburg, issued in 1452. Of the cities under
investigation here, Munich issued its first midwife ordinance in 1488,
Strasbourg in 1500, Frankfurt in 1509, Nuremberg in 1522, the Duchy of
Wurttemberg (where Stuttgart was located) in 1549 and Memmingen in
1578.[32] The first ordinances were reissued and expanded throughout the
early modern period, so they give us a good picture of the ways in which
the concerns of city authorities regarding midwifery changed.

The most striking thing about the ordinances is how little the obstetrical practices they describe and stipulate changed over three hundred years (1450–1750), particularly as this was a period during which theoretical understanding of anatomy and physiology changed tremendously in Germany. As the ordinances become longer and more complex, they did begin to stipulate 'correct' obstetrical procedures in more detail – the earliest ordinances state simply 'she is to handle all to the best of her ability . . . and not attempt to hurry the birth along', while later ones pick up on questions from the midwives' examination and describe how a midwife was to turn a foetus to achieve correct presentation, how she was to recognize whether a foetus is alive or dead and a woman really in labour, and how she is to handle the afterbirth.[33] Once these procedures had been described, however (usually in the mid-sixteenth century), they were simply repeated in all future editions. Thus stipulations on obstetrical practices in the eighteenth century were based on knowledge that was standard two hundred years earlier.

Because there are no case books or diaries of midwives practising in these cities, we cannot tell whether practice changed as little as the ordinances implied, but Audrey Eccles has asserted that in early modern England obstetrical procedures changed much more slowly than those in other fields of medicine, so the ordinances may be reflecting the actual situation.[34] Eccles attributes this slow pace of change to the fact that women very often had set ideas about what they expected a midwife to do, and would not recommend or go back to one who made any changes or did not do what was expected. The fact that her sources describing the lack of change were largely written by male practitioners attempting to woo business away from female midwives make Eccles' conclusions problematic, however. In his work on birthing procedures in England during the same period, Adrian Wilson has discovered that some midwives did accept new techniques and that there was great variance in their level of intervention.[35]

Ultimately, the question as to how much the lack of change in obstetrical procedures described in the ordinances reflected reality is unanswerable, and instead we can best think about what the ordinances themselves imply. They reflect the ideas not of expectant mothers, but of city authorities, who left the procedure for delivery as one of the few aspects of urban life not regulated in great detail. They did this, in my opinion, not because they felt no sense of expertise on the matter – they were perfectly willing to pass detailed regulations regarding other matters about which they knew equally little – but because the way in which a midwife normally handled her clients was a matter between women and thus, in their opinion, not of public concern. Long before the nineteenth century, then, authorities were already paying attention to the gender of those involved in determining whether an issue was public or private, a matter to which I will return in my conclusion.

Emergency baptisms

The lack of specific directives on medical matters in midwife ordinances stands in sharp contrast to the ever-increasing attention paid to other aspects of their role which the authorities clearly deemed public. The earliest ordinances, such as that passed in Munich in 1488, mention one public function explicitly – emergency baptisms – a growing cause of concern for the authorities throughout the early modern period. The Munich ordinance states simply that if a midwife judged a child near death, she was to perform an emergency baptism or she 'would have to answer to God for her laziness and irresponsibility'.[36] A century later, the 1585 Wurttemburg ordinance which covered Stuttgart and the surrounding villages specified that midwives were to go to the pastor of their parish church to learn the proper method of conducting a baptism.[37] By 1688, Strasbourg authorities required midwives to obtain the permission of one of the city's mayors before performing a baptism, as the council thought too many were being performed.[38] Answering to God was apparently no longer enough.

This increasing concern on the part of both religious and political authorities with emergency baptisms resulted in part from changes in the doctrine of baptism in Protestant areas. Catholic doctrine had taught that children who had been baptized by lay people could be rebaptized if there was some doubt that they had been baptized correctly the first time. This second baptism was carried out 'on the condition' that the first one was irregular; it was not considered an actual rebaptism, for rebaptism carried with it the death penalty in Germany at this time, as it meant one rejected the accepted doctrine of infant baptism. Foundlings were also baptized 'on condition', just in case they had already been baptized. In 1531, Luther rejected as casuistry all baptisms 'on condition' if it was known that any baptism had already been carried out, and called for a normal baptism in the case of foundlings. By 1540 most Lutheran areas were no longer baptizing 'on condition', and those who still supported the practice were occasionally branded Anabaptists.[39] It was extremely important, therefore, that midwives and other lay people knew how to conduct an emergency baptism correctly, and most Lutheran cities, such as Nuremberg and Frankfurt, included a long section on emergency baptisms in their general baptismal ordinances.

The rejection of conditional baptism was not the only reason for the increasing control over emergency baptisms, however, for though Catholic doctrine on baptism was reaffirmed at the Council of Trent, Catholic cities also supervised their midwives more closely on this matter, as did Reformed cities, though the opinions of Zwingli and Calvin on conditional baptism were not as strong as those of Luther.[40] In these cases, the cities may have worried that Anabaptist midwives might claim to have baptized an infant when they really had not (thus avoiding the normal church baptism and allowing for a later adult baptism without the crime of rebaptism), but we can also see this as part of the cities' attempts to control one very public aspect of a midwife's responsibilities.[41]

The importance of baptism in all magisterial Christian denominations (that is, excluding radicals like Anabaptists) meant that this was the one sacrament that could not be reserved for the clergy, at a time when both the Catholic and Protestant Churches were becoming more clerically-dominated. But the freedom of a midwife to make the decision to baptize could be and was, at least in theory, restricted, although it is difficult to imagine any midwife actually taking the time to have someone find a mayor if she thought a child was about to die. I have found no cases in which a midwife was actually charged with failing to find the proper authorities before conducting a baptism, which suggests that these laws were followed more in the breach than the observance. Their presence on the books appeased the authorities' sense of discomfort at a lower-class woman having independent power over the destiny of a child's soul, but midwives continued to baptize rather than 'answer to God for [their] laziness and irresponsibility', a phrase which continues to be included in some form in most ordinances into the eighteenth century.

Illegitimate births, abortion and infanticide

In the early to mid-sixteenth century, concerns about public morality and drains on municipal welfare funds combined to lead city authorities to establish a new public function for midwives, but one which they controlled and supervised from the outset. This was the reporting of all illegitimate births, with as many details as the midwife could supply – whether the child was alive or dead, who and where the mother was, and who the father was, if she could find out. (In the eloquent words of the 1605 Strasbourg ordinance, she was to report 'the name of the one that is exclaimed during the pains of birth'.)[42] City authorities did not wholly trust midwives in this matter, however, for they generally required that the 'honourable women' supervise any handling of a birth out of wedlock. By the seventeenth century, at least in the ordinances, a midwife's responsibility to guard public welfare funds might outweigh her duties toward women in childbirth. In the words of a 1688 Strasbourg ordinance:

> When she is called to an unknown person or person out of wedlock who has been overcome by the pains of childbirth, she must then ask her before she gives a helping hand who the father of the child is so that justice is not neglected and children come in to the orphanage who should be taken care of elsewhere.[43]

As guilds in the seventeenth century also became more concerned with the morality of their members, they called on midwives to provide testimony as to whether any child born less than nine months after a marriage was premature or full-term; the father of those judged full-term could be expelled from the guild for pre-marital fornication.[44]

This concern about illegitimate births was not motivated solely by financial or moral considerations on the part of the authorities, however, for the ordinances also make it clear that they recognized that unmarried mothers were more likely to attempt abortion or infanticide. As a late sixteenth-century ordinance from Nuremberg put it: 'Recently evil cases have taken place, that those women who live in sin and adultery have illegitimate children and, during birth or before, purposefully attempt to kill them by taking harmful, abortion-causing drugs or through other notorious means.'[45] Midwives were not only ordered to provide no advice or assistance, but they were not to bury any dead child without informing the council and were in addition to have 'three or four unsuspected female persons' accompany them to the grave of any child.[46] The 1578 Memmingen ordinance required that midwives be even more aggressive in preventing abortion or infanticide:

> When they come upon a young girl or maid or someone else who is pregnant outside of marriage, they should speak to them of their own accord and warn them with threats of punishment not to harm the foetus in any way or take any bad advice, as such foolish people are very likely to do.[47]

If such warnings were not successful, and a woman did attempt or effect an abortion or infanticide, midwives were required to provide testimony and assist in the investigation. In the case of suspected abortion or attempted abortion, midwives were called on to give testimony as to whether the means the mother had used – strenuous physical activity, herb mixtures or other drugs – could in fact have caused an abortion.[48] Though the authorities were intent on stopping abortion, they were also careful to make sure that the child had not simply died of natural causes and the mother was confessing out of fear of torture. Women were occasionally released or given only a light sentence if the method used was not violent or strong enough to induce abortion.[49]

In cases of suspected infanticide, midwives were required to examine the woman to see if she had been pregnant, which generally meant checking whether she had milk, and were often sent out to search for the body of the child. Again their independence in this was limited, for most cities prescribed that a barber-surgeon accompany them, though they recognized that midwives could better assess whether a child had been born alive or stillborn.[50] Barber-surgeons generally assisted in the procedure if an internal autopsy were judged necessary: 'On the report of the sworn midwives as to how they found the dead child with a piece of wood stuck in its mouth, it is recommended that the child be cut open and examined further by the barber-surgeons.'[51] Once the body had been examined, the midwife often reburied it herself in a simple ceremony, a public function which no one noticed, largely, it could be surmised, because the destination of the child's soul could no longer be affected the way it could be by baptism, and because no one would have worried about the type of funeral such a child received.[52]

Midwives were thus given an increased public role in the handling of cases of abortion and infanticide in early modern German cities, as municipal authorities judged that they were the most (or only ones) competent in providing testimony and making diagnoses, and as infanticide became increasingly a matter of municipal concern and punishment. Both Catholic and Protestant areas throughout Europe tried and executed many more women for infanticide at the beginning of the sixteenth century than they had earlier, a trend some historians have seen as related to the rise in witchcraft accusations because both resulted from male fears about 'deviant' women.[53] In some parts of Europe, midwives not only helped investigate cases of abortion and infanticide, but were accused of causing them through natural methods or witchcraft. The *Malleus Maleficarum*, a handbook for witch-hunters written by two Dominican monks, Heinrich Kramer and Jacob Sprenger, and first published in 1486, accused midwives of frequently practising witchcraft; several of the best-known witchcraft trials in Germany were of midwives charged with killing or injuring mothers and infants.[54] In the cities under consideration here, however, witchcraft trials were few or non-existent, and only in the ducal court of Wurttemburg, which included Stuttgart in its jurisdiction, were any midwives tried for witchcraft.[55] Even during the height of the witch-craze, city governments were much more concerned with the honesty, industriousness and competence of the cities' midwives than with their possible diabolic connections; none of the city ordinances mention any specific superstition or magical beliefs or practices.

Midwives also assisted city governments in enforcing other types of moral legislation. As cities enacted more stringent sumptuary codes in the sixteenth century, midwives were required to inform parents about laws which governed baptisms so they would not, for example, spend too much money on the infant's baptism gown or invite too many people to the baptismal feast.[56] As cities worried about the influx of 'foreign' or 'undeserving' poor, midwives were often required to assess whether women requesting food, clothing or free midwifery services were resident and truly needy, both requirements for those seeking public assistance.[57]

88

Conclusions

In some ways, then, midwives provide a counter-example to the general trend of restricting women to the private sphere in the early modern period. I think this can best be explained by two factors. The first is the midwives' class status. Most midwives in south German cities were the wives or widows of artisans, minor city officials, or day labourers and were not wealthy enough to own their own houses but lived in rented accommodation.[58] They were thus respectable, but not solidly bourgeois, a status one can also deduce from the fact that they are referred to by first name only in the diaries of patricians who otherwise label the wives of bourgeois master-craftsmen as '*Frau* So-and-so' and are described in city council minutes as '*Weib*' or '*Mutter* So-and-so' rather than the more respectful '*Frau*'.[59] Those who have discussed the increasing privatization of women's lives have noted that this began with the nobility, was gradually adopted by the middle class (and became, in fact, a mark of bourgeois status) and only very slowly trickled down to the lower classes, for whom it may never have been more than an ideal.[60] Thus, at least in the early modern period, authorities were in part willing to overlook the continuing public role of midwives because no one expected lower middle-class women to remain in their homes.[61]

The second factor is that the financial and moral aims of municipal authorities, particularly regarding infanticide, foundlings and the distribution of public welfare, were strong enough to allow them to overlook their gender and class biases when relying on the testimony of midwives. In theory, women were legally incompetent and morally suspect but, in practice, the word of one woman was enough to convict another, as long as the first woman was a sworn midwife.

In other ways, however, the situation of south German midwives does provide evidence of an increasing split between public and private, and denigration, if not elimination, of women's public roles. The authorities minimized the importance of midwives' roles by keeping their salaries low at a time when other officials' salaries increased, and by restricting their independence by putting them under the authority of the 'honourable women' and the city physician; in the seventeenth century, some cities assumed even more direct control by requiring that a member of the city council be present at all midwives' examinations.[62] The increasing unwillingness of upper-class women to assume the office of 'honourable woman' supports the notion that the privatization of women's lives was occurring at the top of the social scale, and the lack of concrete directives from city authorities about obstetrical procedures indicates that they were willing to consider some matters between women as none of their concern, and thus 'private'.

Evidence regarding midwives thus teaches us to be more cognizant of class status and of discrepancies between theory and practice when we explore the issue of public and private. It also demonstrates that the equation between 'private' and 'domestic', while perhaps valid for the nineteenth century, does not work well in the early modern period. City authorities regarded normal obstetrical care as 'private' because it was something between women, not because it occurred in a domestic setting. As frequently observed, the household in early modern cities was regarded as the smallest political unit and was clearly part of the public realm, but sources on midwifery practice demonstrate that not everything that went on in that household was equally 'public'. Normal deliveries were not considered public and, as we have seen, city authorities gave few specific directives to midwives regarding proper procedures and levels of intervention. If a midwife did something wrong, however, 'whether by doing too little or too much', it became a matter of public concern, and she could be arrested for malpractice, questioned and, if found guilty, fined or removed from office.[63] Why? Because, in the words of the 1578 Memmingen ordinance, 'not only the mother but also the child could be injured by the lack of skill or neglect of the midwife, which touches and affects every housefather in his own house'.[64] In other words, when a child was harmed, the father, the head of that smallest political unit, was also harmed, and the continuation of that household perhaps jeopardized, thereby making the midwife's actions a public matter. I would argue, then, that already by the seventeenth century the sources concerning midwifery provide evidence for regarding gender as more important than location in determining whether something was judged public or private.

Throughout this essay, we have concentrated on official, male opinion as recorded in midwife ordinances, city council records and court cases. Do any of these sources reveal the attitudes of the midwives themselves about the public/private dichotomy? Midwives, of course, did not speak to this issue directly, but in my opinion they did have a sense of themselves as having a public role. Though city councils expressly termed their additional payments to midwives as special gifts, the midwives did not adopt the supplicatory language common for women asking assistance, but instead asked directly for a salary increase or 'the payment of rye and wood which is due to us'.[65] Midwives moving into one of these cities often asked specifically to be granted citizenship – which brought with it public rights and responsibilities for female citizens as well as male – though the councils were willing to let them reside as resident aliens. The Nuremberg city council reported, for example, that 'Katherina, the midwife from Eschenau, is to be informed that she will definitely be granted citizenship at her request if she and her husband will move here'.[66] Midwives in Strasbourg required each new midwife to provide all the others with a 'welcome meal' when she was taken on. The older midwives justified this with the comment that the city council had a similar requirement for new council notaries and ambassadors, officers, the midwives maintained, that were certainly no more important or honourable than midwives.[67] Though these are only hints, they do indicate that at least some early modern midwives recognized that their status was unusual and saw the importance of validating this publicly.

By the mid-eighteenth century, male midwives were beginning to practise in south German towns. Once male practitioners entered the picture, midwifery techniques could no longer be considered a private matter between women, and the city authorities began to regulate procedures of delivery for midwifery practitioners of both sexes more closely. They thus began a process of declaring more and more aspects of pregnancy and delivery public matters, a process that still continues with foetal protection laws and increasing restrictions on birth control and abortion. We often point to the early modern period in Germany, the rest of Europe and the American colonies as a time when very little was considered truly 'private', and see the authorities' regulation of bodily, sexual and moral matters as a sign of the period's rigidity and authoritarianism. This analysis has suggested, however, that the contents of women's wombs were less a matter of public interest then than they are today; our concerns about the negative effects for women of too broad a definition of 'public interest' are not simply historical ones.

Acknowledgements

The archival research for this paper was carried out over several years, and I would like to thank the regents of the Universities of Wisconsin, the American Council of Learned Societies, and the Deutsche Akademische Austauschdienst for their support. The conceptual issues it seeks to raise have been broadened over the years in discussion with friends and colleagues throughout the world. Grethe Jacobson, Heide Wunder, Barbara Duden, Mary Beth Rose, Carole Levin, Lyndal Roper and Natalie Davis have all provided me with ideas and suggestions from their own areas of expertise; such sharing is my favourite part of feminist scholarship.

Notes

1. M.E. Wiesner, 'Early modern midwifery: a case study', *International Journal of Women's Studies*, 6 (1983), 26–43; *idem, Working Women in Renaissance Germany* (New Brunswick, NJ, 1986), 55–73.
2. J. Kelly-Gadol, 'Did women have a Renaissance?', in R. Bridenthal, C. Koonz and S. Stuard (eds) *Becoming Visible: Women in European History*, 2nd edn (Boston, 1987), 197.
3. Ibid., 174–201.

4. C. Klapisch-Zuber, 'The "cruel mother": maternity, widowhood and dowry in Florence in the fourteenth and fifteenth centuries', in *idem, Women, Family and Ritual in Renaissance Italy* (Chicago, 1985), 117–31.

5. M.E. Perry, *Gender and Disorder in Early Modern Seville* (Princeton, NJ, 1990).

6. N.Z. Davis, 'Women on top', in *idem, Society and Culture in Early Modern France* (Stanford, CA, 1975), 124–52.

7. H. Wunder, '"L'espace privé" and the domestication of women in the sixteenth and seventeenth centuries', unpub. paper from seminar for Philippe Ariès, Berlin, 1983.

8. M.E. Wiesner, 'Women's defense of their public role', in M.B. Rose (ed.) *Women in the Middle Ages and the Renaissance* (Syracuse, NY, 1986), 1–28.

9. J. Quataert, 'The shaping of women's work in manufacturing: guilds, households and the state in central Europe, 1648–1870', *American Historical Review*, 90 (1985), 1122–48.

10. M.Z. Rosaldo, 'Women, culture and society: a theoretical overview', and S. Ortner, 'Is female to male as nature is to culture?', in M.Z. Rosaldo and L. Lamphere (eds) *Women, Culture and Society* (Stanford, CA, 1974), 17–42, 67–87; J. Sharistanian, 'Conclusion: historical study and the public/domestic model', in *idem, Gender, Ideology and Action: Historical Perspectives on Women's Public Lives* (New York, 1986), 229–36; S.F. Wempel, 'Sanctity and power: the dual pursuit of medieval women', and S. Stuard, 'The dominion of gender: women's fortunes in the high Middle Ages', in Bridenthal, Koonz and Stuard, *Becoming Visible*, 131–51, 153–74.

11. S.M. Okin, *Women in Western Political Thought* (Princeton, NJ, 1979); J.B. Elshtain, *Public Man, Private Woman: Women in Social and Political Thought* (Princeton, NJ, 1981).

12. J. Landes, *Women and the Public Sphere in the Age of the French Revolution* (Ithaca, NY, 1988); J. Scott, 'Gender: a useful category of historical analysis', *American Historical Review*, 9 (1985), 1053–75; C. Fauré, *Democracy Without Women: Feminism and the Rise of Liberal Individualism in France* (Bloomington, IN, 1991).

13. For a review of the debate about female sovereignty, see C. Jordan, *Renaissance Feminism: Literary Texts and Political Models* (Ithaca, NY, 1990).

14. For municipal midwives in eighteenth-century Germany and Holland, see chs 9 and 10 in this volume by Mary Lindemann and Hilary Marland.

15. Wiesner, *Working Women*; L. Roper, *The Holy Household: Women and Morals in Reformation Augsburg* (Oxford, 1989).

16. Roper, *The Holy Household*; K. Zapalac, *In His Image and Likeness: Political Iconography and Religious Change in Regensburg, 1500–1600* (Ithaca, NY, 1990); M.E. Wiesner, 'Guilds, male bonding, and women's work in early modern Germany', *Gender and History*, 1 (1989), 125–37.

17. Memmingen Stadtarchiv, Ratsprotokollbücher (hereafter RPB), 1510–1625; Nuremberg Staatsarchiv, Aemterbüchlein, Rep. 62, nos 5–139 (1463–1620); Augsburg Stadtarchiv, Baumeisterbücher, 1570–1589; Frankfurt Stadtarchiv, Medizinalia, Ugb. 8a.

18. Memmingen RPB, 1510–1625; Nuremberg Staatsarchiv, Ratsbücher (hereafter RB), 6, f. 57 (1494); 28, f. 311 (1555); 36, f. 238 (1578); Frankfurt Stadtarchiv, Burgermeisterbücher (hereafter BMB), 1500, f. 208; Munich Stadtarchiv, Ratsitzungsprotokolle (hereafter RSP), 1603, f. 176; Strasbourg Archives Municipales, Akten der XXI, 1623, f. 11.

19. Memmingen RPB, 5 Jan. 1571.

20. *Gesetze und Statutensammlung der freien Stadt Frankfurt* (Frankfurt, 1817), 319–20.

21. Memmingen RPB, 1510–70; Memmingen Stadtarchiv, Hebammen, 48, 102, 343, 406; Frankfurt Stadtarchiv, Medizinalia, Ugb. 8a; Munich RSP, 1526. See also ch. 9 in this volume by Mary Lindemann for midwives' complaints in Braunschweig.

22. Nuremberg Staatsarchiv, Aemterbüchlein, nos 5–139 (1463–1620); Memmingen RPB, 1571–1625; Frankfurt Stadtarchiv, Medizinalia, Ugb. 8a, 1499; J.-P. Leffte, 'Aperçu historique sur l'obstetrique de Strasbourg avant la grande révolution', unpub. MD diss., University of Strasbourg, 1952, 13; Augsburg Stadtarchiv, Schätze, no. 42 (1466) and Frankfurt BMB, 1570–89; Munich Stadtarchiv, Kammereirechnungen, 1555–1700.

23. Augsburg Stadtarchiv, Schätze, no. 42 (1466).

24. The ability of patrician men to assert their control over many aspects of urban life in early modern Germany has been noted by a number of observers. See Roper, *The Holy Household*; Zapalac, *In His Image*; H. Schilling, *Aufbruch und Krise: Deutschland 1517–1648* (Berlin, 1988).

25. Nuremberg Staatsarchiv, Amts- und Standbücher (hereafter AStB), no. 101, f. 100; Frankfurt Stadarchiv, Medizinalia, Ugb. 8a, ff. 35–46 (1696–97).

26. Nuremberg AStB, no. 101, f. 100.

27. Memmingen Stadtarchiv, Hebammen, 406, 1740 Hebammenordnung.

28. Memmingen Stadtarchiv, Hebammen, 406, no. 1.

29. Wiesner, *Working Women*, 49–55; A.K. Lingo, 'Empirics and charlatans in early modern France: the genesis of the classification of the "other" in medical practice', *Journal of Social History*, 19 (1985–86), 591–7.

30. Memmingen Stadtarchiv, Hebammen, 406, 1578 and 1740 Hebammenordnung; *Gesetze und Statutensammlung*, 300; Nuremberg AStB, no. 103, f. 323.

31. W. Kallmorgan, *Siebenhundert Jahre Heilkunde in Frankfurt a.M.* (Frankfurt, 1936), 71.

32. Munich Stadtarchiv, Zimilien, no. 41 (Eidbuch, 1488); Leffte, 'Aperçu historique', 15; Frankfurt Stadtarchiv, Eidbuch, vol. II, no. 240 (1509); Nuremberg AStB, no. 100, f. 101; Stuttgart Stadtarchiv, Findbuch, 'Medizin'; Memmingen Stadtarchiv, Hebammen, 406, no. 1 (1578).

33. Quote taken from Munich ordinance. Munich Stadtarchiv, Zimilien, no. 41 (Eidbuch, 1488).

34. A. Eccles, *Obstetrics and Gynaecology in Tudor and Stuart England* (London, 1982), 119–20.

35. A. Wilson, 'The ceremony of childbirth and its interpretation', in V. Fildes (ed.) *Women as Mothers in Pre-Industrial England* (London and New York, 1990), 74.

36. Munich Stadtarchiv, Zimilien, no. 41 (Eidbuch, 1488).

37. Stuttgart, Württembergisches Hauptstaatsarchiv, Polizeiakten, A38, Bu. 1 (1585).

38. Strasbourg Archives Municipales, Statuten, vol. 33, no. 60. For midwives and baptism in eighteenth-century Italy, see ch. 8 in this volume by Nadia Filippini.

39. G. Seebass, 'Das Problem der Konditionaltaufe in der Reformation', *Zeitschrift für bayerische Kirchengeschichte*, 35 (1966), 138–68.

40. R. Kingdon and J.W. Baker, personal communications, Sept. 1991.

41. C.-P. Clasen, *Anabaptism: A Social History, 1525–1618* (Ithaca, NY, 1972), 149.

42. Strasbourg Archives Municipales, Statuten, vol. 7, f. 19.

43. Strasbourg Archives Municipales, Statuten, vol. 33, no. 75.

44. Frankfurt BMB, 1600, f. 253.

45. Nuremberg AStB, no. 100, f. 104.

46. Nuremberg AStB, no. 100, f. 104.

47. Memmingen Stadtarchiv, Hebammen, 406, no. 1.

48. It is important to recognize that the definition of abortion in the early modern period differed from contemporary opinions. Generally in the sixteenth century both popular and learned opinion held that the foetus received a soul only at quickening, not conception, so that the expulsion of a foetus, either intentional or unintentional, before that time was not 'abortion'. Many drugs were advertised as means of 'restoring the menses', with their makers and the women who bought them clearly recognizing that the onset of menstruation would also mean an end to a pregnancy, but neither equated taking such drugs with abortion. Barbara Duden has demonstrated for the late seventeenth and early eighteenth centuries in Germany that though women regarded themselves as probably pregnant before quickening, they did not think of themselves as definitely pregnant, and of the foetus as a human being, and described miscarriages before this time as the expulsion of blood curds or leathery stuff or wrong growths. B. Duden, 'Quick with child: an experience which lost its status', unpub. paper presented at American Historical Association conference, San Francisco, 1989. By the late eighteenth century, however, physicians and political authorities in Germany were increasingly unwilling to let women judge whether the foetus inside them was human or not, and began to view conception, rather than quickening, as the beginning of life. This view triumphed in the nineteenth century, when anti-abortion laws were passed which defined as abortion any intentional ending of a pregnancy, whenever it occurred. For the period considered here, however, abortion meant ending a pregnancy after quickening, that is, after the fourth or fifth month.

49. Nuremberg RB, 12, f. 96 (1522); 69, ff. 545, 548 (1614).

50. Frankfurt BMB, 1520, ff. 2–3; Augsburg Stadtarchiv, Schätze, no. 282.

51. Nuremberg Staatsarchiv, Ratsverlasse, 1141, f. 34.

52. Memmingen RPB, 4 Nov. 1603; Munich Stadtarchiv, Stadtgericht, 865 (1523); Nuremberg RB, 29, f. 354 (1557); 35, f. 125 (1578); 56, f. 507 (1597).

53. E.W. Monter, 'Protestant wives, Catholic saints, and the devil's handmaid: women in the age of Reformations', in Bridenthal, Koonz and Stuard, *Becoming Visible*, 216.

54. J. Klaits, *Servants of Satan: The Age of the Witch Hunts* (Bloomington, IN, 1985), 94–103.

55. Stuttgart, Württembergisches Hauptstaatsarchiv, Oberrat Malefizakten, A209, Bü. 233.

56. J. Baader, *Nürnberger Polizeiordnungen aus dem 13. bis 15. Jahrhundert* (Stuttgart, 1861), 69–70.

57. Ibid. This duty was also often allocated to the 'honourable women'. For sources, see note 22.

58. Memmingen Stadtarchiv, Hebammen, 406; Frankfurt Stadtarchiv, Medizinalia, Ugb. 8a.

59. Nuremberg, Germanisches Nationalmuseum, 'Schuld und Rechnungsbuch Dr. Christoph Scheurl', f. 10.

60. Wunder, '"L'espace privé"'; L.A. Tilly and J.W. Scott, *Women, Work and Family* (New York, 1987), 129.

61. See Wiesner, *Working Women*, esp. 111–47.

62. Strasbourg Archives Municipales, Statuten, vol. 9, no. 80.

63. Freiburg Stadtarchiv, Eidbücher, Rep 3(0), no. 4, f. 26.

64. Memmingen Stadtarchiv, Hebammen, 406, no. 1.

65. Memmingen RPB, 1572, 1584, 1585, 1595 and elsewhere.

66. Nuremberg RB, 3, f. 198 (1481).

67. Strasbourg Archives Municipales, Akten der XV, 1584, f. 121b.

5

From hegemony to subordination: midwives in early modern Spain

Teresa Ortiz

Throughout the early modern period midwives formed one of the most prominent of female occupational groups in Spain. It was the only branch of the medical professions which allowed women total hegemony until the eighteenth century. The history of women's place in the medical professions is one of their gradual exclusion, a process which has continued until very recent times,[1] and one which was no respecter of midwives. Indeed, a complex process of reorganization of the medical professions was taking place in eighteenth-century Spain, which paved the way for, amongst other things, the transformation of the art of midwifery into a male-dominated activity, and the subordination of midwives, who were to become the assistants of obstetric specialists in the nineteenth and twentieth centuries.

Women throughout recorded history have been assisted during childbirth by other women who, in early modern Spain, were designated in Castilian *parteras* or *comadres de parir*,[2] in accordance with the oldest denominations in existence. We can be certain that many women helped their neighbours to give birth without any basis other than that of solidarity of gender and their own experience as mothers.[3] However, it is clear that 'professionals' did exist; women specially prepared to practise midwifery which provided them with a source of income.

This essay will focus on this latter group of women in an attempt to break what can be considered as a major historiographic silence. A bibliographical search has revealed the striking paucity of works whose titles included the term 'midwife' (*comadre, partera, matrona*). My findings are limited to seven short articles, five of which are of a descriptive nature published in midwifery[4] and obstetric journals,[5] while the two others are brief medical-historical notes.[6] More information can be obtained from the abundance of works on the history of obstetrics,[7] medical practice[8] and, more recently, from those on the history of women's work.[9] In all of these, with the exception of the latter, the interest shown in midwives is aside from the main issue and the sources are almost always the same: legal documents and obstetric literature written by physicians and surgeons. Midwives did not publish any works outlining their knowledge in early modern Spain. From these few sources, brief descriptions have been sketched, real or ideal, on the activities of midwives, which have added little to the global view offered in 1795 by the surgeon Juan de Navas in the introduction to his work *Elementos del Arte de Partear*.[10]

The published sources on midwives, therefore, are scarce, which proved to be a handicap when preparing this article. An attempt has been made to overcome this obstacle by re-reading the standard sources, and also by consulting manuscripts of an administrative[11] and fiscal[12] nature, which has facilitated the uncovering of individual midwives, real people, and not merely vague images glimpsed in the works of intellectuals of the period. Some aspects of the professional activities of midwives have been clarified using information acquired from the abundant literature on women's history and local and hospital history produced in Spain in the 1980s, which revealed the value of other sources, such as notarial protocols, city council minutes, censuses and hospital records.

Midwives in the fifteenth to seventeenth centuries

Between the fifteenth and seventeenth centuries the 'art of midwifery' (*Arte de Partear*) was an exclusively female activity. From royalty to commoners,[13] all 'pregnant women and those who have recently given birth, in their need and for their infants, ask for advice from midwives rather than from physicians'.[14] This custom, justified by the necessity of protecting women's modesty,[15] was approved by physicians, who most probably displayed a lack of interest in midwifery, since they believed that 'the midwives' craft is a science or art to work with one's own hands'.[16]

Because of the scarcity of information it is no easy task to sketch a professional and personal profile of midwives between the fifteenth and seventeenth centuries. There must have been many differences between midwives because of the coexistence of various cultures – Christian, Jewish and Morisco – in the peninsula. The diversity of regulations respecting medical practice in the Hispanic kingdoms further complicates the picture. Coupled with the varied practices of midwives, the degree of marginality they suffered depended as much on their cultural background, as on the fact that they were women and at the same time medical practitioners. For example, in the mid-sixteenth century, Morisco midwives were prohibited from practising,[17] and an order was issued to 'female Christian converts that if there was a true Christian midwife, not to give birth with a Christian convert nor with one of her generation'.[18]

I have come across fifteen midwives who, between the sixteenth and seventeenth centuries, practised in different communities in Spain.[19] The marital status of five of them is unknown, eight were married and two were widows. Apart from one, who resided in a coastal village, they all lived in cities. Their status and professional awareness may have been affected by living in urban areas, and by whether they were employed by nobility or commoners. Some midwives gained fame and recognition,[20] highlighted by the fact that their husbands were identified not only by name but also as 'the midwife's husband'.[21]

These women learned their trade working with another midwife, in the same way as craftsmen and the majority of medical practitioners – surgeons, bloodletters, apothecaries, herbalists, spicers and barbers. Only physicians, who were university trained, had a theoretical 'corpus' of knowledge, the transmission of which was regulated by the university. The midwife's knowledge, who 'practising and conversing with another expert midwife would turn out perfect',[22] was of an empirical nature and passed on by word of mouth. They had no universal body of knowledge and their skills were probably as varied as the cultures which existed within the Spanish territory.

In the sixteenth and seventeenth centuries three works on childbirth were published, written in Castilian by the physicians Damián Carbón (1541),[23] Francisco Núñez (1580)[24] and Juan Alonso de los Ruyzes (1606).[25] Carbón's book was the first on childbirth to be published in Spain and the second in Europe after Roesslin's *Rosengarten*, which had been published twenty-eight years previously.[26] Carbón and Alonso de los Ruyzes wrote their books specially for midwives, who were considered to be badly informed and, as Carbón pointed out, 'moved by charity, I will show them in this little work their art and the rules and form that [the said art] must have to be sufficient'.[27] The fact that they were written largely in Castilian bears direct relation to their intended readership. However, such works were not only aimed at midwives. Those of Alonso de los Ruyzes and Núñez were more learned and contained numerous paragraphs in Latin, above all 'the prescriptions, remedies, precepts and grave matters',[28] with the clear intention of being of no use to the *Romancistas* (those who knew no Latin), including midwives.

Midwives for their part had their own remedies, about which little is known, but which were undoubtedly used when they deemed it necessary. We know that Isabel Fernández, a midwife practising in Málaga in 1492, produced some 'medicines' herself which she administered 'if those who give birth with her suffer from any affliction of the womb or other distresses'.[29] María Luna, a Morisco who worked during the mid-sixteenth century in Cuenca, was 'a woman well versed in medical matters and knowledge of herbs and a very good midwife . . . '.[30] Two centuries later (as will subsequently be seen), Luisa Rosado strove to publicize, amongst other things, the effectiveness of a poultice which she had developed herself.

Besides prescribing, midwives, according to the author-physicians, attended all manner of deliveries, normal as well as difficult,[31] and even 'the most inexpert of midwives' knew 'how to carry out a caesarean post-mortem'.[32] Such responsibilities were recognized as being their own, the intervention of the surgeon being limited to cases where the dead foetus had to be extracted in pieces[33] and to gynaecological problems of a surgical nature.[34] The physician only intervened in cases of fever or general ill-nesses during the pregnancy, birth or the puerperium. The midwife's duties continued after the birth and she was in charge of caring for the infant and the mother. The latter was prescribed 'a healthy diet and lifestyle' and the infant had its umbilical cord tied, auditory and nasal orifices cleaned, and was washed and swaddled.[35]

We must ask ourselves what role was played by the works on childbirth written by physicians. Doubts arise as to whether they fulfilled their aim of training midwives. Literacy was not widespread amongst the common women of the sixteenth and seventeenth centuries.[36] Regarding midwives, one of the physicians who wrote for them warned, paradoxically, that hoping that they were learned and studious was 'asking the impossible'.[37] Even supposing that a large proportion of them could read and write, there are still two questions to be answered: first, whether midwives, whose knowledge was of a popular and empirical nature, rooted in the traditions of their own cultures, would feel the need to delve into a medical book; and, second, whether, for the same reasons, they were able to understand the content of texts written by physicians, many of which were intended to instruct but were riddled with references to classical authors, that is, to the physicians' own roots.

It is my belief that physicians, although this was never their claim, actually wrote for themselves, aspiring to possess a new knowledge rather than to devote themselves to it. Given that cultural and social circum-stances did not make their works readily accessible to midwives, putting them forward as advice books for this group was rather rhetorical, and may have been an attempt to overcome the obstacle of morality and customs which placed childbirth within the female domain.[38] It is here that one of the origins of the transformation of childbirth into an aspect of medical science may be found.

Between 1477 and 1523, a decree was in force by virtue of which the *Protomédicos* – the King's physicians and the highest medical authority – examined all medical practitioners, including midwives, who wished to practise, issuing a licence which allowed them to do so.[39] After 1523, the examination and consequently the licence of the *Protomedicato* were only available to physicians, surgeons, apothecaries and barbers. The *Protomédicos* were ordered 'not to bother examining midwives, nor spicers, nor druggists . . . ', thus creating a dividing line between some groups of practitioners and others.[40] This measure did not imply, however, that midwives had freedom to practise, since they continued to fall under the supervision of physicians in most of the kingdoms. Physicians, under orders from the local authority or following corporate decisions, were in charge of granting the right to practise to those midwives wishing to settle in the area.[41] In the Municipal Archives of Málaga there is a record of the examination carried out in 1537 of 'Mari Alvarez, widow . . . , midwife for many years in the city of Valencia and in other places'. Recently arrived in Málaga to carry out her profession, she was examined by the physician Juan Muñoz, who, after 'asking her many questions', decided that she was capable of practising her profession.[42]

In seventeenth-century Zaragoza, the College of Physicians was responsible for the training and examination of midwives. According to its ordinances, they had to be, amongst other things, true Christians, born in Aragón, over 35 years old, and to have served a 4-year apprenticeship with an approved midwife. Classes were offered by the professor of anatomy, as well as the study of a book 'which for this purpose the College will print', but about which we have no information.[43] In the second half of the eighteenth century an attempt was made to introduce a follow-up to this method of training throughout Spain.

Changes in the eighteenth century

During the first half of the eighteenth century control of midwives' work remained in the hands of local doctors and, sometimes, even of priests.[44] In spite of this, in some cities, such as Málaga, midwives retained a high level of autonomy and, in a similar way to the guilds, they examined candidates themselves and ensured that levels of expertise were maintained.[45]

In 1750, a royal warrant delivered by King Fernando VI revoked all previous decrees on medical practice, and once more granted the *Protomedicato* the power to examine midwives, thus combining the Bourbon policy of centralization with the maintenance of the professional interests of physicians and surgeons. It was an attempt to deal with 'the lack of skill of midwives and some men, who to earn a living, have taken up the profession of midwifery'.[46]

A book written by the physician Antonio Medina was published to help midwives prepare for the examination. It contained all the basic knowledge required: anatomy of the female pelvic region, diagnosis of pregnancy, attendance at 'natural' and 'preternatural' deliveries and early post-natal care of the newborn and mother.[47] Although we have no proof of this, it may be supposed that midwives had to study this book on their own. This guided self-instruction was not new and seems to have been as ineffective as it had been in the sixteenth century, probably for the reasons already mentioned, namely cultural estrangement and midwives' low levels of literacy.[48] Measures subsequently adopted to train midwives were more in tune with Enlightenment notions of education, and revealed the inadequacy of this first attempt.

The enlightened believed that education was the means through which technical, scientific and economic progress and also changes in customs could be obtained. This, in turn, would lead to 'public happiness', its generic objective.[49] The other key Enlightenment belief stressed the idea of the 'usefulness' of professional activities and the sciences, and provided the pivot for the entire process of reform which began in the middle of the century.

The medical professions and crafts benefited greatly from this philosophy. Especially worthy of mention is the institutionalization of surgical education in the Royal Colleges of Surgery, both the cause and effect of the steady promotion of surgeons on social and scientific scales.[50] Preparations were made throughout the Enlightenment for the transformation of pharmacy training into a university degree,[51] and in the last decade of the century the first veterinary school was established in Madrid, the embryo of the faculty created in 1835.[52] As far as midwives were concerned, the educational reforms reduced their autonomy and relegated them scientifically and professionally during a lengthy process which lasted throughout the century and which involved other sectors of society. This was reflected in the writings of prominent Church figures on the role of midwives and surgeons at the birth. A gradual change in attitude took place: the Church initially defended midwives but later justified, on both theological and practical grounds, their subordination to surgeons.[53]

The initiatives taken after the first dubious attempt at encouraging self-instruction advocated regulated education and, although some never moved beyond the planning stage, other projects were realized. Amongst the intentions that came to nothing was that of creating two schools for midwives under the auspices of the *Real Sociedad Bascongada de Amigos del País*[54] and the *Regia Sociedad de Medicina y otras Ciencias de Sevilla*,[55] scientific societies of the Enlightenment. Their boards dealt with this matter in 1775 and 1776 respectively. The objective of training women for 'useful' crafts paralleled the work of another institution of the Enlightenment, the *Sociedad Económica Matritense*, which, in 1776, established free schools (*Escuelas Patrióticas*) in the main districts of the city of Madrid to teach the textile trades to girls.[56]

The failure of earlier proposals left the way open for surgeons to monopolize teaching, and the only effective training of midwives began during the last decades of the century, under the auspices and supervision of the new Royal Colleges of Surgery in Barcelona and Madrid, founded in 1760 and 1787 respectively. In 1787, a 'chair of childbirths' (*Cátedra de Partos*) was created for the instruction of surgeons at the Madrid College of Surgery. The statutes laid down that the professor in charge also had to devote himself

100

in the time and hours that he can, without detriment to the teaching of the [male] students of the College, to instruct in one of the rooms of the building, and behind closed doors, the women who wish to learn and have classes.[57]

The 1795 ordinances of the Barcelona College of Surgery also instituted classes for midwives lasting an hour and a half a day for two months, besides practical training in the infirmary or with a trained midwife.[58] It was laid down that 'none of the midwives dwelling in Madrid can henceforth gain the approval of the *Protomedicato . . .* [without having] received instruction from the "professor of childbirths" (*catedrático de Partos*) of this College'.[59]

The knowledge to be imparted at the Colleges of Surgery covered the same points as Medina's book, with the addition of a new duty, never before referred to in midwifery books, that of baptizing newborn infants on the point of death.[60] The first manual of childbirth to appear after the sixteenth century which included both the baptism ritual and instructions on how to perform it was written by the surgeon Babil de Gárate.[61] Increasing attention was paid to this matter in works published during the second half of the century.

Certain requisites which continued well into the twentieth century had to be fulfilled in order to gain admission to these studies. The woman had to be over 25, either widowed or married, in the latter case with written permission from her husband. She had to present a certificate showing 'blood-purity' and to have practised for two years. In addition, she had to present a certificate proving that she was 'respectable'.[62]

Towards the end of the Enlightenment period, this model of education faithfully combined two important aspects of its educational philosophy: the importance of women's education and the need to teach the useful sciences, respecting the principle that each ought to occupy his (or her) rightful position by virtue of his (or her) social background and gender.[63] In addition, it helped surgeons realize their aims of expansion. Although midwives received their instruction at the surgical colleges, their training was different from that of the male surgical students. It was not so rigorous, exclusive to women, and prepared them to a lesser degree.

To obtain the licence from the Barcelona College, without which midwives could not practise in Cataluña, they had to take an examination (*Reválida*) and swear under oath:

not to administer any medicament to women who are pregnant, parturient or puerperal which has not been prescribed by a Latin surgeon or physician; not to work alone at abnormal and difficult births which require special handling, but to call a professor well versed in these operations, if he is close at hand; to carry out a caesarean on those pregnant women who die . . . as long as there is no other to perform it.[64]

101

Officially then, midwives were supposed to withdraw from some of the duties that they had carried out in the previous century, in order to hand them over to surgeons. Women were, of course, not permitted to practise surgery.[65] Although there was no decree which expressly prohibited women from learning surgery, the entrance requirements made their admission to its study impossible. Candidates had to have knowledge of Latin, logic, algebra and physics,[66] knowledge which was practically impossible for women to obtain, except those from the upper class, whose social status would exclude them from midwifery. For middle- and lower-class women, education before 1797 was limited to prayers and needlework, and reading and writing was not taught until after this date.[67]

In turn, it was impossible for a man to become a man-midwife if he was not already qualified in surgery[68] since, in 1750, the 'art of midwifery' had been officially converted into a category of surgery, with the result that the surgeon was also trained in obstetrics. This new concept of midwifery, including the surgical monopoly of its teaching, brought about the expropriation of a knowledge which had belonged to midwives for centuries and which, for cultural reasons related to gender bias, namely illiteracy, lack of power and popular knowledge, they had not been able to retain and develop.

Possibly the only form of resistance open to midwives was to turn a deaf ear, to continue to attend normal and abnormal births, administering external and internal remedies to ease labour,[69] providing mothers and their infants with early post-natal care and performing caesarean sections post-mortem.[70] In addition, they continued to give specialist reports when required by judges on questions concerning matrimony, virginity or inheritance.[71] In many cases, they certainly exceeded the role assigned to them by surgeons. This attitude was based not only on the rebellious character and lively spirit of the midwife, but also on the fundamental problem of the shortage of competent surgeons.[72] With the exception of foreign surgeons and a few others linked to the Court, the evidence points to the fact that rank and file surgeons knew less about childbirth than the reviled midwives. It was in relation to this that, in 1795, Juan de Navas, professor of obstetrics (*catedrático de Partos*) at the Royal Colleges of Surgery of Cádiz and Madrid, warned of 'the decadence of the Art of Midwifery' among surgeons, due to the shortage of members and lack of preparation of those who practised this trade.[73]

The educational reform of midwifery seems, in quantitative terms, to have had little effect on midwives, so that at the end of the century, the presence of trained midwives outside large cities was still rare.[74] Their instruction began very late in the century, in only two centres in the country, which greatly restricted the numbers of women who could attend classes. It is not known whether women in the near vicinity of such centres took advantage of the courses on offer. The only, rather vague, information available is on those who participated in the first course in Madrid; between eight and twelve women attended,[75] who found out about the commencement of these courses from notices displayed in the street advertising free classes.[76] These first Madrid midwives, after obtaining their licence, were fortunate enough to find well paid jobs with the General Board of Welfare (*Junta General de Caridad*). They earned 2,200 *reales de vellón* a year,[77] a large sum of money when compared with average salaries in the late eighteenth century.

Although information on midwives' income is very sparse, there seem to have been many poor midwives, especially amongst those who lived outside cities who, in 1760, were considered by the *Protomedicato* as being 'the most unfortunate people of the villages'.[78] The incomes of some of Córdoba's midwives in 1752 ranged from 120 to 4,000 *reales de vellón*. Averages differed greatly, although in general terms midwives' purchasing power (about 1,200 *reales de vellón*) was half that of Córdoba's physicians and a little lower than that of surgeons (around 1,700 both in Córdoba and throughout the Ancient Kingdom of Granada). Barbers were the poorest paid medical practitioners (about 700 *reales de vellón* in Andalucía).[79] The clear differences in incomes may have depended, as in earlier centuries, not only on their place of work but also on their social status, on the level of competition with other midwives and surgeons, and on the financial position of the women they attended.

By the last quarter of the eighteenth century, surgeons had established legal and educational control over midwives. It also seems to be clear that surgeons held as their own the theory of the 'art of midwifery' – which was beginning to be called obstetrics – but midwives, trained either according to the new canon laws or in the traditional way, had practical experience and assisted the majority of women in giving birth, even at Court.[80] Some of them were endowed with a remarkable professional awareness and an unquestionable capacity for carrying out their work. It was this which morally authorized them to protect their interests and to confront, without reservation, the top professional hierarchies, as is shown in the case of the Court midwife, Luisa Rosado.

Luisa Rosado: a woman proud of being a midwife

Luisa Rosado was born in Toledo – when is not known – and from the summer of 1768 lived at Court, where she worked as midwife for the Royal House for the Abandoned (*Real Colegio de Niños Desamparados*). This institution, founded at the turn of the sixteenth century was, by the eighteenth century, giving shelter to children above the age of 7 or 8,[81] and to poor, disabled women. It also provided free maternity care 'for women who through shame or necessity take refuge there to give birth'.[82]

A short time before arriving in Madrid, Rosado had been practising in Zamora, endorsed by the licence of the 'art of the midwife' (*Arte de Partera*), which she obtained in 1765, after having been examined by the Royal *Protomedicato*. Little is known about her personal characteristics, except that she was of 'medium height'. She was probably also middle-aged, a true Christian and respectable. She gives the impression of being a woman who lived alone and was perhaps a widow like a great many of her fellow midwives.[83] She could read and write and displayed a talent for putting her aspirations and desires for professional advancement on paper, as shown by the documents she addressed to the King and to the Council of Castile – our main source of information.[84] It is clear that she was a determined, ambitious woman, proud of her knowledge and anxious for it to be recognized.

In 1770 she was residing at her place of work, The Royal House for the Abandoned, situated in *calle de Atocha*, near the *Hospital General*.[85] Around this time, Rosado became involved in a complex legal process which lasted over a year, in an attempt – it is not known whether this was successful – to publicize her professional skills. She attempted to achieve her objective by affixing the following notice in the street:

> The Public is informed that Luisa Rosado, midwife examined by the Royal *Protomedicato*, is midwife by the King in the Royal House for the Abandoned and being this very person and none other, lives in the said House for the Abandoned.
>
> The Public is informed that any woman accustomed to aborting for 15 or 20 years is offered a poultice never heard of nor tried in this Court which does not stick to the flesh, and produces such effects, that the foetus is successfully retained for the nine months and the bones strengthened.
>
> Moreover, if by misfortune, as happens every day, the afterbirth, or placenta, is retained in the patient for 20 or 40 hours, even for eight days without her being able to expel it, the said Luisa Rosado will extract it within six minutes without causing discomfort or injury to the parturient although she may be on the point of death, just as she has done before now to others, and will prove this by the presentation of a certificate from Municipal Physicians (*Médicos Titulares*), having acted in their presence with victorious outcome; all of which she offers to perform faithfully and loyally with the help of God Almighty.[86]

In the notice Rosado offered to attend complicated deliveries and to prescribe remedies to prevent miscarriages, both of which were activities purported to be exclusive to surgeons and physicians, and consequently beyond the scope of midwives. The very licence which entitled her to practise clearly warned that she was to be 'accompanied by an approved

104

physician or surgeon at difficult births and that she may not send a pregnant woman for bloodletting nor purging without a physician's order'.[87]

Rosado, however, wished to proclaim herself a genuine expert in her art, all the more provoking because she proposed to do so at Court; probably the place with the highest concentration of man-midwife-surgeons (*cirujanos-comadrones*) in the country. As far as the *Protomedicato* was concerned, the approval of her petition would 'disturb professional surgeons who with a different knowledge know what they must do when difficulty arises . . . '.[88] This was one of the reasons for the rejection of her first petition in March 1770. These fears regarding competition were not unfounded if we bear in mind that midwives still managed more deliveries than surgeons, and that the cases presented by Luisa Rosado in her dossier were complicated births which she attended when another professional, usually another midwife, had failed to deliver the woman. This is especially evident in the case certified by Manuel García del Pozal, physician to the Madrid *Hospital General*, where a woman pregnant with triplets was in labour without the physician or the midwife of the hospital being aware of the situation,

> and seeing the patient so afflicted and in great danger of her life due to the repeated distress, sweating, swooning or fainting she was suffering, they called upon Luisa Rosado, who indeed came and helped her to give birth, and made her produce the infants with such skill, art and diligence, that all those who were present were amazed.[89]

It must be stressed that Luisa Rosado believed in and defended the fact that her knowledge, her 'science',[90] was different from that of surgeons and lay in her natural talents[91] and experience, which she presented with the endorsement of testimonies. At no time did she refer to her training, nor call upon any scientific authority despite the fact that, by this time, works had been written for midwives, most recently in 1750[92] and 1756.[93] She maintained that her knowledge was of an empirical nature, and perhaps for that reason especially useful and beneficial to women in particular and to the people in general.[94] After being rejected by the *Protomedicato*, Rosado twice appealed to King Charles III (in December 1770 and June 1771) arguing along these lines. Her stance was an intelligent one, in tune with the discourse and practice of the science of the Spanish Enlightenment, characterized by the dazzling rise of applied science and empiricism and by the weakening of theoretical reasoning.[95] Her appeal had the desired effect and she obtained permission to display the notices. However, the excess zeal of the *Protomedicato* and its cautious interpretation of the royal approval proved to be a great, perhaps even insurmountable, obstacle.[96]

The Board of the *Protomedicato* belittled her knowledge, alleging that her remedies were inefficient and her beliefs about the movement of the placenta, which appear in some of her briefs, erroneous.[97] Luisa Rosado was of the opinion that the afterbirth moved about the human body,[98] highlighting the popular nature of her knowledge in direct relation to another belief, 'characteristic of the common herd', concerning the roving movements of the uterus, anatomically refuted in 1728 by the famous Spanish physician Martín Martínez.[99] At the end of the century, there were few references to the pathogeny of the process, but the idea which was put on paper, and which we imagine the *Protomédicos* to be in agreement with, was that the remains of the placenta prevented uterine contraction and the expulsion of the lochia.[100] Luisa Rosado's confidence in her own interpretation is striking since, in spite of the clear refutation she received from the *Protomedicato*, she repeated it yet again in a later document.[101]

The retention of the afterbirth was one of the dangers of childbirth in early modern Europe. Some 10 per cent of the complicated deliveries dealt with by the French surgeon Mauriceau in the seventeenth century resulted from this problem.[102] Ventura Pastor, at the end of the eighteenth century, mentions two cases of this nature, 4 per cent of the complicated deliveries he discusses.[103] If we are to believe some of the testimonies of the period, at the beginning of the century 'horrifying, formidable and scandalous ravages [were] wept over in this Court' due to the mishandling of these cases, causing the inversion of the uterus and the mother's death.[104]

Surgeons recommended manual extraction when the placenta had not been expelled. Internal remedies were unanimously rejected. Although there were slight differences of opinion, almost all surgeons advocated commencing gently by pushing on the belly, producing sneezing and retching, or lightly pulling on the cord. If this failed, a hand was to be inserted into the uterus to extract the placenta.[105] Of all the texts on childbirth, those which are expressly aimed at midwives, by Medina (1750) and Gárate (1756), do not anticipate manual extraction. Gárate even recommends an expectant attitude, his experience convincing him that the placenta is always expelled without intervention.[106]

Rosado, rather more active than expected from a midwife, used – as surgeons did – a gentle technique, and 'without any instrument other than her hands placed on the belly, nor more violence in her movements than that produced by her almost imperceptible touch',[107] succeeded, she claimed, in resolving even the most difficult of cases in less than 6 minutes.[108] She cites three cases, supported by witnesses, where she applied her method with remarkable results. One of them concerned a woman who had gone 'four days without being able to expel the afterbirth, until calling upon the petitioner, who arrived and delivered her of it in very few minutes'.[109] On another occasion, which dates back to her period in Zamora, she attended

Francisca Pérez, baker by trade, who after having the afterbirth, or placenta, retained for two days and the labia of the uterus so swollen that it seemed impossible to extract it, on account of the occlusion which the said swelling had made, she delivered her of it with such ease that she had no injury at all. And it was not perceived that this patient throughout the duration of her illness, which was drawn-out, felt any injury to the uterus nor adjacent parts, external or internal . . .[110]

Threatened miscarriages, which Rosado treated with a 'poultice never heard of or tried', were probably a matter more closely linked to medicine than to the 'art of midwifery', since this subject was only dealt with in two treatises at the end of the century. Both suggested identical measures – rest, bloodletting, bathing, mild food and 'temperate' drinks, such as water with orange blossom,[111] or an infusion of barley with a few drops of lemon.[112] The use of a poultice as suggested by Rosado was also contemplated by the author Ventura Pastor, who recommended the application of a napkin soaked in vinegar and common plantain and black nightshade juice.[113] These traditional and well-known remedies, combined with some of the previous ones, produced excellent results in the case of a woman who, after thirteen consecutive miscarriages, succeeded in carrying a baby to full term.[114]

It is not known whether the notice was actually affixed in the streets of Madrid, but in any case Luisa Rosado was not disheartened by her setbacks. In the last brief she addressed to the King in August 1771, she offered to attend the impending delivery of his daughter-in-law, 'in company of the man-midwife chosen to this end, or in his absence and illness'. The daughter-in-law, who was expecting her first child, was Princess María Luisa of Parma, wife of the Crown Prince and future King Charles IV. This petition, undoubtedly daring, expressed the confidence Rosado had in herself and in her profession. She was ambitious enough to attempt to reach the highest echelons of her profession and yet sufficiently cautious to respect the surgeon's authority, without renouncing her own worth.

In the century of the surgeons, Luisa Rosado stood out as an example of a midwife with a clear professional awareness and pride, and a woman sure of herself and of her knowledge. These virtues, which offer a foil to the notion of the professional subordination of midwives and the reassertion of the domestic role of women in the eighteenth century, may not have been so exceptional nor so intrinsic to her character, but rather a manifestation of midwives' resistance and women's determination not to submit to the thrust of science and male power.

Acknowledgements

I am indebted to Maite López Beltrán and to Mikel Astrain for providing me with original, unpublished material and for many important clues; to

Encarnación Santamaría and Carmen Quesada for helping me to gain access to some distant sources. Finally, my most heartfelt thanks go to Alvaro Martínez Vidal for his helpful comments and friendly discussion. This article was translated from Spanish by Linda Hollinger.

Notes

1. On women physicians and other medical practitioners in medieval and early modern Spain, see M. Cabré, 'Formes de cultura femenina a la Catalunya medieval', in M. Nash (ed.) *Mes enllà del silenci: Les dones a la història de Catalunya* (Barcelona, 1988), 31–5; M.E. Perry, 'Las mujeres y su trabajo curativo en Sevilla, siglos XVI y XVII', *VI Jornadas de Investigación Interdisciplinaria sobre la mujer. El trabajo de las mujeres: siglos XVI–XX* (Madrid, 1987), 40–50. On women physicians in the nineteenth and twentieth centuries, see M.C. Alvarez Ricart, *La mujer como profesional de la medicina en la España del S. XIX* (Madrid, 1988); T. Ortiz, *Médicos en la Andalucía del siglo XX* (Granada, 1987), pt 3, chs 18–20, 'La mujer, profesional de la medicina', 179–208.

2. D. Carbón, *Libro del arte de las comadres y del regimiento de las preñadas y paridas y de los niños* (Mallorca, 1541), f. xi calls them *madrinas*.

3. J. Gélis, *L'Arbre et le Fruit. La naissance dans l'occident moderne (XVIe–XIXe siècle)* (Paris, 1984), 173, points out that in 1786 the figure of the *sage-femme* was still unknown in many French regions. J. Ventura Pastor, *Preceptos generales sobre las operaciones de partos . . .* (Madrid, 1795), vol. 2, 324, in one of his observations refers to the case of a woman residing at Court who was assisted in childbirth by her husband and a female neighbour.

4. R. Sánchez Arcas, 'Las comadronas españolas a través de los tiempos', *Surgere*, 144 (1971), 2–19; *idem*, 'Las comadronas españolas a través de los tiempos (conclusión)', *Surgere*, 145 (1971), 2–24; M.J. Cuadri Duque, 'La ciencia y el arte de partear. Antecedentes históricos de la enfermería maternal', *Revista Rol de Enfermería*, 8: 84–5 (1985), 13–16.

5. J.L. Gutiérrez de Alles, 'La instrucción de las comadronas en el año 1750 tutelada en España por el Real Tribunal del Protomedicato', *Tokoginecología Práctica*, 10 (1951), 357–61; R. Sánchez Arcas, 'La sustitución de las matronas por los cirujanos en Europa y España (S. XVII y sucesivos)', *Acta Obstétrica y Ginecológia Hispano-Lusitana*, 18 (1970), 238–48.

6. R. Conejo Ramilo, 'Los cirujanos y las matronas en Archidona durante la Edad Moderna', *Asclepio*, 22 (1970), 125–9; J. Riera, 'Dos parteras sevillanas', *IV Congreso Español de Historia de la Medicina, Granada, abril 1973*, vol. 1 (Granada, 1973), 63–7.

7. M. Usandizaga, *Historia de la obstetricia y la ginecología en España* (Santander, 1944). Studies of the obstetric works of early modern authors include those of A. Castaño Almendral, *La obra tocológica del doctor Babil de Gárate* (Salamanca, 1956); A. Hernández Alcántara, *Estudio histórico de la obra tocoginecológica y pediátrica de Damián Carbón* (Salamanca, 1957); A. Sánchez Martín, *El saber tocoginecológico en la medicina española de la primera mitad del siglo XVIII* (Salamanca, 1958).

8. R. Muñoz Garrido, *Ejercicio legal de la medicina en España (siglos XV a XVIII)* (Salamanca, 1967); L.S. Granjel, *La medicina española del siglo XVIII* (Salamanca, 1969), 86–9.

9. For example, S. Villas Tinoco, 'La mujer y la organización gremial malagueña en el Antiguo Régimen' and V. Fernández Vargas and M.V. López-

Cordón, 'Mujer y régimen jurídico en el Antiguo Régimen. Una realidad disociada', in M.C. García-Nieto (ed.) *Ordenamiento jurídico y realidad social de las mujeres* (Madrid, 1986), 91–104, 13–40; F. López Iglesias, 'Oficios y actividades de las mujeres ovetenses en el Antiguo Régimen', *VI Jornadas de Investigación Interdisciplinaria sobre la mujer. El trabajo de las mujeres: siglos XVI–XX* (Madrid, 1987), 50–6; M. E. Perry, *Gender and Disorder in Early Modern Sevilla* (Princeton, NJ, 1990), 20–9.

10. J. de Navas, *Elementos del Arte de Partear* (Madrid, 1795), 2 vols. The history of the art of midwifery in Spain is located in vol. 1, lxxxvii–civ.

11. For example, that of the Board of the *Protomedicato*. A catalogue of interest is that of G. Albi, *El Protomedicato en la España Ilustrada: Catálogo de documentos del Archivo General de Simancas* (Valladolid, 1982), where the papers were found on which the last part of this article is based.

12. The *Catastro de Ensenada*, a population and property census carried out in a great many of the provinces of the Spanish Peninsula between 1752 and 1756, is an excellent source.

13. Some references to the birth experiences of queens are to be found in E. Junceda Avelló, *Ginecología y vida íntima de las reinas de España* (Madrid, 1991).

14. Carbón, *Libro del arte de las comadres*, ff. xi, v.

15. Ibid., ff. x, xi.

16. Ibid., 'Epístola'.

17. L. García Ballester, *Los moriscos y la medicina* (Barcelona, 1984), 103. This measure would be related to the Moslem custom of circumcising new-born male infants.

18. Ibid., 116. M. Palacios Alcalde, 'Formas marginales de trabajo femenino en la Andalucía moderna', *VI Jornadas de Investigación Interdisciplinaria sobre la mujer. El trabajo de las mujeres: siglos XVI–XX* (Madrid, 1987), 84, cites an *auto-da-fé* carried out in 1516 against a midwife, a 'Christian convert from the Jewish faith' (literally 'new Christian from a Jew'). [Translator's note: in early modern Spain there was a distinction between those who were *cristianos viejos* (literally old Christians translated as 'true Christians') and *nuevos* (new Christians translated as 'Christian converts'). The former, unlike the latter, had neither Jewish nor Moslem blood.]

19. Riera, 'Dos parteras sevillanas'; Palacios Alcalde, 'Formas marginales', 84; Junceda Avelló, *Ginecología*, 41, 74, 80; Archivo Municipal de Málaga (hereafter AMM), Libro de Actas Capitulares (hereafter LAC), vol. 1, ff. 173v–174, 24 June 1492 (information supplied by Professor Maite López Beltrán from 'Espacio público y espacio privado: el trabajo extradoméstico en Málaga en el tránsito a la modernidad', in B. Villar (ed.) *Los espacios de las mujeres en el Antiguo Régimen. Inercias y cambios* (Málaga, forthcoming)); M. Birriel, 'Datos sobre los oficios de moriscos de la costa de Granada (1561)', *Actes du IV Symposium International d'Études Morisques sur: Métiers, vie religieuse et problématiques d'histoire morisque* (Zagohuan, 1990), 43–9; M.C. García Herrero, 'Administrar del parto y recibir a la criatura'. Aportación al estudio de la obstetricia bajomedieval', in *Aragón en la Baja Edad Media. Homenaje al profesor Antonio Ubieto* (Zaragoza, 1989), vol. 8, 283–92 idem, *las mujeres en Zaragoza en el S. XV* (Zaragoza, 1990), vol. 2, 288, 291.

20. The historiography has concentrated on those closest to the Court. Junceda Avelló, *Ginecología*, 74, 80, 84, cites, amongst others, Quirce de Toledo, head midwife of Isabel of Portugal, wife of Carlos V.

21. F. Bejarano Robles, *Libro de los repartimientos de Málaga* (Málaga, 1985), 93, 103, makes two references to such individuals. (Information supplied by Maite López Beltrán.)

22. Carbón, *Libro del arte de las comadres*, f. xii.

23. Ibid.

24. F. Núñez, *Libro del parto humano en el cual se contienen remedios muy útiles y usuales para el parto dificultoso de las mujeres* . . . (Alcalá, 1580). A 1683 edition has been used here. This was one of the most widely consulted books in the seventeenth and first half of the eighteenth centuries, passing through six known editions, the last four forming part of G. Ayala's book, *Principios de cirugía* (Madrid, 1693, 1705, 1716 and 1724). See A. Hernández Alcántara, *La obra tocológica y pediátrica de Núñez de Coria* (Salamanca, 1960), 5–6.

25. J. Alonso de los Ruyzes de Fonteche, *Diez privilegios para mujeres preñadas* (Alcalá, 1606). The chapter 'Privilegio octavo, para elegir comadre', ff. 110–61, is a short midwifery manual.

26. Usandizaga, *Historia de la obstetricia*, 107–18; Hernández Alcántara, *Estudio histórico*. A facsimile edition of Carbón's book has been published in Spain by Galloso-Wellcome (n.p., n.d.), with an introduction by P. Laín Entralgo.

27. Carbón, *Libro del arte de las comadres*, 'Epístola'. The third author, Núñez, *Libro del parto humano*, does not mention who the book is intended for although, throughout his work, the midwife is the central figure in childbirth.

28. Alonso de los Ruyzes, *Diez privilegios*, 'Al lector'.

29. AMM, LAC, ff. 173v–174.

30. L. García Ballester, *Historia social de la medicina en la España de los siglos XII al XVI* (Madrid, 1976), 133.

31. Carbón, *Libro del arte de las comadres*, ff. xii, v; Núñez, *Libro del parto humano*, on ff. 20v–25, explains the handling 'by the midwife' of cases where the delivery 'is not natural'; Alonso de los Ruyzes, *Diez privilegios*, f. 108 and ff.

32. Núñez, *Libro del parto humano*, f. 59. Alonso de los Ruyzes, *Diez privilegios*, was not so optimistic and believed that a midwife was rarely trained to extract a dead foetus, a task which should be performed by a surgeon. For midwives and caesarean section in Italy, see ch. 8 in this volume by Nadia Filippini.

33. Carbón, *Libro del arte de las comadres*, f. xl.

34. Núñez, *Libro del parto humano*, ch. iv.

35. Alonso de los Ruyzes, *Diez privilegios*, ff. 107v–164; Carbón, *Libro del arte de las comadres*, ff. xiv, v.

36. C. Larquié, 'La alfabetización de los madrileños en 1650', *Anales del Instituto de Estudios Madrileños*, 17 (1980), 250–1. For literacy amongst English midwives, see chs 2 and 3 in this volume by David Harley and Ann Giardina Hess.

37. Literally 'asking for pears from an elm tree'. Alonso de los Ruyzes, *Diez privilegios*, 108–13.

38. Merry Wiesner considers that in Germany Roesslin's *Rosengarten* would be widely known amongst midwives. M.E. Wiesner, 'Early modern midwifery: a case study', in B. A. Hanawalt (ed.) *Women and Work in Pre-Industrial Europe* (Bloomington, IN, 1985), 94–103, esp. p.100. See also ch. 10 in this volume by Hilary Marland for the use of midwifery texts by Dutch midwives.

39. M.E. Muñoz, *Recopilación de las leyes, pragmáticas reales, decretos y acuerdos del Real Protomedicato. Hecha por encargo del mismo Real Tribunal* (Valencia, 1751), 107; *Novísima Recopilación de las leyes de España* (Madrid, 1805–7), libro VIII, tit. X, ley I.

40. Muñoz, *Recopilación de las leyes*, 109–10; *Novísima Recopilación*, libro VIII, tit. X, ley II. This is quoted by many authors, amongst them Navas, *Elementos del Arte de Partear*, vol. 1, lxxxviii–ix and Muñoz Garrido, *Ejercicio*, 69–70.

41. Muñoz, *Recopilación de las leyes*, 314–16, referring to the Kingdom of Valencia; Navas, *Elementos del Arte de Partear*, vol. 1, lxxxix, to the Kingdoms of Seville, Aragon, Valencia, Navarre and the Principality of Catalonia.

42. AMM, Escribanías de Cabildo, legajo 2, ff. 458v–459, 15 May 1537. (Information supplied by Maite López Beltrán from her article cited in note 19.)

43. Navas, *Elementos del Arte de Partear*, vol. 1, xci–xcii. See also J. Blasco Ijazo, *Historia del Colegio de Médicos de la provincia de Zaragoza, 1455–1961* (n.p., 1961), 21.

44. In the first quarter of the century, the laws of Navarre stated that midwives wishing to practise had to be examined by the municipal physician and the parish priest, the latter being responsible for their moral rectitude. J. Ramos Martínez, *La salud pública y el Hospital General de la ciudad de Pamplona en el Antiguo Régimen (1700–1815)* (Pamplona, 1989), 309. For the intervention of priests in the appointment of midwives in eighteenth-century Italy, see ch. 8 in this volume by Nadia Filippini.

45. Villas Tinoco, 'La mujer', 100–1.

46. Muñoz, *Recopilación de las leyes*, 309–14; *Novísima Recopilación*, libro VIII, tit. X, ley X.

47. A. Medina, *Cartilla nueva, útil y necesaria para instruirse las matronas, que vulgarmente se llaman comadres, en el oficio de partear* (Madrid, 1750).

48. It seems that by the eighteenth century more women could read and write. The acquisition of these skills was dependent on their geographical base and social background. Literacy levels were much higher amongst men. See A. Viñao Frago, 'Alfabetización e Ilustración: Difusión y usos de la cultura escrita', *Revista de Educación* (1988), special no., 298.

49. A. Domínguez Ortiz, *Carlos III y la España de la Ilustración* (Madrid, 1988), ch. 7, 'La enseñanza. La cultura', 161–86; M. Vico Monteoliva, 'Utopía, educación e Ilustración en España', *Revista de Educación* (1988), special no., 483–4.

50. See A. Lafuente, J. Puerto Sarmiento and M.C. Calleja Folguera, 'Los profesionales de la Sanidad tras su identidad en la Ilustración española', in J.M. Sánchez Ron (ed.) *Ciencia y sociedad en España: de la Ilustración a la Guerra Civil* (Madrid, 1988), 71–92; M.E. Burke, *The Royal College of San Carlos* (Durham, NC, 1977).

51. J. Puerto Sarmiento, 'La profesión farmacéutica: del gremialismo al corporativismo', in J.L. Peset (ed.) *La ciencia moderna y el nuevo mundo* (Madrid, 1985), 395–421; M.C. Calleja Folguera, *La reforma sanitaria en la España ilustrada* (Madrid, 1988).

52. C. Sanz Egaña, *Historia de la Veterinaria Española* (Madrid, 1941).

53. This is a hypothesis which is being developed together with Alvaro Martínez Vidal in a forthcoming study of relationships between priests, surgeons, midwives and the art of midwifery in early modern Spain. See ch. 8 in this volume for a comparison with eighteenth-century Italy.

54. C. Undabeitia Lajusticia, 'Empresas sanitarias en la Bascongada. Preparación de las matronas', *Actas del Primer Congreso de la Sociedad Vasca de Historia de la Medicina, Bilbao, 1985* (Bilbao, 1985), 205–9.

55. A. Hermosilla, *Cien años de medicina sevillana* (Sevilla, 1970), 234–5.

56. M.V. López-Cordón, 'La situación de la mujer a finales del Antiguo Régimen (1760–1860)', in R. Capel (ed.) *Mujer y sociedad en España. 1700–1975* (Madrid, 1982), 93–5.

57. *Real Cédula de S.M. y Señores del Consejo, en que se aprueban y mandan observar las ordenanzas formadas . . . para el Colegio de Cirugía establecido en Madrid . . .* (Madrid, 1787), 28.

58. *Ordenanzas de S.M. que deben observarse por el Real Colegio de Cirugía de Barcelona . . .* (Madrid, 1795), 153–4, 231.

59. *Real Cédula*, 29; *Ordenanzas de S.M.*, 159.

60. *Real Cédula*, 28–9; *Ordenanzas de S.M.*, 155–6.

61. B. de Gárate y Casabona, *Libro nuevo cuyo título: Nuevo y natural modo de auxiliar a las mugeres en los lances de los partos . . .* (Pamplona, 1756), 156. The subject of baptism will be dealt with in the research project cited in note 53. For midwives

and baptism in early modern Germany and eighteenth-century Italy, see chs 4 and 8 in this volume by Merry Wiesner and Nadia Filippini.

62. For requirements for midwives, see Archivo General de Simancas (hereafter AGS), legajo 1544, Sección Guerra Moderna, 1763; *Estatutos y Ordenanzas que S.M. manda observar a los Colegios y Comunidades de Cirujanos establecidos en Barcelona, Cádiz . . .* (Barcelona, 1764), tit. XII; *Novísima Recopilación*, libro VIII, tit. X, ley XI, cap. 9.

63. J. Varela, 'La educación ilustrada o cómo crear sujetos dóciles y útiles', *Revista de Educación* (1988), special no., 245–74.

64. *Ordenanzas de S.M.*, 156–7. The same terms appeared in the licence issued by the *Protomedicato* and in books written for midwives in the eighteenth century.

65. We know, however, of one woman 'surgeon' who practised at this time. She was French and devoted herself to ophthalmology and was not trained in any of the Spanish colleges of surgery. P. de Demerson, 'Una mujer cirujano en tiempos de Carlos III', *Anales del Instituto de Estudios Madrileños*, 9 (1973), 415–26.

66. Burke, *The Royal College*, 80.

67. M. López Ortega, 'La educación de la mujer en la Ilustración española', *Revista de Educación* (1988), special no., 324; López-Cordón, 'La situación de la mujer', 93.

68. *Novísima Recopilación*, libro VIII, tit. X, ley X, cap. 3.

69. In 1773 Isabel Cortés, midwife of Archidona (Málaga) prescribed and administered medicines to sterile women and those who had recently given birth, and was consequently denounced by the town physicians and banned from repeating such activities. Conejo Ramilo, 'Los cirujanos y las matronas', 129. Around the same time Luisa Rosado was applying poultices to expel the placenta (see the following section).

70. As was the case with María Pirizié, a French midwife who practised in La Luisiana (Seville) in the second half of the century. P. de Demerson, 'La cesárea postmortem en la España de la Ilustración', *Asclepio*, 28 (1976), 207–8.

71. Muñoz, *Recopilación de las leyes*, 310; Medina, *Cartilla nueva*, 21–2. For the midwife as expert witness in England and Germany, see chs 2, 3 and 4 in this volume by David Harley, Ann Giardina Hess and Merry Wiesner.

72. The 1795 ordinances of Barcelona College envisaged midwives performing these functions when an expert surgeon was not available. *Ordenanzas de S.M.*, 157.

73. Navas, *Elementos del Arte de Partear*, vol. 1, III.

74. Ibid., II.

75. The first figure is given by Burke, *The Royal College*, 99. The second is from E. Salcedo y Ginestal, *Obras de Don Antonio de Gimbernat* (Madrid, 1926), vol. 1, 257.

76. Burke, *The Royal College*, 99.

77. Salcedo y Ginestal, *Obras de Don Antonio de Gimbernat*, 257.

78. On account of this, the sum of money midwives had to pay to obtain their licence from the *Protomedicato* was reduced from the proposed 500 *reales de vellón* to 100, and was free for poor midwives. AGS, Sección Guerra Moderna, legajo 1543, 27 March 1760. Information supplied by Mikel Astrain, from 'La medicina del mar. Sanitarios y Sanidad Naval al servicio del Rey: De Utrecht a Trafalgar, *c.* 1712–1805', unpub. PhD thesis, University of Granada, 1992.

79. The information on Córdoba is from A. López Ontiveros, *Córdoba 1752 según las Respuestas Generales del Catastro de Ensenada* (Madrid, 1990), 175–9, 233, that on the Kingdom of Granada from T. Ortiz, C. Quesada and M. Astrain, 'Las profesiones sanitarias en el Reino de Granada según el Catastro de Ensenada (1751–1754)', Granada, unpub. paper, Diputación Provincial, 1990, 131.

80. According to the analysis of the sixty-five observations included in Ventura Pastor, *Preceptos generales*, vols 1–2, 77 per cent of deliveries were attended in the first instance by midwives.

81. C. Rubio Pardos, 'La calle de Atocha', *Anales del Instituto de Estudios Madrileños*, 9 (1973), 96; J. Soubeyroux, 'El encuentro del pobre y la sociedad: asistencia y represión en el Madrid del S. XVIII', *Estudios de Historia Social*, 20–21 (1982), 21, 46.

82. Archivo Histórico Nacional, legajo 51444, Sección Archivo Antiguo del Consejo de Castilla, quoted by Domínguez Ortiz, 'La Galera o cárcel de mujeres de Madrid a comienzos del S. XVIII', *Anales del Instituto de Estudios Madrileños*, 9 (1973), 278. See also Soubeyroux, 'El encuentro del pobre y la sociedad', 90.

83. We have data on the marital status of only seven midwives: five were widows, one was married and one single. Ramos Martínez, *La salud pública*, 80, 306–7.

84. AGS, Sección Gracia y Justicia, leg. 989, ff. 687–708. Many of these documents have been reproduced, with an introductory study, in T. Ortiz, 'Luisa Rosado, una matrona en la España de la Ilustración', *Dynamis*, 12 (1992), 323–47.

85. Rubio Pardos, 'La calle de Atocha', 96–7.

86. AGS, Sección Gracia y Justicia, leg. 989, f. 695.

87. AGS, Sección Gracia y Justicia, leg. 989, f. 689.

88. AGS, Sección Gracia y Justicia, leg. 989, f. 694.

89. AGS, Sección Gracia y Justicia, leg. 989, f. 703.

90. AGS, Sección Gracia y Justicia, leg. 989, f. 687.

91. AGS, Sección Gracia y Justicia, leg. 989, ff. 687, 704, 705.

92. Medina, *Cartilla nueva*.

93. Gáratea, *Libro nuevo cuyo título: Nuevo y natural modo de auxiliar a las mugeres en los lances peligrosos de los partos . . .* (Pamplona, 1756).

94. AGS, Sección Gracia y Justicia, leg. 989, ff. 687, 688, 702.

95. A. Lafuente and J.L. Peset, 'Las actividades e instituciones científicas en la España ilustrada', in M. Sellés, J.L. Peset and A. Lafuente (eds) *Carlos III y la ciencia de la Ilustración* (Madrid, 1988), 53.

96. AGS, Sección Gracia y Justicia, leg. 989, ff. 701–2.

97. AGS, Sección Gracia y Justicia, leg. 989, f. 693.

98. AGS, Sección Gracia y Justicia, leg. 989, ff. 687–687v, 701.

99. M. Martínez, *Anatomía completa del hombre* (Madrid, 1728), 184–5. (Information supplied by Alvaro Martínez Vidal.)

100. J.B. Matoni, 'De los estragos que causan las secundinas retenidas, y sus respectivos auxilios, leída en la Regia Sociedad de Sevilla . . . en 10 de marzo año de 1780', 1780, MS; P. Vidart, *El discípulo instruido en el Arte de Partear* (Madrid, 1785), 52–4. These are the only works where references have been found to the pathology of the retention of the afterbirth.

101. AGS, Sección Gracia y Justicia, leg. 989, f. 701, junio de 1771.

102. M. Laget, 'La naissance aux siècles classiques. Pratique des accouchements et attitudes collectives en France aux XVIIème et XVIIIème siècles', *Annales E.S.C.*, 32 (1977), 970, makes an exhaustive analysis of this author's observations and the figure provided has been calculated from her information. Laget studies 594 observations, of which 358 are miscarriages and the rest (236) complicated deliveries. Twenty-five of these were due to the retention of the afterbirth.

103. Ventura Pastor, *Preceptos generales*, vols 1–2. He cites forty-nine cases of complicated deliveries out of a total of sixty-five observations.

104. D.M. Zapata, *Dissertación médico-theológica* (Madrid, 1733), 78. Zapata attributed this to rough handling by midwives. F. Perena, *Conclusiones breves y claras*

teológico-médico-legales contra la disertación . . . que dió a luz Diego Mateo Zapata (Madrid, 1733), however, believed that the problem lay not in rough, but in inexpert, handling.

105. See P. Petit, *Cuestiones generales sobre el modo de partear y cuidar a las mujeres que están embarazadas o paridas* (Madrid, 1717), 30–2, 65–7; Zapata, *Dissertación médico-theológica*, 78, 89–90; Medina, *Cartilla nueva*, 66–8; Gárate, *Libro nuevo cuyo título*, 93, 130–3; J. Raulin, *Instrucciones sucintas sobre los partos, para la utilidad de las comadres* (Zaragoza, 1772), 54–5; F. Mauriçeau, 'Aforismos', in A. Levret, *Tratado de partos* . . . (Madrid, 1778), vol. 2, 349; Matoni, 'De los estragos'; *idem*, 'De las precauciones que exige la operación de extraer las secundinas después del parto', *Memorias Académicas de la Real Sociedad de Medicina y demás Ciencias de Sevilla*, 3 (1785), 1–19; Navas, *Elementos del Arte de Partear*, 145–6; Ventura Pastor, *Preceptos generales*, vol. 1, 211–17; Vidart, *El discípulo instruido en el Arte de Partear*, 52–5.

106. Medina, *Cartilla nueva*, 66–8; Gárate, *Libro nuevo cuyo título*, 93–6. Gárate claims (p. 133) to know of the case of a woman who did not expel the placenta for eight years, remaining healthy during the whole period.

107. AGS, Sección Gracia y Justicia, leg. 989, f. 704.

108. AGS, Sección Gracia y Justicia, leg. 989, f. 687.

109. AGS, Sección Gracia y Justicia, leg. 989, f. 705. The two other cases are on f. 690v.

110. AGS, Sección Gracia y Justicia, leg. 989, f. 690v. This is the testimony of a physician from Zamora, certifying this and other interventions by Luisa Rosado.

111. Ventura Pastor, *Preceptos generales*, vol. 1, 318–19. An observation of a case is to be found on p. 385.

112. Vidart, *El discípulo instruido en el Arte de Partear*, 132.

113. The Latin names are '*Plantago Major L.*' and '*Solanum Nigrum L.*' respectively. P. Font Quer, *Plantas medicinales. El Dioscórides renovado* (Barcelona, 1973), 583–5, 724–5.

114. Ventura Pastor, *Preceptos generales*, vol. 1, 385.

6

The politick midwife: models of midwifery in the work of Elizabeth Cellier

Helen King

Elizabeth Cellier lived and worked in London, in the latter years of her practice during the 1670s and 1680s in the parish of St Clement Danes. There are enormous difficulties in studying her life and work; her interests and publications straddle the two fields of midwifery and politics, but the evidence is almost entirely centred on two periods of political unrest. In the first, 1678–81, the Popish Plot and its aftermath, her role was primarily political; in the second, 1687–88, in the months before the Glorious Revolution, she issued detailed proposals for a college of midwifery. For each period, allegations have been made that she was not responsible for the ideas which circulated under her name: contemporaries claimed that the astrologer Gadbury, or unnamed Jesuits, wrote her political broadsheets, while it has been suggested that the prime mover behind the college of midwives was one of the Chamberlen family of obstetricians, who used Cellier as a front because midwives would only unite behind another midwife.[1]

The most recent writer on Cellier, Margaret George, sets her in the context of 'the new, seventeenth century female self-conscious self-involvement' and labels her as 'Cellier the professional';[2] yet, despite the attempts of midwifery historians,[3] we know almost nothing about her professional practice. I propose here to use her work – and the many pamphlets denouncing her alleged political activities – primarily as a source for illuminating enduring positive and negative images of the midwife. I would further argue that the separation of her roles into first plotter, then midwife, is misleading. She was, as her contemporaries called her, the Popish Midwife; her Catholicism and her midwifery are deeply linked.

In her own words, Cellier was 'born and brought up under Protestant Parents', but converted to Catholicism after seeing her parents persecuted for their loyalty to the king (EC6:1).[4] Her second marriage was to the French Catholic merchant Peter Cellier.[5] Elizabeth Cellier is first heard of in the context of the Popish Plot of 1678 and the Meal Tub Plot of 1679; in the latter, it was in her meal tub that the incriminating lists of plotters and meeting places were found on 26 October.[6] To quote Ronald Hutton, 'It has been said that history is played out once as tragedy and once as farce. If so, the "Popish Plot" of 1678 was certainly the former and the "Meal Tub Plot" of 1679 as clearly the latter.'[7] The context of these so-called plots is well known. After the conversion to Roman Catholicism of the then heir to the throne, James, became known in 1673, rumours grew of a plot, led by the Jesuits but also involving the French and the Irish, in which the King – Charles II – and the Protestants in London would be murdered and popery in England restored. In 1678 the notorious liar Titus Oates 'revealed' just such a plot to Sir Edmund Berry Godfrey, a justice of the peace. On 17 October 1678, Godfrey was found dead: 'the case remains utterly mysterious'[8] since Godfrey appears to have been both hanged and run through with a sword (EC3). Was it suicide dressed up as murder, or murder ineptly disguised as suicide (EC10)? It was generally – conveniently – assumed that he had been killed by Catholics but, in view of the boost given by the murder to the credibility of Oates's conspiracy claims, it is possible that Oates was himself involved.[9] Further information given led to the imprisonment of five Catholic lords and the execution of a number of Jesuits and Catholic laymen.

Oates's stories of a 'Popish Plot' were believed because people wanted to believe them; they resonated with powerful underlying fears.[10] It may be something of this climate which lies behind two references to Cellier in the London Sessions Records for 10 April 1678. On 27 March recognizances – promises to keep the peace – were taken from John Atterbury, Thomas Rogers and George Sturman to the effect that Susanna Atterbury should appear at the Sessions of the Peace to be held on 8 April. This relates to an incident on 26 March in the parish of St Martin Ludgate, in which it was alleged that John Atterbury and his wife Susanna, with John, Sara and Elizabeth Atterbury, presumably their children:

> did assemble and congregate riotously, routously and unlawfully to the disturbance of the King's peace, and, being then and there assembled, did assault, strike, wound and maltreat one Elizabeth Cellier, the wife of Peter Cellier, so that it was despaired of her life, to the grave injury of the same Elizabeth Cellier.[11]

All pleaded not guilty, but John senior and his wife were found guilty of assault – but not of riot – and each fined 20s.

Cellier first became involved in the 'plots', on her own account, as a charitable visitor to the Catholics in Newgate in January 1679 (EC6:3). According to the Earl of Peterborough, however, she was acting as the agent of the Countess of Powis, whose husband was one of the five Catholic lords: 'an ingenious woman', Cellier 'from the Calling of a Midwife had opportunity of frequenting domestically many considerable Families'.[12] On one of her visits Cellier says that she heard someone crying out in pain; the turnkey said it was a woman in labour, Cellier offered her assistance, but was then told that it was a Catholic being tortured. Her main informant was Thomas Willoughby, real name Dangerfield, who also claimed that the Popish Plot had been dreamed up by a Presbyterian group led by the Earl of Shaftesbury (EC4).[13] Delighted by anything which could end the accusations against the Catholics, Cellier paid Dangerfield's fines and proceeded to support him while he gathered further information to support his claims; such information was concealed in Cellier's meal tub, where it was found by the Middlesex justice after Dangerfield turned against his patron.

London, at this time 'self-consciously the major Protestant city in Europe',[14] had a significant Catholic population who attended mass at the royal chapels and 'at those of the French, Spanish, Portuguese, Venetian and (later) Florentine representatives';[15] the main fear was, however, not so much of local Catholics as of 'foreigners'.[16] Cellier, a Catholic married to a Frenchman, was thus in the wrong place at the wrong time. On 11 June 1680 she was tried for treason, but acquitted (EC1); on her release from custody she published 'Malice Defeated' (EC6), in which she made a number of allegations against the State, in particular claiming that the Catholics in Newgate were being tortured. At a second trial at the Old Bailey on 11 September she was found guilty of libel and sentenced to pay a fine of £1,000, with one year in jail and three sessions in the pillory, some of her pamphlets to be burned on each occasion (EC2).

She is certainly one of the most colourful figures in the two so-called plots. Not only the many broadsheets published in 1680 and 1681 attacking her, but also her own speeches and publications, relish the potential of her dual role as midwife and alleged Catholic conspirator. Her opponents play with her identity as a Catholic and a woman. A pamphlet of 1680 circulated under Cellier's name by her enemies claims that she intends to bring Britain under 'the power of the Tripple Crown' with herself as 'Archbishopess of this *Island*' (EC3). In 'The Scarlet Beast Stripped Naked' she is presented as the second Pope Joan who 'dropped her untimely Bastard in Procession to *Angello*' (EC4). She is also represented as hoping to be made Saint Cellier so that she will be able to sell pieces of the pillory in which she was placed as holy relics (EC8), and comforts her printer by telling him he too will be canonised 'when we have a *Romish Successor*' (EC9).

But, even more than a woman, she is a midwife. This provides far greater scope for attackers, with Cellier presented as saying, 'I must be my own Midwife and deliver myself of this damned plot' (EC8) and a reference in the Calendar of State Papers for 23 July 1681 to pamphlets 'begot ... by ... two convict priests now in Newgate, and midwived into the world by the assistance of their fellow prisoner, the infamous Mrs Cellier'.[17] The account of her trial at the Old Bailey for printing 'Malice Defeated' includes a description of how she distributed it to many booksellers, telling each 'that he had the *Maiden-head* on't, and was the first Man she ever offer'd it to' (EC3). In his reply to 'Malice Defeated', Dangerfield savages Cellier's reputation, attributing to her numerous love affairs, including one with a Negro servant and another with a Spaniard whom she instructed in 'the School of *Venus*, &c.'. Dangerfield draws on the image of midwife as drunken gossip using her knowledge of female anatomy to satisfy women's lusts, accusing Cellier of making money 'with the help of her moving hand'.[18] A verse attack on Cellier from the same year includes the lines,

> You're skill'd, what Natures Fabrick is below,
> And all the secret Arts of Gropeing know,
> Sexes defect with *D-do* can supply . . . (EC7)

However, these allegations should be read beside the medical theories of the period: following a practice dating back to the Hippocratics, but best known through the work of Galen, it was believed that women as well as men produced a seed which needed to be expelled regularly.[19] Galen described the application by a midwife of 'the customary remedies' to the vulva of a woman with retained seed. It is in this tradition that seventeenth-century medical works such as Riverius's *The Practice of Physick* advise marriage as a cure for conditions involving intense sexual desire, but add that, in circumstances in which this advice cannot be put into practice, 'the Genital Parts should be by a cunning Midwife so handled and rubbed, as to cause an Evacuation of the over-abounding Sperm'.[20]

Another attack on Cellier's political involvement is represented as coming from Mother Creswell, 'the most noted bawd of the Restoration'.[21] Before inviting her round to share 'a Bottle of Rhenish or two' 'Lady Creswell' addresses Cellier as 'Dear daughter' and refers to the suspicious timing of midwives' work, saying to Cellier, 'our Concerns are most in the Night-watches' (EC5). The allegation that midwives drink heavily is found elsewhere in accusations against Cellier (for example, the postscript to EC9), but should not be taken seriously. Manuals such as Poeton's *The Midwives Deputie*[22] advise the deputy to avoid 'wine or strong drink', while Doreen Evenden's recent thesis demonstrates conclusively that 'London midwives in the Tudor–Stuart period were not incompetent and poor. Midwives were highly skilled and thoroughly experienced through their participation in a system of unofficial apprenticeship.'[23] Evenden argues that it is only the many centuries of bias in favour of male professionals which have led to the labelling of midwives in this period 'as generally incompetent illiterates';[24] much the same could be said about accusations of drunkenness.[25]

Cellier is also accused of consorting with the astrologer John Gadbury, and indeed with the Devil (EC1). As I have already mentioned, other pamphlets alleged that Gadbury wrote many of the works which appeared under her name[26] or blame the Catholic priests with whom she was associated, calling her 'our Wonderful witty thing of a Mid-Wife, or a priest got into her Belly, and so speaking through her' (EC4). Mention of the Devil recalls the image of the midwife-witch, best known from the work of Thomas Forbes.[27] David Harley has recently re-examined the sixteenth- and seventeenth-century sources on witchcraft and has shown that, far from being accused of witchcraft, midwives were more likely to appear in the role of expert witness, using their knowledge of the normal female anatomy in order to detect witches' marks.[28]

Midwife as drunken bawd, user of incantations, consort of the Devil himself; such allegations take on a new life when applied to the Popish midwife, as negative images of the midwife meet violent anti-Catholicism. Yet it is the victim of such slanders, Elizabeth Cellier, who is credited with a scheme for a college of midwives published in 1687 (EC11), the very existence of such a scheme having been taken as further evidence to support the general validity of the 'ignorant midwife' model. There are hints that Cellier's intentions were already known – and were a further cause of amusement to her enemies – in 1680. A pamphlet of that date circulated under her name is signed, 'From our Colledge this last of *May*, &c.' (EC3). The postscript to a broadsheet of 1681 links the college back to the image of the drunken midwife: 'The *Muses* of our *Colledge* being got Tipsy in Drinking the old HEALTH . . . ' (EC9).

After 1681 no more is heard of Cellier until 1687 apart from a cryptic reference in a letter from the Earl of Rochester to the Marquess of Ormonde on 4 September 1684: 'What your Grace hath sent me, concerning Mrs Cellier's piety, I know no use that is to be made of it, but as of news, when I hear anything of it from other hands, that you had sent me.'[29] However, the accession of James II in 1685 meant that England had a Catholic monarch, and the focus of Protestant unease moved even more to the question of the succession. James's marriage to Mary of Modena in 1674 had produced four babies – all of whom died – and four miscarriages. It is then appropriate that the Popish Midwife makes her comeback during 1687, the year in which Mary of Modena was confirmed as yet again pregnant. It was also in 1687 that the College of Physicians gained from James II the right to license the printing and publishing of books on physic and surgery, together with the right to suppress 'Illiterate and illegal practitioners of the art of physic' in London and for 7 miles outside it. In November of the same year the College wrote to all bishops announcing that it would henceforth be censoring all books on physic.[30]

The Treasury Papers record, on 10 May 1687, the king's mercy to Elizabeth Cellier in regard to the sentence imposed on her in 1680.[31] In the following month Cellier published her proposals for a college of midwives

(EC11). In November Mary of Modena was confirmed as two months pregnant, and a newsletter of 26 November alleged that Cellier's proposals had been approved.[32] I have been unable to find any other evidence for this, but Cellier herself claimed that James had agreed in September 'to unite the Midwives into a Corporation, by His Royal Charter, and also to found a *Cradle-Hospital*, to breed up exposed Children' (EC12). In January 1688 'A day of thanksgiveing upon the occasion of the queens being with child'[33] was proclaimed, and on 16 January Cellier published 'To Dr . . . an Answer to his Queries, concerning the Colledg of Midwives' (EC12).

Unsuccessful attempts to form the City of London midwives into a corporation had been initiated by members of the Huguenot Chamberlen family in 1616 and 1634.[34] It was in their interests to present the London midwives as untrained, ignorant and downright dangerous, and they asked that training be improved through anatomy lectures and other instruction to increase their skill. Cellier proposed a corporation of 2,000 midwives 'practising within the limits of the weekly Bills of Mortality', the first thousand paying £5 admittance plus £5 per annum, the second thousand 50s. From this money and from charitable donations a Hospital would be founded 'under a Governess, a female Secretary and twelve Matron-assistants' to protect and educate foundlings. It was to have 'twelve lesser Houses in the greatest Parishes' 'where any woman can be taken in', delivered of her child – who would be sent to the main hospital – and given one month's maintenance. These lying-in houses would of course give scope for practical midwifery instruction.[35] In addition, lectures and discourses were to be given to the midwives – by a man. On lecture days, 'once a Month at least', all midwives would assemble to hear the 'principal Physician, or Man-Midwife' and to report any 'extraordinary occurrents' in their practice to the Governess. Copies of the lectures would be sold, but any licensed midwife could read them at the College. Apart from the Physician, 'no men shall be present at such publick Lectures, on any Pretence whatsoever, except such able Doctors and Surgeons, as shall enter themselves students in the said Art', paying £10 admittance and £10 per annum. From these enrolled males the Governess, Secretary, twelve Matrons and twenty-four assistants would choose the principal Physician by ballot, 'the Governess three Balls and the Secretary two Balls' (EC11).

What was the significance of these proposals? The Governess clearly has a central role; thus Spencer sees the scheme as 'a monopoly intended mainly for [Cellier's] own benefit'.[36] Yet Cellier's own principal interest, as expressed in the 1688 pamphlet defending her scheme, seems to lie with the Foundling Hospital side; 'to prevent the *Many Murders, and the Executions which attend them* . . . so many *Innocents* as would otherwise be lost' (EC12). The Physician also has a key role, perhaps supporting the suggestion that a Chamberlen lay behind these proposals. The most likely member of the family must be Hugh senior, who in 1687–88 lived in the same parish – St Clement Danes – as Cellier.[37] In March 1688 he was in trouble with the College of Physicians for practising physic without a licence, some of his patients having died; in 1689 he went on to propose his own scheme for a 'New Establishment of Physick' with seven colleges encompassing physicians, surgeons and apothecaries.[38]

In terms of midwifery education, how would the system proposed by Cellier differ from what was in existence? In the seventeenth century there was 'usually little formal instruction' for midwives,[39] but this does not mean that there was little knowledge. Wilson suggests that most midwives in this period 'set up practice on the basis of having seen some deliveries in the capacity of gossips and probably buying a "midwife's book" for elementary instruction'.[40] Such books, despite their use of the vernacular, their prefaces defending the revelation of women's 'secrets' and their imagined audience of literate women reading the book to their illiterate sisters, only combine antiquarianism, irrelevance, salaciousness and the blindingly obvious. Much of the material tells us very little about practical midwifery[41] and far more about 'the nature of medieval male curiosity about women's sexuality'.[42] Indeed, some writers of this period suggest that books in the hands of the otherwise untrained are positively dangerous; in particular, Percival Willughby's *Observations in Midwifery*, written around 1670, compares the woman who trusts a young midwife who 'hath read a little in a midwife's book' to 'an unadvised passenger, that will hazard his safety with a Pilot, that never went a sea voiage, but, by reading of bookes, or crossing the Thames, or some small river, makes himself a Pilot'. Such young midwives use their books merely to impress their clients, by showing them the pictures.[43]

In this situation, Willughby recommended the 7-year apprenticeship system which he attributed to the London midwives.[44] Pelling has argued that the history of medical education has in general paid insufficient attention to apprenticeship.[45] Even outside the formal system, women were trained as a deputy to an experienced midwife, sometimes a family member;[46] 'divers do practise without Licence, and some are Deputies to others'.[47] Doreen Evenden has recently analysed over five hundred testimonials from senior midwives, fellow deputies and satisfied clients presented by London midwives to Church officials in order to obtain a licence between 1661 and 1700. These show that a period well in excess of seven years was often served, under highly skilled midwives; matriarchal ties existed between two or three generations of midwives, and information and advice passed rapidly through the networks thus created.[48]

In place of this traditional and highly effective women's network, Cellier's proposals would set up a hierarchy headed by the Governess, to whom 'extraordinary occurrents' were to be reported. Was Cellier's problem that, as a Catholic, she was largely excluded from the unofficial midwives' networks? Unfortunately we do not know whether her own training was based on the deputy system or on books, except that she clearly had access to a copy of Guillemeau's *Child-Birth*. However, as a Catholic midwife, it could be argued that her status was reduced after 1662, when the Act of Uniformity returned the right to license midwives to the Church of England. Before 1643, since a midwife could baptize *in extremis*, the Church took a central role in the regulation of the profession.[49] According to Cellier, between 1643 and 1660, as a result of the abolition of the hierarchy, midwives were no longer licensed by the Bishops, but were instead controlled by the Company of Barber-Surgeons. The archives of the Barber-Surgeons do not support this claim.[50] Guy argues that, in London at least, during these two decades 'The emphasis dramatically shifted from moral virtue and ecclesiastical function to professional competence'.[51] This claim has been challenged by Evenden, who demonstrates that ecclesiastical licensing took competence as well as good character into account, while its costs in money, time and energy deterred women from applying unless they were serious practitioners.[52] There is no evidence that Cellier was ever licensed,[53] but she would in theory have been able to obtain a licence until 1662. This is not to say that she would not have practised, since Church licensing was not always rigidly enforced[54] and even records of presentments for practising without a licence in this period show that, while some women were excommunicated or fined, others were given the licence after being duly sworn.[55] However, the oaths taken by midwives emphasize the importance of performing baptism into the Church of England. The form of the oath given in the *The Midwives Deputie* specifies 'That you shall not be privy or consent that any popish priest or other party shall in your absence or in your company or of your knowledge or sufferance baptize any child by any Mass, Latin service, or prayers, other than those appointed by the Laws of the Church of England'.[56] Most versions of this oath merely say 'any priest'; the form 'any popish priest' is noteworthy. However, rather than suggesting that a personal grudge against ecclesiastical licensing lay behind Cellier's proposals, I would argue for a deeper sense of exclusion from midwives' networks; if Cellier only worked with the Catholic community in London, a licence based on an oath to baptize babies into the Church of England would have been a positive hindrance.[57]

In her 1688 pamphlet, 'To Dr . . . an Answer to his Queries, concerning the Colledg of Midwives', Cellier argues for the antiquity of professional, collegiate, teaching organizations of midwives over those of physicians. This theme also surfaces in Cellier's political involvement of 1679–81, where 'Lady Creswell' urged her to confine her interests to midwifery, since 'You have an honest calling, and though I say it, a very ancient one, and was of great esteem in all Ages of the World' (EC5). In 1688 Cellier claims that Shiprah and Puah in Exodus 1: 15–16 and 20–21 were 'the Governesses and Teachers of other Midwives' (EC12).

But in this pamphlet Cellier goes much further than in her published proposals for a College and Foundling Hospital, arguing that midwives used to practise all branches of physic for women. She says that there were colleges of female physicians in pre-Roman Britain in the time of the Druids, and that in London there were colleges of women centred on a temple of Diana. In order to prove her thesis about the antiquity, not just of midwifery, but of the collegiate organization of midwifery, Cellier uses a number of passages taken from Guillemeau's *Child-Birth, or the Happy Deliverie of Women* (1612). This is an interesting choice of source, in view of one of the few pieces of evidence for the books used by – as opposed to written for – midwives in this period, Edward Poeton's *The Midwives Deputie,* which dates from the 1660s or 1670s. When the midwife in this manuscript asks what books her deputy has read, the answer is *The Byrth of Mankynde* – a translation of the *Rosengarten,* which ran into ten editions between 1504 and 1604, becoming 'the standard work' on childbirth[58] – and Guillemeau. Having read these two, the deputy is described as being 'well furnished, if you understand what you have read, and remember what you understand'.[59]

The central story which Cellier takes from Guillemeau[60] is that of the first midwife, Agnodike. The Latin mythographer Hyginus, who preserves variants of myths which do not survive elsewhere, tells her story in a section headed 'Who discovered/invented what'. He claims that women in classical Athens were forbidden to study medicine, but Agnodike bypassed the ban by cutting her hair, donning male apparel and becoming the student of Herophilus. She then practised as a man, until one day when she heard of a woman 'that had long languish'd under private Diseases' (EC12). When Agnodike offered her help, the woman declined assistance from any man. In reply Agnodike lifted her clothes, revealing herself to be a woman. The male doctors, finding their clientele dwindling, accused Agnodike of seducing her patients, and the women of feigning illness in order to enjoy the young doctor's attentions. Brought before the courts to defend herself, once more Agnodike lifted her clothes to expose her true sex. This only led to the charge being altered from seduction of patients to breaking the law forbidding women from studying medicine; for Cellier, does this echo the events of 1680, when she was tried first for treason and then for libel? Agnodike's women supporters then arrived and told the assembled men, in the words of Hyginus, 'You are not husbands but enemies, for you condemn she who discovered health for us.' The Athenians then are supposed to have changed the law to permit freeborn women to study medicine.

In an earlier article[61] I discussed the popularity of this thoroughly unreliable account in the history of medicine, in which Agnodike has been seen variously as the first midwife, as a midwife fighting to recover the ancestral rights of her sex or as a precedent for women in medicine in general. For Cellier, Agnodike supplies not only a historical precedent of a midwife fighting for her professional rights, but also a personal role model who makes sense of her own earlier experiences. As I have indicated, in some instances Agnodike's story resonates with Cellier's own life: for example, the two trials. At other points in the story, Cellier embellishes Guillemeau's version to make it more relevant to her. Thus she attributes the passage of a law that 'no Woman should study or practise any part of Physick on pain of Death' to 'some Physicians being gotten into the Government' – a reference to the power of the College of Physicians? – and to 'Miscarriages happening to some Noble Women about that time' – recalling the reproductive history of Mary of Modena. She adds an additional named character, 'Agisilea one of the Areopagites wives', with whom it is alleged that Agnodike committed adultery; this may relate to the attacks on Cellier's own moral character made by Dangerfield. A particularly transparent case of rewriting the myth occurs in her description of Agnodike's first trial, where Cellier notes '*there being Witnesses to be found then* (as of late Years, that would swear any thing for Money)'; at Cellier's trial in June 1680, the jurors who acquitted her demanded payment, which she refused, while at the September trial some of her defence witnesses changed their stories or never appeared (EC2).

Cellier also attacks the book-learning of doctors as opposed to the practical experience of midwives. She describes the 'Women of this Age, who are so sensible and impatient of their Pain, that few of them will be prevailed upon to bear it, in Complement to the Doctor, *while he fetches his Book, studies the Case, and teaches the Midwife to perform her work*'; this is, Cellier says, like Phormio 'who having never seen a Battel in his Life, read a Military Lecture to *Hannibal* the *Great*'.[62] This is a common response of threatened midwives; compare not only Jane Sharp's 'it is not hard words which perform the act',[63] but also the petition of the London midwives in 1634 stating that Peter Chamberlen cannot teach midwifery 'because he hath no experience in itt but by reading'.[64]

What is going on here? Why Cellier's insistence that midwifery 'ought to be kept as a Secret amongst Women as much as is possible' and her scorn for men 'pretending to teach us midwifery', when the 1687 scheme envisaged the replacement of female networks with a hierarchy, and a man-midwife as Director? If the scheme was indeed the work of a physician seeking to control midwives, is 'To Dr . . . ' Cellier's revised opinion of this physician? Cellier appeals to a higher authority, James himself, for, 'Where the Word of a King is, there is Power.' His reward for granting her requests will be that God will give him 'a Prince by his Royal Consort' who will 'lead to Battel the soldiers wich the Hospital will preserve for him' (EC12). She reminds the anonymous doctor that for the last four years she has been claiming that 'Her Majesty was full of Children, and that the *Bath* would assist her Breeding'; now this is proved true. Thus in January 1688 Cellier pins her hopes on the succession.

A London Catholic with a French husband was not a good thing to be in 1680: despite a Catholic monarch, January 1688 was hardly a better time to be a London Catholic midwife with French connections. On 31 January the body of the husband of a French midwife, Mary Awbry or Hobry, was found 'mangled' on a dunghill in Holborn. His arms and legs were found in 'the common shore [sewer] under the Savoy'.[65] Denis Awbry appears to have been a violent, impecunious man who, on the night of 27 January, came in drunk at 5 a.m. and 'acted such a violence upon her Body in despite of all the Opposition that she could make, as forc'd from her a great deal of Blood'. After he fell asleep, Mary strangled him, dismembered his body and then, with the aid of her young son, scattered the parts around London. Mary confessed to the murder, and many people had heard her say prior to this night, 'Il faut que Je le Tue.' On 2 March she 'was burnt in Leicester Feilds [sic] for killing her husband'.[66]

The '*Plain* and *Naked* narrative' published in pamphlet form describing this notorious case names her son as 'John Desermeau', while some witnesses call her 'Madam Desermeau'. On her own testimony, Mary had married Awbry 'about four years since'. One of the two French midwives in London known to have been regulated by the Church of England was Mary Des Ormeaux, licensed in 1680 after swearing that she was conformable to the Established Church, and mainly serving the French community in London.[67] Is this then the same woman? The description of her trial makes it clear that she speaks no English, and the witnesses who state that they have used her services as a midwife are all of French extraction; she is described as 'the French midwife'. The account of the crime gives some insight into a midwife's life in the period; for example, she is called to a woman 'ready to fall in Labour', stays the night, leaves when it has proved to be a false alarm, but returns daily to check on progress.

If the two women are in fact one and the same, then Mary's religious position is unclear. In order to be licensed she needed to show herself 'conformable' to the Church of England. Yet in the pamphlet account of her trial she is asked,

> How it came to pass that she, being of the Communion of the Church of *Rome*, came to throw the Quarters of her Husband into a House of Office at the *Savoy*, which was a way to bring so great a Scandal upon the Religion she professed, by laying the Murther at the Door of the Professors of that Religion?

After 1661, the Church of the Savoy was used by French Huguenot families in the Covent Garden area, many of whom fled from France after an edict of 28 February 1680 declared that Protestant women should be attended only by Catholic midwives. The licensing of Mary Des Ormeaux in 1680 may at first sight appear to fit into this pattern. However, if she is to be identified with the Mary Desermeau/Awbry of 1688, it is not so straightforward. The reference to the Savoy is not to the French Huguenot church, but to the short occupation of a section of the Savoy Hospital by the Jesuits, in 1687–88.[68] By 1688 – possibly as a result of the marriage to Denis Awbry, whose first present to her was 'a little Office of our Blessed Lady' – Mary, like Elizabeth Cellier, was a Catholic.

On 10 June 1688 a son was born to Mary of Modena, although his parentage was immediately doubted – thus ensuring the Catholic succession, but leading to the arrival of William of Orange. Cellier and her College are not heard of again.

I would argue that the highly public existence of Elizabeth Cellier as plotter and midwife, far from advancing the reputation of seventeenth-century London midwives, has had the effect of distorting our image of their competence.[69] Her political involvement gave free rein to her opponents to resurrect negative images of the midwife as drunken bawd, and the 1687 scheme has only provided further ammunition for those who see the midwife of this period as an ignorant, unskilled woman in need of proper training.

Where the Cellier of the 1687 scheme has absorbed the image of midwives as a danger to the health of mother and child, and supported male professionals and their model of medical hierarchy, the Cellier of the 1688 'To Dr . . . ' attacked physicians and argued for female solidarity, and the reclaiming for women of 'women's secrets' which books such as the *Byrth of Mankynde* had claimed to reveal for the ultimate good of women. Which is the true Cellier? It may be relevant that Hugh Chamberlen senior's prosecution by the College of Physicians was in March 1688, and possibly Cellier wanted to distance herself from him before this occurred. Thus, perhaps, neither is the true Cellier; rather, once more she shows her instinct for survival, shifting her allegiance to preserve her own interests.

Appendix 1: Publications by or associated with Elizabeth Cellier (with British Library reference)

EC1. 'The triall of Elizabeth Cellier, at the Kings-bench-barr, on Friday June the 11th 1680'. BL 1605/104.
EC2. 'The tryal of Elizabeth Cellier, the Popish Midwife, at the Old Bailey, September 11 1680'. BL 1475.c.2.(36).
EC3. 'The Complaint of Mrs Celiers and the Jesuits in Newgate, to the E of D [i.e. the Earl of Danby] and the Lords in the Tower, concerning the Discovery of their new sham-plot.' ?1680. BL 1897.c.20.(18**).
EC4. 'The scarlet beast stripped naked, being the mistery of the meal-tub the second time unravelled.' 1680. BL T.1*.(105).
EC5. 'A letter from the Lady Creswell to Madam C. the Midwife, on the publishing her late Vindication . . . also A Whip for Impudence . . .' 1680. BL 1881.c.3(28).

ROUTLEDGE

11 New Fetter Lane
London EC4P 4EE
Telephone: 071-583 9855
Fax: 071-583 4519

We have much pleasure in sending you
the accompanying book for review

Title: **Art of Midwifery**

Author: **Marland**

ISBN: Hb **0 415 06425 2**

Pb

Publication Date: **17.6.93**

Published Price: £ **50.00** Hb

£ Pb

A copy of the review would be greatly appreciated.
Reviews should not appear in the press prior to the
date of publication.
For further information please contact:

Cecilia Gregory

EC6. 'Malice Defeated, Or, a brief Relation of the Accusation and Deliverance of Elizabeth Cellier'. BL T.96*(1.).

EC7. 'To the praise of Mrs Cellier the Popish Midwife: on her incomparable book.' 1680. BL C. 20.f.2.(133.).

EC8. 'Mistriss Celier's Lamentation for the loss of her liberty.' 1681. BL 1881.c.3.(34).

EC9. 'A true copy of a letter of consolation sent to Nat. the Printer . . . from the Meal-Tub Midwife . . .' 1681. BL 700.1.24.

EC10. 'The new Popish sham-plot discovered, or The cursed Contrivance of the Earl of Danby, Mrs Celier, with the Popish Lords, and Priests, in the Tower and Newgate, fully detected in villanously suborning Witness to swear that Sir Edmund-bury Godfrey wilfully murdered himself.' 1681. BL T.3*.(49).

EC11. 'A Scheme for the Foundation of a Royal Hospital', E. Cellier, June 1687 in J. Somers, *A Collection of Scarce and Valuable Tracts* 1752, vol. 2, ff. 243. BL 184.a.14.

EC12. 'To Dr . . . an Answer to his Queries, concerning the Colledg of Midwives', E. Cellier, 16 January 1688. BL 1178.h.2.(2.).

Notes

1. J.H. Aveling, *English Midwives. Their History and Prospects* (London, 1872, repub. ed. by J.L. Thornton, 1967), 63–85; J.R. Guy, 'The episcopal licensing of physicians, surgeons and midwives', *Bulletin of the History of Medicine*, 56 (1982), 541; J. Donnison, *Midwives and Medical Men*, 2nd edn (London, 1988), 25–7.

2. M. George, *Women in the First Capitalist Society* (Brighton, 1988), 6–7, cf. 112.

3. For example, J.E. Gordon, 'Mrs Elizabeth Cellier – the "Popish Midwife" of the Restoration', *Midwife, Health Visitor and Community Nurse*, 11:5 (1975), 139–42.

4. Major pamphlets are referred to using codes beginning EC. A full list, including British Library (BL) reference, is given in Appendix 1.

5. She may have been *his* second wife if he is the 'Peter Celier', merchant of the parish of St Martin Orgar, on a list of reputed Catholics in London dated 19 March 1657; at this date Peter Celier has a wife, 'Margarett'. 'Margaret Celleir' appears as a witness to a marriage in the Chapel Royal at St James's on 14 October 1668. H. Bowler, *London Sessions Records 1605–1685* (London, 1934), 132; J.C.M. Weale (ed.) *Registers of the Catholic Chapels Royal and of the Portuguese Embassy Chapel 1662–1829*, vol. 1, *Marriages, London Catholic Record Society*, 38 (1941), 10.

6. 'Thomas Dangerfield's Particular Narrative of the Late Popish Design', (1679), 26.

7. R. Hutton, *Charles the Second, King of England, Scotland, and Ireland* (Oxford, 1989), 383.

8. Ibid., 360.

9. George, *Women in the First Capitalist Society*, 113.

10. J. Scott, 'England's troubles: exhuming the Popish Plot', in T. Harris, P. Seaward and M. Goldie (eds) *The Politics of Religion in Restoration England* (Oxford, 1990), 118.

11. Bowler, *London Sessions Records 1605–1685*, 202–3.

12. R. Halstead, *Succinct Genealogies of the Noble and Ancient Houses* (London, 1685), 434–5; R. North, *Examen: or, an Enquiry into the Credit and Veracity of a Pretended Complete History* (London, 1740), 256–64.

13. J. Miller, *Popery and Politics in England 1660–1680* (Cambridge, 1973), 175.
14. Scott, 'England's troubles', 118.
15. Miller, *Popery and Politics in England 1660–1680*, 21.
16. Scott, 'England's troubles', 119.
17. Calendar of State Papers (Domestic), 1 Sept. 1680–31 Dec. 1681 (ed. F. H. Blackburne Daniell, 1921), 370.
18. T. Dangerfield, 'Thomas Dangerfield's Answer to "Malice Defeated"' (London, 1680), 17–18.
19. [Hippocrates], *Diseases of Women*, 2.201 (Littré 8.384); Galen, *On the Affected Parts*, 6.5 (Kuhn 8.420).
20. L. Riverius, *The Practice of Physick* (London, 1655), 419.
21. R.A. Erickson, '"The books of generation": some observations on the style of the British midwife books, 1671–1764', in P.-G. Boucé (ed.) *Sexuality in Eighteenth-Century Britain* (Manchester, 1982), 90, n. 2.
22. E. Poeton, *The Midwives Deputie*, undated MS, BL, Sloane 1954, 5v.
23. D. Evenden-Nagy, 'Seventeenth-century London midwives: their training, licensing and social profile', unpub. PhD diss., McMaster University, 1991, iii. See also ch. 1 in this volume by Doreen Evenden.
24. Ibid., 7. See also D.N. Harley, 'Ignorant midwives – a persistent stereotype', *Bulletin of the Society for the Social History of Medicine*, 28 (1981), 6–9 and ch.2 in this volume by David Harley.
25. Indeed, midwives are not the only medical practitioners attacked in the political pamphlets. Thomas Dangerfield mentions one of Cellier's two daughters, who married a Mr Blaredale, a Catholic apothecary in Arundel Street who supplied six grains of opium dissolved in syrup of gillyflowers to make a certain William Strode talk; however, it only made him 'somewhat drowsy'! After a second failure, Cellier blamed the apothecary 'for not ordering the compound aright', 'Thomas Dangerfield's Particular Narrative of the Late Popish Design', (1679), 54, 5.
26. Ibid., 26.
27. T.R. Forbes, 'Midwifery and witchcraft', *Journal of the History of Medicine*, 17 (1962), 264–83.
28. D. Harley, 'Historians as demonologists: the myth of the midwife-witch', *Social History of Medicine*, 3 (1990), 1–26.
29. Historical Manuscripts Commission: Calendar of the Manuscripts of the Marquess of Ormonde, KP. NS, vol. VII, 269–70. Should we understand by this that she was considering a reversion to the Protestant faith at this time?
30. H.J. Cook, *The Decline of the Old Medical Regime in Stuart London* (Ithaca and London, 1986), 204–6.
31. Calendar of State Papers: Treasury Books, vol. 8.3 (1685–89), 1352.
32. Historical Manuscripts Commission: Report on the Manuscripts of the Marquess of Downshire, vol. 1.1, 278:

> Mrs Celliere, the celebrated *quondam* midwife, is said to have obtained a patent that those of her profession shall be incorporated and pay each 5l. *per annum* which shall go towards the charge of a College of Infants or Foundlings, whereby there will be less pretence for doing violence to bastards.

33. N. Luttrell, *A Brief Historical Relation of State Affairs from September 1678 to April 1714*, vol. 1 (Oxford, 1857).
34. Aveling, *English Midwives*, 20–4, 34–40; Donnison, *Midwives and Medical Men*, 25–6.
35. Donnison, *Midwives and Medical Men*, 31.

36. H.R. Spencer, *The History of British Midwifery from 1650 to 1800* (London, 1927), 147–8; Evenden-Nagy, 'Seventeenth-century London midwives', 366.

37. Aveling, *English Midwives*, 145.

38. Ibid., 152–4.

39. Forbes, 'Midwifery and witchcraft', 264.

40. A. Wilson, 'Participant or patient? Seventeenth-century childbirth from the mother's point of view', in R. Porter (ed.) *Patients and Practitioners: Lay Perceptions of Medicine in Pre-Industrial Society* (Cambridge, 1985), 136.

41. Evenden-Nagy, 'Seventeenth-century London midwives', 27–30.

42. J.F. Benton, 'Trotula, women's problems, and the professionalization of medicine in the Middle Ages', *Bulletin of the History of Medicine*, 59 (1985), 50–1; Erickson, '"The books of generation"', 74; M.H. Green, 'Women's medical practice and health care in medieval Europe: Review essay', *Signs: Journal of Women in Culture and Society*, 14 (1989), 462, n. 86; F. M. Getz, 'Charity, translation, and the language of medical learning in medieval England', *Bulletin of the History of Medicine*, 64 (1990), 1–17.

43. P. Willughby, *Observations in Midwifery*, ed. H. Blenkinsop (Warwick, 1863), 72–3, 341.

44. Ibid., 73, cf. 206.

45. M. Pelling, 'Medical practice in early modern England: trade or profession?', in W. Prest (ed.) *The Professions in Early Modern England* (London, 1987), 90–2, 97.

46. Wilson, 'Participant or patient?', 136; Donnison, *Midwives and Medical Men*, 21.

47. C. Goodall, *The Royal College of Physicians of London Founded and Established by Law, and An Historical Account of the College's Proceedings against Empiricks and Unlicensed Practisers* (London, 1684), f. 465.

48. Evenden-Nagy, 'Seventeenth-century London midwives'. See chs 1, 2 and 3 in this volume by Doreen Evenden, David Harley and Ann Giardina Hess for training networks amongst English midwives.

49. Guy, 'The episcopal licensing of physicians, surgeons and midwives', 538.

50. Evenden-Nagy, 'Seventeenth-century London midwives', 18.

51. Guy, 'The episcopal licensing of physicians, surgeons and midwives', 541.

52. Evenden-Nagy, 'Seventeenth-century London midwives', 74.

53. Ibid., 12.

54. Wilson, 'Participant or patient?', 136.

55. T.R. Forbes, 'The regulation of English midwives in the sixteenth and seventeenth centuries', *Medical History*, 8 (1964), 239; Donnison, *Midwives and Medical Men*, 20.

56. Poeton, *The Midwives Deputie*, 8v.

57. Evenden-Nagy, 'Seventeenth-century London midwives', 129.

58. A. Eccles, 'The early use of English for midwiferies 1500–1700', *Neuphilologische Mitteilungen*, 78 (1977), 380; P. Slack, 'Mirrors of health and treasures of poor men: the use of the vernacular medical literature of Tudor England', in C. Webster (ed.) *Health, Medicine and Mortality in the Sixteenth Century* (Cambridge, 1979), 248.

59. Poeton, *The Midwives Deputie*, 9v.

60. J. Guillemeau, *Child-Birth or, the Happy Deliverie of Women* (London, 1612), 80–1.

61. H. King, 'Agnodike and the profession of medicine', *Proceedings of the Cambridge Philological Society*, 32 (1986), 53–77.

62. Cicero, *De orat.*, 2.18. This is apparently taken from N. Culpeper, *A Directory*

for Midwives (London, 1651), 172: 'I have not medled with your Callings nor Manual Operations, lest I should discover my Ignorance like *Phormio* the Phylosopher, who having never seen Battel, undertook to read a Military Lecture before *Hanibal*, the best Soldier in the World'.

63. J. Sharp, *The Midwives Book, or the Whole Art of Midwifery Discovered, Directing Childbearing Women How to Behave Themselves in their Conception, Bearing and Nursing of Children* (London, 1671), 3–4.

64. Cited in Aveling, *English Midwives*, 40; Donnison, *Midwives and Medical Men*, 26–7.

65. Unless otherwise attributed, all references to the Mary Awbry case are from Anon., 'A Hellish Murder Committed by a French Midwife on the Body of Her Husband . . .' (London, 1688), BL 112.c.3.

66. Luttrell, *A Brief Historical Relation of State Affairs*.

67. Evenden-Nagy, 'Seventeenth-century London midwives', 220.

68. R. Somerville, *The Savoy. Manor: Hospital: Chapel* (London, 1960), 78–9.

69. For a contrast with another highly public midwife, France's Mme du Coudray, see ch. 7 in this volume by Nina Gelbart.

7

Midwife to a nation: Mme du Coudray serves France

Nina Gelbart

Mme Angélique Marguerite Le Boursier du Coudray was unique, for she was a political midwife, a public figure. Most work to date, whether prosopographical or biographical, gives us an insight into midwives whose experiences were rather like those of others, who functioned in the private sphere and whose examples can be generalized. Martha Ballard of *A Midwife's Tale*, for instance, was a kind of 'everywoman', in the sense that each town had one or several such practitioners. This is not to say that Ballard was a common or ordinary person – in fact she was exceptional in the number of deliveries she attended and in keeping a record – but rather that her work, her comings and goings, her functions in the town and the way she was regarded and counted on, were patterns that repeated and played themselves out in the lives of many other contemporary New England midwives. The importance of Martha Ballard's story is precisely that it is representative of a broader phenomenon: it suggests the general contours of the lives of colonial women cast in this role. Hers mirrors the experience of many, perhaps hundreds, of others.[1]

Mme du Coudray, on the other hand, was a singular phenomenon, officially charged with a patriotic mission. Selected in 1759 by King Louis XV to travel throughout France teaching midwifery to the entire nation, she was from the beginning exclusively chosen to perform this duty. The monarch, who along with most demographers of the day feared that France's population was shrinking dangerously fast, might have designated a corps of women to undertake the obstetrical mobilization of the countryside. But the task was given to Mme du Coudray alone, and her travels in this capacity went on for nearly three decades. Of course she was not entirely free to choreograph her own movements; numerous ministers of state, court doctors, royal intendants and the King himself shaped and controlled her travels at various junctures, and involved themselves in the populationist politics of her crusade. Yet the fact remains that Mme du Coudray had an unprecedented opportunity for autonomy, a greater chance to write her own lifescript, a larger solo performance, than almost any other female save royalty in early modern Europe.[2]

We get a glimpse of this woman's character in her earliest known letter, a circular sent to the thirty intendants, or King's men, whose job it was to implement the royal will throughout the French provinces. The date is August 1760, and the national midwife, dispensing with the traditional 'Monseigneur' by which intendants are accustomed to being addressed, opens with a businesslike 'Monsieur'. She informs them she has written a childbirth textbook, the *Abrégé de l'Art des Accouchements*. She has also invented a machine, an obstetrical model of a mother's pelvis, with a foetus inside that can be extracted from every conceivable position, and upon which midwifery students can practise manoeuvres allowing them to deliver in even the most difficult circumstances. She mentions that the King has given her a <u>*brevet*</u> commissioning her to disseminate this teaching method everywhere. In three short months peasant women will learn all that is necessary, even novices who have no previous knowledge of the art, because the machine prepares them to deal with all eventualities more efficiently than real life experience, for in nature one has to wait a long time to encounter difficult births and might never be presented with all potential problems. Mme du Coudray urges the recipients of her letter to consider the necessity of training women from the villages in order to put an end to rampant infant mortality and also to the deformities resulting from botched deliveries, which she considers even worse than death itself. Men must learn also; she will gladly instruct local surgeons as well. She presents herself as a patriotic servant of the state, empowered with the awesome task of <u>averting the depopulation catastrophe.</u> She urges the intendants to demonstrate their devotion to France, and to humanity. She will 'second' them with her establishment. 'My zeal showed me the way, and the same motive animates me to share it.'[3]

This is an astonishing letter in every respect, but especially coming as it does from a hitherto unknown woman. The tone is bold, never apologetic. She speaks as an equal, avoiding the deferential form of address. That she has authored a medical book shows an absence of hesitation to enter the almost exclusively male world of scientific print culture; the number of published midwifery manuals by women at this time was very small. Her aggressive use of the obstetrical model, including her exaggerated claim to have invented it, represents an innovative tactile pedagogy designed to bridge the gap between her elite training, through private apprenticeship in Paris, and the unlettered provincial audience she needed to reach. And in a sense she *had* invented her particular kind of mannequin, for though miniature models of wax, glass, ivory and wood had existed for some time, life-size malleable ones made of fabric and leather do seem to have been of her own devising.[4] Her matter-of-fact offer to teach surgeons as well as women shows her upending, with unselfconscious ease, the usual medico-political hierarchy which always placed males on top in the position of dispensing expertise. But most significant is the way in which Mme du

Coudray steps boldly into the public sphere of authority, adopts a tone of familiarity, treats the intendants as peers whom she takes into her confidence and whom she trusts to recognize the gravity of the national situation and the urgency of sharing in and facilitating her work. From the very start, then, Mme du Coudray shames the men with whom she has to deal out of their complacency and obliges them to enter into professional co-operation with her so that together they may save the *patrie*. Where did the 45-year-old sender of this letter get her vision, her energy, her confidence to undertake this mission singlehandedly? It is an awesome, lonely task. She is splendid in her isolation, but what motivates and fuels her? Is it a particularly magisterial manifestation of what Margaret Mead has referred to as 'post-menopausal zest'?[5]

The first trace of her that I have been able to discover is in 1745 when, at the age of 30, practising in the capital, and using simply the name Le Boursier, she spearheaded a group of forty Parisian midwives petitioning the *Faculté de Médecine* for better anatomical instruction. These women complained that the city surgeons, who were supposed to invite them to dissections and supervise their licensing examinations after their 3-year apprenticeships, had stopped performing either of these functions. As a result they felt inadequately prepared, and to add insult to injury many illegal matrons with no training at all were hanging up shingles and claiming to be as worthy of a clientele as anyone else. Since a large part of the grievance here was unauthorized practice by female quacks, it cannot be seen as a banding together of midwives in a gender-sensitive camaraderie. But it can be understood as a moment of intensely shared work identity, resulting from a fear that their professional integrity had been violated.[6] The doctors were being called upon by the petitioners to help midwives re-establish the boundaries of their field, and to enhance their education. That Le Boursier, whose signature appears toward centre top on a page with thirty-nine others, should experience this threat to her livelihood as an outrage and organize others to see it in that light, is perhaps an early indication of her strong sense of self. This act of petitioning, after all, is a refusal to remain silent in the face of intellectual starvation and professional jeopardy.[7]

There is other evidence, too, that Le Boursier had an unusually high and healthy self-esteem. When she took on apprentices, she charged one of the steepest fees for the 3-year training programme in the entire community, 300 *livres* just to instruct her protégé. Most midwives charged only 100 or 200 *livres*, and threw in room, board, light, heat and laundry in a sort of package deal. But Le Boursier insisted that her trainee live on her own and clothe and feed herself, coming to her only on rounds when she was called to a birth or when she presided over one in her home.[8] She seemed not to need or want a boarder or companion as did so many of her colleagues. While we must resist the temptation to read hints of her future into her past, these indications suggest that this woman had an independent, no-nonsense streak, a desire early on to distinguish herself from the crowd of two hundred Parisian midwives, and no fear of showing her impatience with problems or of doing things according to her own formula. It should not altogether surprise us, then, that in 1751 she suddenly turned her back on this scene, dropped everything, and accepted an invitation to Auvergne to instruct peasant girls in the town of Thiers.

How exactly this came about is impossible to establish, but Le Boursier had clearly made a superior reputation for herself in the capital, for it was her name that came up at court when the *seigneur* of Thiers and his wife looked into the matter and requested a recommendation.[9] The area around Clermont had been alerted to the national concern about depopulation by its very enlightened intendant, La Michodière, and he had summoned a succession of Paris-trained midwives to help, none of whom had stayed very long in the unwelcoming Auvergnat terrain. Le Boursier, however, was made of sterner stuff. She seemed ready for autonomy and adventure. Having left Paris behind her without apparent regret, she resolved not to let any obstacles stand between her and her new determination to forge out on her own. As she approached middle age, her vigour increased.

For the next eight years she taught the women of this forbidding, impoverished region, developing a deep commitment to them and an even deeper gratitude, because it was they who opened her eyes, kindled her ambition, gave form and substance to her calling. It was they who, through their candid stories and lamentations about miscarriages, stillbirths, hideous scars and premature infertility, first alerted her to the alleged blood and gore of rural delivery practices, to the atmosphere of terror and death that hung over these brave matriarchs for whom burial of their offspring followed their birth with gruesome regularity.[10] In the capital she had known nothing of this; even poor women who could not afford private midwives had access to the renowned *salle des accouchées* in the *Hôtel Dieu* where they received expert care.[11] No, the kind of carnage, the tales of woe she was hearing for the first time, seemed to her to be the special curse of a countryside devoid of trained practitioners. She had been safely insulated from all this, but had now lost her professional innocence. Henceforth she would devote herself to remedying this frightful situation.

During the 1750s while she laboured in Auvergne, teaching hundreds of students gratis and with astounding success, news of her rare talent and charisma came to the attention of the powers in Versailles. She had written her *Abrégé*, a transcription of her lessons, which was approved by the booktrade censors in the capital. She had deployed her obstetrical machine, for which she requested and received approbation from the Royal Academy of Surgery in Paris.[12] By all reports her teaching was spectacular, and she must have begun to picture a grander stage for her performance. Around this time she started calling herself Mme Le Boursier du Coudray, soon after that simply Mme du Coudray, and next *veuve* (widow) du Coudray, for reasons we can only guess at. Perhaps she really did marry during these years, though that seems improbable, because her husband is never once referred to in her hundreds of letters, is never with her on her travels, and she has no children of her own. Indeed she appears to positively savour the unattached, nomadic life, and goes through the next three decades entirely unencumbered by any concept of anchor or home. It is more likely that she invented this spouse when she moved to the provinces, for, whereas numerous Paris midwives were maiden ladies or *filles majeures*, in the countryside it was considered a necessary badge of honour and experience for a midwife to be married, and preferably to be a mother as well. Our midwife would work to change all this eventually, but when first launching into her new career it no doubt seemed best to conform to custom. The surname du Coudray with its noble particle even gave her a touch of class which she may have felt would serve her in good stead. She obviously saw pseudonymity as a creative way of forging a new identity.[13] She would fabricate an aristocratic name for her adopted niece later on; clearly she considered role-playing not only fair game, but enabling. The name was new and the mission was new and she would grow into these stories even as she spun them. This kind of inventiveness would make up for the fact that she was a childless woman. It gave her true personal fulfilment and justified her becoming the national midwife and matriarch, claiming all born babies as hers, saving subjects for France and souls for God and humans for humanity, making birthing on a grand scale her very business.[14]

On 19 October 1759 the King officially authorized du Coudray to take her teaching beyond Auvergne, to spread her knowledge everywhere 'throughout the realm', and he guaranteed that she would be able to do this without interference from anyone.[15] The *brevet* made it sound so easy, but in fact no sooner did her trainees return to their villages than they encountered all manner of resistance, resentment and hostility from older matrons who hated the new fangled 'experts', from local surgeons who thought all women incompetent regardless of their 'schooling', and from pregnant women who out of loyalty and habit preferred to use the traditional helpers or to deliver with no special assistance at all other than the mutual aid extended by friends, relatives and neighbours.[16] Du Coudray herself certainly did not find the path clear, despite the *brevet*'s brave rhetoric about royal protection, and it is the story of the various obstacles she needed to overcome, and her attempts to do so, that will constitute the remainder of this chapter.

Moulins was her first stop once she left Auvergne to begin her national tour. The intendant Le Nain was enthralled by her, and felt lucky and proud to be the first to secure her services, for, after all, every intendant had received the letter in which this royal ambassadress announced herself to the world, but Le Nain had had the perspicacity to snatch her up before she got too far afield. Impressed that Frère Côme, the unorthodox but brilliant and celebrated lithotomist, was an ardent backer of du Coudray, Le Nain threw himself into making her stay in his region a success. So thrilled was he with how well things went, from the recruiting of suitable students in the parishes to the mechanics of the many months of lessons themselves, that he printed a *Mémoire*, a guide for all his fellow intendants so that they might also implement her teaching stint successfully in their regions.[17] Young women were selected by the priests in surrounding villages and came to the town where the class was offered. Each course took approximately 2 to 3 months, meeting 6 days a week all morning and afternoon, so that every student, in conjunction with the lessons on anatomy, had ample opportunity to practise taught manoeuvres on the mannequin. These women, receiving a special certificate upon graduating, then returned to their hamlets to practise their new profession. Another class was offered for male surgeons who would become teacher-demonstrators, would purchase one of du Coudray's machines, and would then be able to give refresher courses in perpetuity after the midwife's departure. A more expensive silk version of the mannequin would be bought and kept on display in the *Hôtel de Ville* of each town, to function as a model when the others wore out from use and needed to be repaired.

Heady from her triumphant stay in Moulins, where du Coudray had by all accounts taken like a born performer to the teaching stage, she quickly gathered both momentum and confidence. She had by 1763 moved on to Bourgogne, had taught to enthusiastic groups in Autun, Bourg-en-Bresse and Chalons-sur-Saône, and had begun to see the dramatic difference her courses could make.[18] Full of boldness, she sent off an extremely aggressive letter to the intendant of Bordeaux, Boutin, who reacted badly to her brazen self-promotion. It was her first serious diplomatic blunder. Inexperienced in provincial politics and unaware of regional sensitivities, she had tactlessly implied in her letter that Versailles considered the Gironde particularly backward and therefore especially needful of her services.[19] Boutin felt this was not for her to judge. Deeply affronted, he refused to accept her offer to teach there. What he failed to realize, of course, was that you could not turn down the King's midwife and get away with it. Mme du Coudray, for one, would hold a grudge against him and his region's officials for years, considering them stupid, entirely benighted because of their incapacity to recognize the urgency of her mission. And the King's royal ministers would not forgive Boutin either.[20] He was the first to thwart the monarch's scheme and he would pay the price in humiliation, spending most of the next decade apologizing to and pursuing the insulted midwife, grovelling to make her forgive him and bring her renowned expertise to his province. It gave her enormous satisfaction to humble him as an object lesson to others who might not pay her the proper respect.

In 1764 du Coudray moved on to Limoges, Tulle and Angoulême, where the intendant Turgot was already demonstrating the liveliness and open-ness to innovation that would soon catapult him to positions of higher power. Recognizing at once the extreme national significance of what the midwife was doing, he drummed up support for her in the surrounding parishes, brooking no argument. He had, however, little patience with du Coudray's lofty opinion of her own importance, and no doubt his suspicion of her as a powerful female rubbed off on some of the sub-delegates. 'You will perhaps find her person ridiculous enough with the high estimation she has of herself', wrote Turgot.[21] And the sub-delegate of Angoulême echoed that attitude:

> She has her imagination so full of the superiority of her talents that she often puts to the test the most resolute patience by the explan-ation she is always ready to make of her merits and the recitation of her honours . . . so that whoever does not render her similar homage appears in her mind as a mere automaton, having nothing human but the shape.[22]

Yet both men were clearly impressed with her abilities and her seriousness of purpose, and consequently they helped rather than hindered her efforts. The essential thing, in their eyes, was that she was extremely competent and gave useful lessons. She, meanwhile, may or may not have been aware of their laughing behind her back, but did not deign to react to it, because far greater worries preoccupied her, especially the retirement of Bertin, one of her most helpful ministerial supporters. Bertin, however, assured her that many at Versailles besides himself believed in her and her work, and that she need not fear that her cause would be forgotten with his departure, though he did recommend that she make it a practice to secure letters of accomplishment, or recommendations, from all the intendants in whose regions she had taught and would teach.[23] These testimonials of her successes instructing provincial students in the art of midwifery would be her insurance, her validation, her passport to continued future teaching engagements, her job security. They gave a new flavour to her interactions with the intendants, for however impatient she might be with some of their apparent prevarications or obtuseness, she was beholden to them for their endorsement. They in turn depended on her, because she had to report to the court any administrative obstacles thrown in her path, and relay favour-able or unfavourable reviews of her stay in each region. The resulting dynamic was complex, and seems to have led most often to a creative tension that kept both the King's men and the King's midwife on the level of good, co-operative behaviour. Though not always.

The mid-1760s brought a new Controller General, the frugal Jansenist Laverdy, on to the scene. He liked du Coudray and thought that she should have a guaranteed annual salary. But as he could not tap the royal treasury – France was desperately trying to recover from the financial blows of the Seven Years' War – he tried to have the provinces pitch in and put together an 8,000 *livres* pension for her. It was the provinces, he argued, that reaped the benefits of du Coudray's labours, for her students fanned out into the countryside bringing enlightened obstetrical practice to even the most isolated, backward areas. He also calculated that if she spent 3 to 6 months in each region she could efficiently cover or 'do' the whole of France in six or seven years.[24] Laverdy was a keen mathematician and an efficient, crisp administrator but he did not take into account human nature. The provinces refused to chip in and finance a service many of them did not feel the need for. This was also a time of increasing resentment in the countryside against what the regions perceived as oppressive royal will. Furthermore, du Coudray herself was a middle-aged woman with emotional and physical requirements, especially the need to rest between exhausting spells of teaching. She was not a machine and did not function by precision clockwork. What Laverdy thought might require seven years was to take well over two decades.

Du Coudray headed north in the winter of 1765 to Poitiers. The intendant there, de Blossac, appreciated her a great deal, but commented that it was rote learning, practised routine, that made her instruction so effective for her students. 'They know how to deliver like a cobbler knows how to make shoes. That is all that is necessary.' He suggested to another intendant that he try to engage her sooner rather than later, for surely her zeal and industry, so admirably demonstrated just now for him, could not last forever.[25] The local newspaper, the *Affiches de Poitou*, began to report on du Coudray's courses; she was soon to become a favourite feature article in the provincial press wherever she went.

Next she pressed west to the Atlantic coast, Niort, Les Sables d'Olonnes, La Rochelle and Rochefort, where she gave a special course to the royal naval surgeons, demonstrating the employment of obstetrical instruments which women were not permitted to use, and teaching them how to perform caesarean sections. She moved with alacrity through this exclusively male curriculum, and even invented some accessories for her machines, such props as clear and red fluids, representing the amniotic waters and blood, which she deployed through a series of sacs and sponges to make the childbirth practice on the mannequins much more realistic. These 'grand operations' as she called them would soon become a standard part of her teaching of women students too, for she was always seeking to upgrade her performance.[26]

On 18 August 1767 the King finally awarded her an annual salary of 8,000 *livres* to be paid by the royal treasury, in lieu of Laverdy's provincial donations which had never materialized. The war had ended a few years earlier and the tight grip on funds had relaxed somewhat. In addition, there was a promise of a 3,000 *livres* retirement pension when du Coudray could no longer travel.[27] This was an epiphany for the midwife. She was to use the money to pay for her transportation, though the towns and cities where she taught would continue to provide furnished and fully equipped lodging, light and firewood. Somehow, however, in her eagerness to broadcast this new vote of confidence from her monarch, she boasted overmuch and confused some intendants and city officials into believing that they no longer needed to provide anything for her but a classroom. She was travelling by now with an entourage of four or five, so housing for the ménage was expensive. Having bragged too loudly about the King's largesse, she now had to spend a lot of time and energy disabusing regional administrators of their false impression that she came free.

Orleans, Blois, Chartres, Montargis – du Coudray seemed indefatigable. She arranged her route by writing to several intendants at a time, announcing her proximity, explaining her available dates, and juggling the possibilities, playing them off against each other until one eventually worked out.[28] Poor Boutin was still struggling to get her to relent and come to Bordeaux but, still stubbornly refusing, she moved instead to Bourges in the dead of winter, 1768. Here things went very badly, at least from the point of view of her comfort. So miserly was the city that the 53-year-old midwife, denied candles and logs, threatened to close down her course and hibernate if Bourges would not provide adequate heat and light. Laverdy, ever watchful and thrifty, was actually part of the problem. Although he still supported her, he worried about the company that now travelled with her and the added financial burden that housing *them* put on the towns. Observers reported that her team was comprised of two surgeons, an apprentice who helped with the demonstrations, a chambermaid and a lackey. The intendant of Bourges, Du Pré de St Maur, hastily came to her defence, however, assuring Laverdy that this troupe of helpers was entirely necessary if she was to teach classes of one hundred women at a time.[29] But while the intendant was supportive in principle, he was absent during her visit and she needed to endure the shabby treatment of his underlings. She wrote in no uncertain terms to St Maur about the indignities she was being subjected to. 'I confess to you, Monsieur, that if all the city corps had been this same way, it would have given me a furious disgust for my mission.'[30] Horrified and deeply embarrassed, St Maur reprimanded and disciplined the town officials and put things to rights for the midwife and her team.[31] Ever resilient, du Coudray proceeded to do some of her most impressive teaching to date. It was here that she trained the remarkable Mme Jouhannet, one of her prize students, who went on to found her own clinic.[32] Frère Côme explained that du Coudray had immediately invested nearly half of the King's newly promised pension in a set of twenty-six engravings for the second edition of her *Abrégé*.[33] The drawings broke away from the anatomical conventions of the time, and were made by a new technique of multi-chrome colour printing.[34] They were thus extremely costly to produce, but rather than pocket the recently allotted funds the midwife reinvested them in her mission, using them in good faith and demonstrating her genuine devotion to her calling.

From Bourges she went on to Issoudun and Châteauroux, extremely concerned because the promised royal stipend had not yet arrived, worried that Frère Côme, who had become a sort of unofficial impresario directing her travels and her monies from Paris, might have forgotten her or fallen ill.[35] Perhaps because these anxieties tried her forbearance, she got uncharacteristically prickly at the next stop, Perigueux in the beautiful Dordogne, refusing to give a copy of her book to the town *syndic* who did not appear to treat her with adequate reverence.[36] But despite this uppity mood she finally allowed Frère Côme, who soon sent the awaited payment and reassured her that he was well and loyal, to persuade her to relent and go to Bordeaux. He managed to smooth things over – a diplomatic coup in which both Boutin and the midwife saved face – and put her in touch with the intendant's special secretary, Duchesne, a man of immense charm who was to become du Coudray's first close friend and confidant since the start of her travels. Just before arriving in Bordeaux she had had another rather frustrating stop in Agen, where the students were undistinguished, the food bad and boring and the officials so foolish in her eyes that they even defied the intendant's orders and refused to purchase one of her machines, one of her 'monuments to humanity' as she immodestly called them.[37] So, with her ego bruised, she arrived in Bordeaux in the spring of 1770 and indulged herself in Duchesne's soothing friendship. This was a watershed in her travels. She knew she had basically completed her rounds in central France and would now launch the second part of her odyssey which would take her farther afield to the outskirts of the country, to areas with which she was not at all familiar. For this she needed to be both physically and psychologically fortified. Duchesne's special support and camaraderie gave her a new kind of sustenance and set a precedent. Henceforth she would admit to a need for this kind of affection. Du Coudray had denied herself emotional intimacy up to this point, perhaps because she wanted to establish her professional power and prove her mastery of the monumental job with which she had been entrusted. But now there was little doubt about her competence, and she could afford to relax and acknowledge the importance of such bonds. She had shown herself to be a consummate voyager. Here we see that a journey within was taking place as well, a recognition of vulnerability and need.

Bordeaux was not only the scene of her first important friendship. It was also the place where she began to confront her own mortality. The young apprentice travelling with her was her so-called niece, 15-year-old Marguerite Guillaumanche who would later claim to have been 'raised' by her 'aunt' and must therefore have been travelling and learning with her already for some time.[38] This niece had her first serious suitor in Bordeaux, a wealthy but unscrupulous scamp who insinuated himself into the household for a time as a surgeon-disciple of the midwife and began the flirtation. Du Coudray disliked him instinctively but knew no sanctimonious lecturing or preaching would dissuade the flattered adolescent girl as effectively as seeing the young man's true stripes. Sure enough, he soon stole some items and went to sell them at a county fair. The niece saw the light, the thief was disgraced, and the aunt, though pleased to be rid of the feckless youth, suddenly began to worry about her niece's future should she die.[39] She seems to have pushed this problem to the back of her mind – she does not dwell on it in the letters – though it probably made her regard another new member of her group in a different light. Jean-Pierre Coutanceau, a surgeon considerably older than the rogue, had accompanied the team from Bordeaux to Auch and Montauban in the winter of 1771. The midwife liked him far better and started almost immediately to refer to him as her 'provost' and pass on to him many teaching and demonstrating responsibilities.[40] She was extremely busy now filling back orders for machines, which she and her entourage produced themselves, so the extra helping hand was appreciated. Also, unaccountably, the government had decided to print and distribute at its own expense a rival childbirth text by a man named Raulin. This must have been disturbing to du Coudray. She had never fancied that she had a monopoly on the subject of birthing, but the market she counted on to buy her *Abrégé* was now being tempted by a free volume of no particular merit that she could see, though it had a rousing endorsement by the Sorbonne Faculty of Theology of its special section on baptism![41] The midwife was gradually beginning to have her hegemony challenged. The support of the intelligent and loyal Coutanceau was at least some comfort.

The year interval from spring 1771 to June 1772 did nothing to set her mind at ease. It was a low point for her, a time of enforced wandering as a rootless fugitive who could find no place to alight. She travelled from Montauban to Grenoble during that year, trying to set up her teaching establishment in Toulouse, Montpellier, Narbonne and Marseilles, but these regions would not allow her to settle.[42] Undoubtedly mortified by these rejections, the midwife wrote no letters to her friends during these bleak months. We next hear from her happily ensconced in Grenoble where the intendant was treating her royally. She was thriving, her health and morale restored. She joked, bossed, pushed and charmed; her relief at being welcome and valued again was almost palpable.[43] Attempts to go next to Lyon did not work out, but she moved north to Besançon where once more things went smoothly. Here she got involved especially deeply with her students, many of whom were Lutheran, and had come from their villages with grossly inadequate funding. She lent them money (which she knew full well she would never get back), offered moral support, intervened in their family feuds, testified for them at their trials. She struck deals with the parish priests, promising to put in a good word for them with the archbishop if they in turn agreed to boycott all midwives at baptisms who were not her graduates.[44] Du Coudray took to calling her niece Mlle de Varennes during this period. The young woman was of the most humble peasant extraction – her parents came from the tiny hamlet of Talende in Auvergne and could not sign their names – but it must have served the midwife's purposes to have the world believe that she was noble.[45]

In 1773 the group moved to Châlons-sur-Marne where the intendant, Rouillé d'Orfeuil, was extremely attentive, advertising du Coudray's visit on large posters, offering free lodgings in town to her students and incentives to their husbands including exemption from such hated taxes as the *taille* and *corvée*. He ordered twenty-three machines for the major towns in his generality, and created such positive feeling about the midwife's courses that surgeons almost came to blows in their scramble to be chosen for the class in which she trained demonstrators.[46] Here in Châlons du Coudray also solidified a second very close friendship with the man supervising her stay, one St Etienne.[47] She adored him and his family and merrily reported back to them for years after her departure about all her ups and downs, certain that they would care and would want to be kept informed.

The next stop, Verdun, was far less pleasant. There were 108 students and the whole teaching team was in a state of collapse from exhaustion. She had made a side-trip to Metz to see a display of some of the rival mannequins now being produced in Paris, yet another source of competition. Her plans for subsequent travel had been bungled by the intendant Calonne, and Besançon had still not paid up for the machines. What is more, one of the surgeon disciples travelling with her was proving himself to be totally incompetent.[48] In general the mood of the midwife and her ménage was melancholy. Luckily the next two stints, Neufchâteau and Nancy, proved to be uplifting. Du Coudray found another good friend in the person of Neufchâteau's sub-delegate, Royer. The students there were so appreciative that a mass of thanksgiving was dedicated in the midwife's honour. And a romance had finally blossomed between Coutanceau (whom du Coudray trusted with more and more of the teaching, so that he had begun to amass his own fan mail) and her niece.[49] Seeing the seriousness of the couple's intentions, the midwife needed to provide a dowry and so hastened to Paris to secure her niece officially as her conjoint and heir. She negotiated such advantageous terms for the niece's eventual takeover of her mission that she waxed rhapsodic in her letter to Royer explaining these events. She felt, as she put it, like 'Queen of the ministers', so regally had she been treated at court.[50] Fortunately this euphoria sustained her through a depressing course in Amiens where the administrators were apathetic, beggars rampant, and where her spirits might otherwise have sagged. Instead, buoyed up by her recent triumph in the capital, du Coudray pressed her friends to get her story into the national *Gazette de France*. It was all very well and good that provincial papers published articles on her teaching everywhere she went. But these had only local interest and distribution. She now craved a broader audience, a reading public that stretched through the entire kingdom.[51]

Meanwhile the couple had posted marriage banns announcing their betrothal in numerous cities as the team moved to Dunkerque, then Lille. Here in Flanders du Coudray's efforts came to the attention of the Comte de Nery. He sang her praises to the Austrian empress Maria Theresa whose daughter Marie Antoinette, after years as dauphine, had just become France's queen. A voyage was arranged across the frontier to Ypres, du Coudray's only extraterritorial venture, where she taught with great success despite the protests of the conservative, misogynistic medical faculty at Louvain.[52] On 28 February 1775 Marguerite Guillaumanche, aged 19, married Jean-Pierre Coutanceau, aged 37, in the parish church of St Nicolas in Ypres, having been given special dispensation by the priest in Lille. Why they chose to marry during this brief trip beyond the French borders is unclear, but their enthusiastic students provided an elaborate procession to the church and a cheerful wedding feast after the ceremony.[53]

Du Coudray could easily have stayed longer in the Austrian Flanders, and Holland was making overtures as well, but she felt duty bound to honour her French commitments, the next of which was in Caen.[54] The *curés* here adored her, thought she was heaven-sent, and the intendant Fontette was especially solicitous, frequently attending her classes, no doubt grateful that she had turned down international fame to come, as promised, to him. Paying special attention to her teaching methods, he applauded her determination to recruit the youngest students possible. This was, indeed, one of du Coudray's great innovations, her creation of a youthful, vigorous group of trained professionals in contradistinction to the old matrons, young women who had years of service to the state ahead of them, who could thus make the teaching investment worthwhile. Fontette also staunchly defended her *Abrégé* after the government again endorsed another rival work, this one by the doctor DuFot, which it now distributed free along with Raulin's volume.[55] However disturbed she may have been by this continuing erosion of her literary territory, du Coudray had something else, a more personal matter, on her mind. She was writing frantically to both Rouen and Rennes trying to set up a long stay at one of these cities, for the new bride had lost no time getting pregnant, was expecting around Christmas time, and the midwife wanted to be quietly and comfortably settled for the last months of the young woman's term.[56]

A baby boy was born to the niece and nephew in Rennes on 28 December 1775.[57] Unfortunately Mme Coutanceau was unable to breast-feed the child and a wet-nurse was reluctantly added to the entourage which now numbered eight or nine and had begun to resemble a caravan.[58] Du Coudray far preferred women to suckle their own infants, and in the *Abrégé* spoke at length about the importance of maternal milk. Barring that, it was imperative to choose the wet-nurse with tremendous care. Pages were devoted to this selection procedure. The woman du Coudray picked to nourish this baby, the closest she would ever have to a grandchild, was no doubt thoroughly scrutinized to fit all requisite criteria.[59]

Gout had begun to plague the midwife, and other difficulties now presented themselves in rapid succession. In Nantes during the summer and fall of 1776 the teaching was gruelling. Coutanceau had to double up lessons because the students had been sloppily recruited and were unusually 'dense'.[60] In addition, du Coudray had by now come to the realization that ministerial support for her was waning, a point brought painfully home by the printing and distribution of other obstetric books 'at the government's orders'. Sensing that a conspiracy might be forming against her, she went to Paris to leave all her letters and credentials there in safe keeping, perhaps in the hands of the loyal Frère Côme, or with another professional friend, the surgeon Sue. Then she headed for Evreux – arrangements to teach in Rouen had fallen through because accommodation for the large household could simply not be found – where a crisis of a different kind occurred. An ugly rumour circulated that du Coudray had extorted money from her students and pressured them into buying her a clock, and an even uglier letter purporting to be from Frère Côme maligned her and her course of instruction. The sub-delegate, who knew, trusted and admired the midwife, was certain that the letter was forged by the same ruthless parties who had spread the other rumours. He tracked down and punished the guilty, but not soon enough to prevent considerable damage, for du Coudray was beside herself and for some time inconsolable. The very idea that Frère Côme might betray or abandon her was more than she could tolerate.[61] Around the same time, a doctor in Paris, Alphonse LeRoy, published a slanderous broadside against her. It must have seemed like the sky was crashing in on the 62-year-old midwife, and a weaker, less organized person might have given up entirely. But she had foreseen this, in outline if not in precise detail, had sensed the winds blowing against her, had understood that at the very least it would be hard for the government to sustain its exclusive commitment to her for so long. Luckily she had armed her allies in Paris, for they now produced a vindication of her, the printed *Lettre d'un Citoyen*, tracing the history of her mission, singing her praises and providing numerous testimonials to her greatness from doctors, surgeons, intendants, sub-delegates, syndics and priests throughout France, and from past royal ministers and the King himself in Versailles. This brochure, a dramatic reminder of her great service to the country and an admonition against national amnesia and ingratitude, was distributed in large numbers free of charge in Paris. It was in direct response to LeRoy's scandalmongering, and helped dispel any unflattering impressions left by the Evreux episode.[62] But it also dealt with the larger significance of the midwife's contribution. This spectacular defence of her person and her professionalism renewed du Coudray's belief in herself and what she was about. There were still many years of fight left in her.

The midwife made a second trip to Paris that year, 1777, to meet and win over the new finance minister Necker. She could no longer leave anything to chance, and this latest changing of the guard convinced her that she should present herself in person. She also befriended his influential wife, Mme Necker, an avid supporter of hospitals and public health projects. But an emergency summons from Coutanceau, who had gone ahead to open classes in Le Mans, obliged her to drop her business in the capital and go rushing to his aid.[63] The intendant of Le Mans, de Cluzel, was a strange character. After appearing altogether indifferent to the recruitment of students for many years, he suddenly decided to entice them by offering to *pay* them to take the course! Other intendants had done what they could to provide living expenses, but now de Cluzel had promised an extra stipend. No one had ever tried this before. The result was a stampede. Hundreds of women inundated Le Mans from near and far. Pandemonium reigned, and the cavalry had to be called in to restore order. Coutanceau was clearly in over his head. Du Coudray came to the rescue, set up a system of triage to get the course down to teachable size, though even at 130 it was still her largest crowd ever. She dazzled them with her performance, brought to bear all kinds of extra motivating tricks to keep the enormous group riveted on what she had to show and tell them. It must have exhilarated even as it exhausted her, for she had been able to whip things into line where her younger relatives had failed. She was, indeed, spell-binding, and still the strongest of them all.[64]

The following spring confirmed this, when her niece suffered some sort of breakdown and needed to take the waters at Fourges-les-Eaux. Her departure from the teaching team at this time of huge crowds was an enormous hardship, as was the financial burden of her journey with a servant and her stay at the resort. Du Coudray was forced to drum up additional business in the form of more orders for machines to cover the new, unanticipated expenses.[65] Despite her ability to muster more energy than the younger generation in a catastrophe, du Coudray was now, inevit-ably, slowing down too, feeling older and wearier after the pyrotechnic display in Le Mans. In Angers, her next stop, where she taught 140 students, breaking all enrolment records, she insisted for the first time on being provided with living quarters near her classroom, for she no longer wanted to be carried long distances bumping along in a chair. Walking was out of the question, but even being transported through the city's rutted streets was now too uncomfortable.[66] And before opening classes in Tours, she visited a friend in the outskirts of the city. This is the only known instance of time for socializing being taken out of her rigorous schedule. She must have badly needed the rest.

Perhaps the tedium of her business was finally affecting her. Whatever the reason, she now did something entirely unprecedented, agreeing to give classes to male students at the Royal Veterinary School at Alfort. With no detectable sense of outrage or even discomfort, she acquiesced in treating human birthing as a variation of animal husbandry, likening women to so many cows.[67] After all du Coudray's years of service to the State, it seems almost as if babies as a product were becoming indistinguishable from other chattels, as if what she had been doing all along was, literally, just delivering the goods.

From Alfort the midwife worked hard to secure a steady post for the Coutanceau family. Her attention focused increasingly on them. At 65 she still had ambitions of her own, especially for a 'grand voyage' to Languedoc and Provence where she had been turned away a decade earlier, and which remained areas she had not 'done'. She considered this unfinished business, a great gap in her coverage of the nation, and she wrote repeatedly to Versailles and royal officials in the Midi, or south of France, in her attempt to work this out so that she might achieve a sense of completion. Meanwhile, she finally secured a position for her niece and nephew in Bordeaux, and Coutanceau went ahead to get things started, followed several months later by his wife.[68] Du Coudray, now on her own and still waiting for a go-ahead, decided to make her way south anyway, teaching again in Bourges, then in Auxerre, then in Belley where she had a strong contingent of enthusiastic students, both male and female, from Savoy. When plans for the great trip fell through once again, the midwife must have understood, finally, that it was time to retire. Resigning herself to this, she did no more public teaching after 1783, but shuttled for many years between Bordeaux and Paris trying to help out the Coutanceaus in a variety of ways.

And they badly needed her assistance, though they showed considerable initiative once on their own. Mme Coutanceau, out from under the shadow of her aunt for the first time, worked aggressively in Bordeaux in her effort to realize a dream, the setting up of a maternity clinic there.[69] In 1784 she published a textbook of her own, undertook an extensive round of teaching throughout Guienne, and – unlike her aunt – fought hard to keep men out of the profession, to secure the territory of professional midwifery exclusively for women.[70] Perhaps it was her belligerency on this latter issue that brought the inordinate wrath of the local surgeons down upon her; they tried systematically to undermine the Coutanceaus and even managed to turn some royal ministers against them. For a while it looked as if they would soon be out of business. The couple was grateful for their aunt's connections in the capital which helped to neutralize this menace, but du

Coudray's influence had its limits. And France had once more sunk into bankruptcy. All hopes for getting additional financial support for the Bordeaux hospice were dashed. After elaborate negotiations in Versailles, du Coudray finally had to divert some of her own hard-earned retirement pension to support her niece's operations, for the royal treasury was not about to come up with extra funds. An official document was drawn up outlining this new financial arrangement.[71] It cost France nothing, and du Coudray willingly made the sacrifice when it became clear that no more monies were forthcoming. At least her efforts had done away with the immediate threat to their establishment.

The royal treasury, in fact, was soon to be rendered obsolete by the advent of the Revolution. The Bastille fell while Mme Coutanceau was preparing to teach in the little town of Castillones, and within a few months the universe of the two midwives changed drastically. From whence, if anywhere, would their payments come? Who was actually running the country? How soon would they need to hide the taint of their close association with the monarchy? Mme Coutanceau tried as best she could to ride the political tide. She made a trip to Paris and delivered a request for financial support to the National Assembly, outlining the importance of her work and revealing that her distinguished aunt had saved the life of their hero Lafayette, so it was incumbent upon them to repay the favour.[72] This visit resulted in nothing more than a vague endorsement from one of the Assembly's committees, but no funding. In July 1791 du Coudray, by now quite infirm and living in Bordeaux with her younger relatives, called her notary to her and gave power of attorney to a pharmacist she knew in Paris, Noel Seguin, whose task it became to collect her overdue back pay and her current pension payments. Wishful thinking! Mme Coutanceau eventually asked M. Seguin to do the same for her, but also to no avail.[73] Funds had dried up; the two women and their lives' work seemed forgotten in the revolutionary upheavals. Yet they somehow went on with their duties while political events unfolded in the background. The Coutanceaus did finally get their own hospice granted to them by the city of Bordeaux, on the very day that Charlotte Corday murdered Marat in Paris. They needed to outfit their clinic entirely out of their own pockets,[74] and feed their patients as well. Their altruism and philanthropic efforts were heroic and became part of Bordeaux lore. Mme Coutanceau could rightfully boast that she had become the first female founder and director of a provincial maternity hospital, and she remained in that capacity, despite widowhood and precarious health, until well into the 1820s.

Du Coudray lived to be 79 years old, succumbing finally on 17 April 1794 or 28 Germinal Year II, during the Terror.[75] The guillotine had by then come to Bordeaux, and the city was being squeezed in one of the infamous 'forced loans' through which the revolutionary government sought to raise money from the provinces to fight its foreign wars.[76] She was, in fact, with two tax collectors when she died, and, though we cannot be certain, it might have been the strain caused by their interrogation that finally broke her spirit. She had only recently been awarded a certificate of '*civisme*' attesting to her patriotism, measured by willingness to contribute to the national coffers. But that did not suffice. Contributions were expected to continue on a regular basis and collectors had been sent from the capital to make sure this occurred. The old midwife was, technically, on the royal ledger books, the recipient of a large pension that put her in a high tax bracket, but of course she had been paid nothing for years. It must have been awkward, if not impossible, trying to explain this discrepancy to the tax men during their visitation. And she probably still possessed some of the plaques and gifts she had received on her travels – she may indeed have been cashing them in one by one and living off their worth. But here too there was a problem, for these objects, emblematic of the monarchy, stood as blatant reminders of her erstwhile royalism and may have put her in mortal danger. She could not declare them openly to the Paris collectors. In short, things had doubtless been harrowingly tense for du Coudray ever since the dreaded Committee of Public Safety had dispatched its representatives to Bordeaux. She left no testament or formal succession, and no inventory after death was made of her possessions. Perhaps in the end she had been robbed of everything, or perhaps this was just a symptom of the near total disruption of notarial practice during the Terror. In any case the great midwife exited unsung, upstaged by the political cataclysm that brought down the curtain on the regime in which she had starred.

Yet she achieved a kind of immortality. Her motto, *Ad Operam*, proudly emblazoned above her portrait, had inspired her to accomplish great feats. She had spread obstetrical enlightenment by creating a truly revolutionary pedagogy, a felicitous mix of medical theory, hands-on technique and psychological sensitivity. In the several surveys conducted of provincial health practices by the Royal Society of Medicine in the 1780s, and again by the National Assembly in 1790–91, Mme du Coudray was the only individual teacher named in the otherwise impersonal printed questionnaire, and a staggering two-thirds of all midwives practising had studied with her or with one of the demonstrators she had trained.[77] We cannot be sure that she had any inkling of the scope, the sheer breadth of her influence. But I suspect she did, and that she foresaw it from the very start, and that it was the force propelling her to keep going, spurring her on 'to work'.

Notes

1. L. T. Ulrich, *A Midwife's Tale: The Life of Martha Ballard, Based on Her Diary, 1785–1812* (New York, 1990). Another 'exceptional' midwife, in terms of her record-keeping, the large number of deliveries she attended and her status as a

recognized expert in difficult and protracted labours, was Vrouw Catharina Schrader, who practised in Friesland in the Netherlands between 1693 and 1745. See H. Marland, M.J. van Lieburg and G.J. Kloosterman, *'Mother and Child were Saved': The Memoirs (1693–1740) of the Frisian Midwife Catharina Schrader* (Amsterdam, 1987). For examples of collective studies, see M.E. Wiesner, 'Early modern midwifery: a case study', *International Journal of Women's Studies*, 6 (1983), 26–43, and chs 4 and 9 in this volume by Merry Wiesner and Mary Lindemann. For another highly 'public' midwife, England's Elizabeth Cellier, see ch. 6 in this volume by Helen King.

2. I am presently completing a book-length biography of Mme du Coudray, *Delivering the Goods: The Midwife Mission of Mme du Coudray in 18th Century France*, which will cover in detail what this article can only sketch.

3. Archives Départmentales (henceforth AD) du Cher, C319, f. 24. Most of the documentation for this story can be found in the C series of provincial archives throughout France.

4. See J. Gélis, 'La formation des accoucheurs et des sages-femmes aux XVIIe et XVIIIe siècles: evolution d'un matériel et d'une pédagogie', *Annales de Démographie Historique* (1977), 153–80.

5. Much interesting work has been done on the middle-aged vigour of professional women. See scattered references to this in C. G. Heilbrun, *Writing a Woman's Life* (New York, 1988). Florence Nightingale and Elizabeth Blackwell spoke of this in their correspondence especially with regard to women in medicine. See L.A. Monteiro, 'On separate roads: Florence Nightingale and Elizabeth Blackwell', *Signs*, 9 (1984), 520–33. On Margaret Mead, see M.C. Bateson, *Composing a Life* (New York, 1989).

6. For a comparison with similar issues in eighteenth-century Braunschweig, see ch. 9 in this volume by Mary Lindemann.

7. See Archives Nationales (henceforth AN), Minutier Central (henceforth MC) XV, 640 (29 juin 1745). These are notarial archives. See also (for fuller context) *École de Médecine: Commentaires de la Faculté*, vol. XX, 953–74.

8. See AN, MC LXXV, 617 (22 janvier 1751). I have compared the terms of this agreement with about forty other midwife apprenticeship contracts signed before notaries in the same year.

9. See *Lettre d'un Citoyen amateur du bien public, a M***, pour servir de défense à la mission de la dame du Coudray, qui forme des Sages-femmes par tout le Royaume, de la part du Roi, attaquée dans un écrit public* (Paris, 1777) l, and AD du Puy de Dome, C1404, f. 4.

10. Although all of this is documented in the archives at Clermont, du Coudray gives a summary of it in her textbook, the *Abrégé de l'Art des Accouchements* (Paris, 1759). See, in particular, the dedication to the intendant Ballainvilliers (who replaced la Michodière shortly after her arrival but was at least as supportive), and the 'Avant Propos'.

11. For an enthusiastic contemporary review of the *Hôtel Dieu* from a usually severe critic of his times, see L.S. Mercier, *Tableau de Paris*, ed. Desnoiresterres (Paris, 1853), 'Sages-femmes', 215–18. See also M. Fosseyeux, *L'Hôtel Dieu de Paris au 17e et 18e siècles* (Paris, 1912), 286–95.

12. See the *Abrégé*, later editions of 1769, 1773, 1777 or 1785, for copies of the various approbations from the academy, censors' reviews and *brevets* from the King honouring her work.

13. See the interesting thoughts on this in J. DeJean, 'Lafayette's ellipses: the privileges of anonymity', *Publication of the Modern Languages Association* (Oct. 1984), 884–902, and C. Hesse, 'Reading signatures: female authorship and revolutionary

law in France 1750–1850', *Eighteenth Century Studies*, 22 (1989), 469–87.

14. For thought-provoking discussions of childlessness, see A. Rich, *Of Woman Born: Motherhood as Experience and Institution* (New York, 1977), 252–7.

15. See the full text of this in *Lettre d'un Citoyen*, 5–6.

16. For the problems faced by du Coudray's students and 'graduates', see, for example, AD du Puy de Dôme, C1400, ff. 12, 15, 17–19, 21–33. These same sorts of difficulties were encountered nearly everywhere. For popular resentment of the trained midwife in Italy, see ch. 8 in this volume by Nadia Filippini.

17. See Le Nain's *Mémoire sur les cours publics d'accouchements*. Le Nain would continue to sing du Coudray's praises to other intendants for years to come. See, for example, AD d'Ille-et-Vilaine, C1326, f. 2.

18. See AD de la Côte d'Or, C363 and E3383.

19. AD de la Gironde, C3302, f. 4.

20. AD de la Gironde, C3302, f. 13. See also f. 10.

21. AD de la Gironde, C3302, f. 8.

22. AD de la Gironde, C3302, f. 6.

23. AD du Puy de Dôme, C1405, f. 9.

24. See AD de l'Orne, C301 and AD d'Ille-et-Vilaine, C1326, ff. 3, 4.

25. See AD de la Vienne, C62 and AD d'Ille-et-Vilaine, C1326, f. 6.

26. See AD du Doubs, 1C598 and AD Charente-Maritime, D10, f. 87.

27. AN O^1 111, f. 226.

28. See, for example, AD du Cher, C319, f. 27.

29. AD du Cher, C319, f. 43.

30. AD du Cher, C319, f. 58.

31. AD du Cher, C319, f. 60.

32. AD du Cher, C319, f. 137.

33. AD du Calvados, C981 (20 mars 1768).

34. For a fuller discussion of these illustrations, see N. Gelbart, 'Delivering the goods: patriotism, property and the midwife mission of Mme du Coudray', in J. Brewer and S. Staves (eds) *Changing Conceptions of Property in Early Modern Europe* (forthcoming).

35. AD du Cher, C319, f. 299.

36. AD de la Gironde, C3302, f. 36.

37. AD de la Gironde, C529, f. 11 and C3302, ff. 32, 33.

38. The 'niece' was born in 1755 in Clermont, but du Coudray was nowhere in the picture – not as relative, godparent or presiding midwife. So their exact relationship, if any, remains a mystery. See AD du Puy de Dôme, 3E113 dep Fonds 1.78, régistre de baptême.

39. AD de la Gironde, C3302, ff. 39–40.

40. See AD Tarn-et-Garonne, Archives Communales de Montauban, 27GG1, letters dated 21 décembre 1770 and 6 janvier 1771; AD Ille-et-Vilaine, C1326, f. 33.

41. This was Raulin's *Instructions succinctes sur les accouchements en faveur des sages-femmes des provinces faites par ordre du ministre* (Paris, 1770).

42. AN H1092, ff. 122–3, 143, 147–8, for example, show Montpellier's intendant St Priest giving her the brush-off.

43. AD de la Gironde, C3302, f. 49. See also Archives Municipales de Grenoble, GG carton 239; AD de la Drome, C1/34; Archives Municipales de Crest, GG17 (6 avril 1772).

44. AD du Doubs, 1C598 (letters dated 18 mai 1772 through to 24 octobre 1772).

45. *Affiches de Franche Comté*, 23 octobre 1772.

46. For an example of surgeons vying with each other for selection, see what occurred in nearby Troyes. AD de l'Aube, C1167. My thanks to the archivist Benoit

Van Reeth for his help with these documents.
47. AD de la Marne, C355, ff. 144, 138, 150.
48. AD de la Marne, C355, f. 142.
49. AD de Meurthe-et-Moselle, C314, ff. 56, 102; AD des Vosges, 1C43, ff. 27, 58; *Affiches, announces et avis divers pour les trois evêchés et la Lorraine, ou Affiches de Metz*, 1773, 204.
50. AD des Vosges, 1C43, f. 63.
51. AD de la Marne, C355, f. 145.
52. See Vanhamme, 'Documents concernant l'enseignement de l'obstetrique et le problème de la maternité aux Pays Bas autrichiens', *Bulletin de la Commission Royale d'histoire*, 108 (1943), 41–59. See also at the Bibliothèque Royale de Bruxelles, Archives Générales du Royaume, Conseil Privé autrichien, liasses 1224 and 1227.
53. AD du Nord, Commune de Lille, Paroisse St Catherine, mariage. See also J. Cordonnier-Vander Mursel, *Ephemerides Yproises*, 431.
54. See *Lettre d'un Citoyen*, 14–15.
55. AD du Calvados, C981–C990, assorted unnumbered folios; AD d'Ille-et-Vilaine, C1326, f. 13.
56. AD de la Seine Martime, C95, f. 37 and AD d'Ille-et-Vilaine, C1326, f. 21.
57. Archives Municipales de Rennes, Paroisse St Sauveur, naissances.
58. AD des Vosges, 1C43.
59. See *Abrégé*, 139–44.
60. AD d'Ille-et-Vilaine, C1326, f. 30.
61. AD de la Seine Martime, C95, ff. 68, 74 and C97, f. 100.
62. For the full title, see note 9.
63. AD d'Indre-et-Loire, C355 (11 janvier 1778). An interesting correspondence with Mme Necker can be found in AD de la Gironde, 5M552.
64. AD d'Indre-et-Loire (5 février 1778).
65. AD d'Indre-et-Loire (23 avril 1778).
66. AD d'Indre-et-Loire, C356 (10 juin 1778).
67. See *Almanac Vétérinaire*, 1782–90, nouvelle édition (Paris, 1792), 32–3.
68. See *Archives Historiques de la Gironde*, vol. 25 (Bordeaux, 1887), 438–9, and AD de la Gironde, C3303, f. 2.
69. See AD de la Gironde, C3303 and C3304.
70. See her *Elements de l'art d'accoucher* (Bordeaux, 1784), 'Avertissement' and 334–56.
71. See AD de la Gironde, 5M552 (10 juillet 1784).
72. See AN, F[16] 936, 'Mémoire de la dame Coutanceau, sagefemme'.
73. AN, MC II 754 (23 août 1791) and II 757 (10 février 1792).
74. See AD de la Gironde, 3E 13277 (6 avril 1793) where Mme Coutanceau explains that she has been paid nothing since 1790.
75. AD de la Gironde, 4E 785.
76. On Bordeaux during this period, see R. Brouillard, *Des impositions extraordinaires sur le Revenu pendant la Révolution (contributions patriotiques, emprunts forcés) et de leur application dans la commune de Bordeaux* (Bordeaux, 1910); F. G. Pariset, *Bordeaux au 18e siècle* (Bordeaux, 1968); R.M. Brace, *Bordeau and the Gironde 1789–1794* (Ithaca, 1947).
77. See J. Gélis, 'L'Enquête de 1786 sur les "Sages-femmes du Royaume"', *Annales de Démographie Historique* (1980), 299–343, and T. Gelfand, 'Medical professionals and charlatans. The Comité de Salubrité enquête of 1790–1791', *Histoire Sociale/Social History*, XI (1978), 62–97.

[handwritten annotations at top of page:] Political fragmentation but : religious unity / state & church are of the same ?? / Enlightenment : change : modernity? science / Divergence b/w ??? state/ **8** religion. / Men-M, rare in Italy

The Church, the State and childbirth: the midwife in Italy during the eighteenth century

[handwritten margin notes:] Competition / different in Italy ; / aimed at control / rather than competition. / Italy stands out for ??? (p 168)

Nadia Maria Filippini

Attempts at reconstructing a picture of a typical eighteenth-century Italian midwife and her place in society are beset with a multitude of problems. In addition to a fundamental difference between the towns and the country-side that obtained throughout the peninsula, political fragmentation com-plicated the picture since, at that time, Italy consisted of numerous states. This lack of unity resulted in different policies regarding the populace and the adoption of varied demographic strategies and medical regulations. As a consequence, midwifery practice too was subjected to a multitude of laws and decrees. In such a varied and fragmented society, the figure of the midwife emerges in many different and sometimes contradictory guises.

Alfonso Corradi, an eminent historian of nineteenth-century Italian obstetrics, attributes the weak penetration of the figure of the man-midwife into the birthing chamber and the almost exclusive monopoly of women in the field of obstetrics – which makes Italy so different from other European countries – to the 'multiplicity and differentiation of laws' and to an 'absence of any agreement on disciplines'.[1] His explanation could well be too simple; above all, he does not take into account the role of the Catholic Church, both as a 'unitary' political and organizing force, and as a normative presence which was particularly strong in the area of childbirth. However, Corradi did point out an important aspect of midwifery in the eighteenth century: its extreme diversity, an aspect receiving little notice in recent studies (which have generally been confined to narrow local areas) in which such differences have often been ignored, when they should have been emphasized and questioned.[2]

Bearing these qualifications in mind, I shall endeavour to outline some characteristics of the eighteenth-century Italian midwife. I will not attempt to present a unitary picture, which without doubt would be forced and distorted in some of its features. I shall concentrate on northern Italy where numerous studies have been conducted in recent years. The choice of period is by no means accidental. The eighteenth century, and in particular its second half, was a time of important changes: in many

152

regions, the State intervened directly in the training of midwives, as well as in the creation of rules and the division of labour. This was especially due to the pressure exercised by an ever-increasing number of '*chirurghi-ostetricanti*' (obstetric surgeons). At the same time, the Catholic Church intensified its traditional control, thus causing a great deal of tension in relations between secular and religious institutions. Differentiation between midwives became more marked, while conflicts between those who participated in this process and those who refused to be part of it or who were excluded became more open and sharp. Focusing on this period allows us to locate both traditional aspects and elements of continuity and new or changing features represented by the figure of the midwife.

The '*comare levatrice*', a central figure in the Italian community

Towards the middle of the eighteenth century Giovanni de Grevembroch (1731–1807), a painter and acute observer of the Venice of his time, published his now famous book entitled *Gli Abiti dei Veneziani di quasi ogni età con diligenza raccolti e dipinti nel secolo XVIII* (*Venetian Dress for all Ages, Diligently Collected and Painted, for the Eighteenth Century*).[3] All sorts and conditions of people are included in this enormous array of portraits. The midwife, '*La comare levatrice*', is represented, and we see her in the street on her way to a birth dressed in sombre colours, a shawl over her head as became a woman of her age, stepping out, proud and decisive, followed by a porter carrying her wooden birthing chair on his shoulders. She appears too, in another illustration, the baptism scene. As Grevembroch points out, she is the only woman admitted to the ceremony: she has the responsibility of bringing the new-born child to church. Grevembroch also gives summary details of what her craft involves and the number of midwives in the city – about one hundred according to official data, but really many more, he claims. Even one hundred is a good distribution for a city of 150,000 inhabitants and an average birthrate of 5,000 per annum.[4]

In the precise language of the painter, then, we learn about the salient features of the eighteenth-century midwife, in both her professional and social roles. She 'walks abroad', she is an oft-seen, immediately recognizable figure as she goes about her quarter of the town. Her art is essentially a manual one. She carries no instruments. The only sign of her trade is the birthing chair. Her ties with the Church involve baptism but, as we shall see, this duty was aimed more generally at keeping an eye on female sexual morality.

To shed further light on the features of a typical midwife, and in particular her social background, we can avail ourselves of a variety of sources, pictorial, folkloric and archival, in particular medical and court records, parish registers, baptismal rolls and reports of canonical visits.

Despite their fragmentary nature, because they generally relate to a variety of individual situations, these are more valuable than legal normative texts, in so far as they often contain very vivid descriptions of the lives and activities of midwives.

The midwife was a mature woman, she was married or widowed and had borne children; her social background was humble, and she came from those classes whose members 'lived by [the] fruits of their daily toil', and it is under this category that she is usually entered in the census.[5] This categorization held for the city as well as the countryside: in both contexts, the midwife's skill, reputation and social standing derived from experience, experience in the double meaning of that term which, on the one hand, described the possession of traditional wisdom and lore and, on the other, referred to direct and personal empirical practice. The midwife's esteem in the community was founded on these qualities, and these qualities established her communication with the woman she attended. Two Italian words for the midwife of the eighteenth century, *comare* and *mammana*, were both derived from mater or mother. And, when all is said and done, 'mothering' is what her task entailed. Mercurio Scipione, the author of *La Comare o Ricoglitrice* (1596), one of the earliest midwifery manuals in the Italian vernacular, described her as 'like a mother' (*'come una madre'*).[6] Like a mother, she had conceived, carried and given birth to children, and as a mother she could help, comfort and advise. The rural midwives were all 'advanced in years to the point of seeing this as the chief qualification for the job'.[7] This was also one of the first points to emerge from an enquiry held in the Duchy of Milan around mid-century, while the midwives rolls in many city archives confirm the fact that a midwife had to be either married or a widow, of a fairly advanced age and with long professional experience. When registration on the midwives rolls was made compulsory by the health authorities, all the applicants fitted these criteria. Those listed on the Verona Roll of 1755 (one of the oldest extant) were all married, with decades of experience behind them (a minimum of 16 years and maximum of 30). The same tendency was repeated in the Venice rolls several decades later.[8]

Daughters, daughters-in-law, nieces, grand-daughters, sisters and sisters-in-law of midwives were the most likely apprentices in the profession, as was true for all other female crafts: skills were passed on, but all within the network of female relations. The reputation of the *'maestra'* (teacher-midwife) was all-important and apprenticeship, based on active co-operation and work sharing, lasted many years. In petitions for registration on the midwives roll made to the Venetian Health Authority (one of the most famous and efficient), the question of the length of apprenticeship arises time and again. One Venetian midwife wrote in 1771:

For eighteen years I, Giacomina Marcaina, daughter of Orsola Bobbi, midwife of Giudecca with the approval of the Above Eminent

Magistracy, have assisted my mother in the above-mentioned profession. My mother herself is now advanced in years, being 79, and is
present at nearly all the births.[9]

Some of the *maestra* midwives had more than one apprentice, and almost
certainly drew occasionally on the help of such as servant girls, neighbours
and co-tenants, giving the magistracy much cause for complaint.[10]

The midwife's sphere of activity was not limited to pregnancies and
births. It also included female maladies, especially those related to sexuality. It
was the *levatrice* whom women consulted about irregular menstrual cycles,
breast-feeding, sterility, rape or venereal disease. Evidence for this comes
principally from criminal proceedings rather than health records. The
midwife was always present at such trials, as for those for infanticide, called
in either by the plaintiff or by the court.[11]

When Caterina Brighenti of Venice discovered that her 7-year-old daughter
had a strange discharge she immediately took her to the midwife, who
confirmed not only that the child had been raped but also that she had
contracted a venereal disease. These facts were reported immediately to the
magistrates who ruled on such offences (*Esecutori contro la Bestemmia*), as
recorded in the minutes of the trial.[12] When Anna Perina Galvan began to
have strange pains and 'swelling' of the stomach, she called in the doctor but,
in fear that she might be pregnant, she also consulted the midwife, who did
something that is typical of her role and importance. Once she was sure that
the as yet unmarried girl was pregnant, she persuaded her to speak to her
family, and accompanied her to calm troubled waters.[13]

The main activity of the midwife, however, was to deliver children and
assist during labour. For this she had two instruments at her disposal. One
was the birthing chair, the other her own hands. The use of birthing chairs
is documented throughout Italy, to the point of their being the very symbol
of the midwife's craft. In an attempt to protect the profession, the
Magistratura della Sanità (health magistrature) in Venice passed a law pro-
hibiting other women from 'bringing in or leaving such chairs in the
house'.[14] Abbot Emanuele Cangiamila from Palermo in Sicily, wrote that
the midwife would seat the woman in labour on a special chair made for
births, called a *banco*; he is loud in his praise of their usefulness.[15] The stool
most commonly in use, according to one Venetian doctor, was a kind
of 'wooden armchair with two strong lateral supports and a strong back',
with a hole in the seat.[16] The woman was seated on the chair throughout
labour while the midwife crouched at her feet. According to Bernardino
Ramazzini, this was a tiring and uncomfortable position for the midwife,
which made her work more difficult than that of other European midwives.

In England, France, Germany and other countries, perhaps the
midwives suffer less in that the woman giving birth to her child stays

155

in her bed, and not on these seats with holes in them, as in Italy, so that she [the midwife] goes home all aches and pains, cursing the art that she has taken on.[17]

In the countryside, where these chairs were scarce to say the least, women gave birth on their feet or seated on another woman's lap. Apart from the other required characteristics, then, the Italian midwife had to be strong.[18] Her art was essentially manual; her main tools were her hands, since the care she provided was essentially based on massage, pressure and the administration of 'aromatic and warming remedies, generous wines, and broth enriched with freshly laid eggs'.[19] The notion behind this was that an absence of contractions or an excessively protracted labour were usually due to a lack of adequate nutrition; childbirth was, therefore, an effort to be aided with proper sustenance and nourishing food, a not altogether incorrect deduction at a time when the poor were almost universally underfed.

In difficult births the midwife resorted to bleeding, a practice which is very well documented.[20] Grevembroch describes how she applied, or re-quested the application of leeches, but, above all, the midwife intervened with a variety of manual operations, dilating the cervix and turning the foetus inside the uterus. Such practices were widely known and used by midwives, long before obstetricians formally codified them and claimed them as belonging to their own sphere of competence.[21]

The use of instruments to extract a dead child was probably not foreign to midwives, and there is evidence that they carried out this practice in the countryside. The Milan Medical Commission speaks of 'roughly made hooks' which, it appears, midwives used in extreme cases to pull out a dead foetus,[22] but, by the eighteenth century, this practice had all but died out in the towns, where a surgeon would be called in.

Once it had been brought into the world, the baby was washed, swaddled, dressed and made comfortable. In rural districts these tasks were followed by the cutting of the fraenulum under the tongue.[23] In the days following the birth, the midwife also took care of the mother; she 'put her back into shape' and 'applied leeches and other remedies'.[24]

This meant several days work for which there was no fixed tariff. Pay-ment, as Grevembroch says, varied 'according to the quality and conditions of the family'.[25] A midwife's earnings depended on the kind of customers she served, and the quarter where she worked; the midwife was morally bound to give her help free to needy families. 'Charity', in fact, was one of the gifts required of a midwife and her own social esteem was measured by it.[26] Apart from this, however, there was the matter of personal fame and prestige, differentiating one midwife from another and taken very much into account when it came to payment.

The midwife was a well-known figure in her quarter of the town or village. She walked the streets, went about her business in her neighbourhood, was seen by all. Everybody knew her house. In the towns, her sphere of activity nearly always encompassed the part of town in which she lived. From an enquiry based on the Venetian baptismal rolls for the year 1786, it was found that the majority of births were attended by midwives in their own quarters. This is an indication of direct acquaintance between the midwife and her customers.[27] Her very presence was enough to set people thinking of pregnancy and birth. The large and bulky chair she carried around with her did nothing to keep her work secret. For this very reason, when a woman wished to keep her pregnancy quiet, it was she who went to a midwife, and not the local one, when the time came to give birth. Given the lack of maternity hospitals, but even after their institution, the midwife's house often continued to function as a private clinic, especially for unmarried women who wanted to hide their 'sin'. This practice continued well into the nineteenth century in most Italian cities, despite repeated attempts by various governments to bring it to an end after the institution of maternity wards.[28] After the birth the midwife herself took the child to the hospice for abandoned children. In fact most of the children entering these institutions, legitimate or illegitimate, were consigned to them by the midwife. This was one of her duties; it was a particularly delicate one and she was paid well for it.[29]

Two other areas of her work were hidden from the public eye, contraception and abortion. Many women must have turned to her for information and intervention, expert as she was in pregnancy and the use of herbs. All the priestly admonitions, all the legal warnings to have nothing to do with such practices, stemmed from the necessary secrecy of this work; obviously any quantitative evaluation of it is impossible. It is hard to say just how many of the embryos pushed into cracks in the church walls or thrown into the cemetery (St Mark's was one of the traditional places for this) resulted from the interventions of the midwife. What is certain is that when her intervention was discovered, the punishments meted out were exemplary. She was excommunicated in public before the authorities and populace, then led off to serve her sentence.[30]

The midwife was expert in women's and new-born infants' illnesses; she was in absolute charge at births and she knew all there was to know about family secrets, illegitimate births and abandoned children, consigned to institutions. The midwife was an important, indeed central, figure in town life. It is no wonder, then, that first the Church and then the State tried to control her activities and make her a pawn in their own search for power.

Ecclesiastical control

In the days immediately following a birth, the midwife, the godfather and a crowd of relatives would take the child to church to be baptized. Out of all the women folk, this task was strictly reserved for the midwife. The mother went to church only after the ritual forty days' purification, to receive a solemn blessing following the impurity of birth, as was required by the Council of Trent (and was still required in the early years of our own century).[31]

The midwife's presence at the ceremony was highly symbolic. She had helped the child to come into the world and now she stood by it at its new birth (the spiritual and eternal one), its true birth into the Catholic culture, the birth that would open the gates of heaven and bless the child's entry into the civic community. She, who had welcomed it at its physical birth, now solemnly delivered it into the hands of the priest, to become a true 'child of God'. The midwife's presence in church is telling. It stands for her co-responsibility for the child's eternal salvation and at the same time her recognition of religious authority as the chief point of reference in her own activities.

Besides its importance as a sacrament, the ritual of baptism provided a valued opportunity for the priest to keep in touch with the midwife, so he could gather information about her activities and maintain some control, albeit indirectly, over the sexuality of his women parishioners. He could learn who the midwife's customers were and assess the scope and range of her activities. He could question her on her practices, as well as on matters of parenthood and on 'illegitimate' pregnancies, and check on the presence and movements of other midwives in his parish. Here too, the juridical records give us interesting insights into the community of midwives in the eighteenth century, particularly with regard to illicit unions and illegitimate births. The records of trials concerning the deflowering of virgins not only show how much credence was given to the midwife in such cases, but also the pressure that the parish priest could bring to bear. On 29 July 1794, a Venetian midwife delivered the child of one of these unfortunates. She took the baby to be baptized and declared, as was the practice, that the child was illegitimate of parents unknown. This the parish priest duly entered in the baptismal roll of the church, but later he must have drawn the midwife aside, and found out who the baby girl's parents were and the events surrounding the affair. This has come down to us through the court records of the ensuing lawsuit. A similar case was reported in Verona, where a priest found severe anomalies in the administration of the sacrament by a midwife. She had attempted to baptize infants during birth to calm the mothers. Again, another midwife, it was claimed in court records, had not used the exact words of the rite.[32]

Since the Counter-Reformation the Church had accorded the midwife special attention, endeavouring to give her role a specific outline within the Church's institutional structure. The social importance of the midwife and her part in the life of the community made her an important pawn in the post-Tridentine process of the Christianization of society, since the midwife was not only the one who administered the sacrament of baptism, but was also a well of information about female sexuality in the community. Baptism and morality were cornerstones of Counter-Reformation ecclesiastical policy. Doctrinal differences concerning the significance of baptism and the unredeemed souls of new-born infants had made both the practice and the diffusion of this sacrament an affirmation of orthodoxy and a battle against heresy, as Jacques Gélis has rightly pointed out.[33] The Church was also tightening its grip on female sexuality on the symbolic level of the observation of the '*iperdulia*' (higher veneration due to the Madonna),[34] and this process too was to involve the midwife.

It was of fundamental importance, then, that the midwife be brought under control, and the Church did not hesitate to engage in a hard fight to obtain this, with indictments and persecutions. As appears from the records of Inquisition trials in the sixteenth and seventeenth centuries, especially in the border areas of northern Italy, suspicions of witchcraft that had traditionally weighed on midwives were often tied in with accusations of magical practices and baptismal abuses.[35] In addition to repressive action, the Church aimed to exercise an educational role: various synods made it the duty of parish priests to instruct their midwives. This injunction became universal in the *Rituale Romanorum* of Pope Paul V (1614), a text which laid down the practice of sacraments, while supervision of the midwives' work in a given district was to be carried out by the bishops in their pastoral visits.[36] The obvious corollary to obligatory instruction was obligatory morality and religious staunchness; since this instruction involved the administration of a sacrament, the choice of who was to be a midwife passed into the hands of the clergy.[37]

By the eighteenth century this institutionalization was all but complete. By then, the midwife was a woman who not only enjoyed the approval of the parish priest but who was often chosen by him. In the countryside it was decidedly the priest who nominated the midwife. He did so from the altar after high mass on Sunday.

> It is the priest of the parish who selects the oldest woman or the one who is freest of obligations of husband and children. He instructs her in the formula of baptism and then announces her name from the altar for all the people to hear.[38]

Such control was not so easy in the towns where the population was more mobile. Here the Church moved in a more indirect way, issuing an official attestation of the right to administer sacraments. The Archiepiscopal Curia also carried out periodical checks on the midwives practising in the various dioceses. Fiocca informs us that in Rome, for example, these were implemented by Cardinal Vicario in the seventeenth century.[39]

During the eighteenth century this periodic check became more stringent in the fight against the practice of abortion and during the campaign for caesarean section post-mortem. Rigorist-Jansenist currents formed the background to open debate over recent discoveries in genetics, and a new understanding and interest in the field of infancy. Discoveries in embryology at the end of the seventeenth century had not only brought previous scientific ideas into doubt, but had also questioned the theological beliefs connected with them, thus leading to a reconsideration of animation and the beginning of life, as well as of the lot of unredeemed souls. De Graaf and Leeuwenhoek's discoveries of follicles and spermatozoi, using the recently developed microscope, and the examination of embryos, made the formation of the embryo, logically, a continuous process from the moment of conception. Regarding the implications as to when the human embryo could be considered to acquire a soul, the opposing theories of the 'ovists' and the 'animalculists' came together.[40] The new discoveries were obviously very much in favour of the thesis that animation and conception were simultaneous and not several days apart as Aristotelian tradition stated. Thus abortion, voluntary or spontaneous, each for their own reasons, took on a particularly grave aspect. It was no longer seen as a matter of a 'flux of blood' or of a still amorphous mass, but as the loss of an already present life and with it, therefore, a soul, something that set the rigorists and Jansenists to preaching hellfire and damnation sermons. The death of a pregnant woman at this point was just as disquieting, in that, dying, she was taking an unbaptized infant to the grave with her.

The eighteenth century, then, saw an intensification of the fight against abortion. Greater attention was paid to the practice of baptism. These movements once again, crossed the path of the midwife.[41] In 1679 Pope Innocent XI issued a decree condemning the 'laxity' which upheld later animation of the human foetus (that is, at birth) and the admissibility of abortion in the case of unmarried women. In 1732 Cardinal Lambertini (later Pope Benedict XIV) delivered a notification stressing the importance of accurate instruction for the midwives of the parish; 'that they should be *well* instructed in the administration of Baptism in cases of necessity'.[42]

What was being asked of the midwife was not only to know the formula of baptism in cases of necessity, but also to know how to baptize a several-months-old foetus, to know how to behave in cases of monstrosity and, above all, to recognize the difference between the so-called 'false germs' or fleshy masses in discharges of blood and an aborted foetus. This question attracted a great deal of theological and scientific debate.[43]

In 1746 a priest, Girolamo Baruffaldi, wrote a scientific and religious book of instruction, a catechism for midwives, that was used throughout Italy and eventually adopted in various schools of midwifery. Its title was *La Mammana istruita per validamente amministrare il Santo Sacramento del*

Battesimo in caso di necessità alle creature nascenti ('The Midwife Instructed in Administering the Holy Sacrament of Baptism in Cases of Necessity to Children During Birth'). In his foreword Baruffaldi called

> upon those women who want to become midwives to study or have themselves taught accurately and methodically not only to know which are the difficulties of Birth . . . but, God-willing, also the surest way to make them Christians since among Christians that midwife who be not learned in the circumstances of that faculty is not perfect.[44]

In 1745 the Sicilian theologian Cangiamila published his *Embriologia Sacra* with the subtitle 'The Office of Priests, Doctors and Superiors Concerning the Eternal Salvation of Children in the Womb'. This was a vast and learned work of four volumes, in which the abbot pleads for the adoption of a series of measures, one of which is caesarean section on women who have died while still carrying their child, even in the early stages of pregnancy. This is a task Cangiamila would refer to the surgeon but, where necessary, even to the midwife, and he enjoins the ecclesiastical and civil authorities to prepare her adequately for the task and to supply her with the necessary instruments. This was implemented in the Kingdom of Sicily by Charles III in 1749. Cangiamila's book enjoyed enormous success in the Catholic world, was approved by Pope Benedict XIV, ran through many editions and was translated in all the Catholic countries. Its content found echoes in many other works of its kind in the years that followed.

The midwife was, according to Church directives, to become a more responsible and competent figure. She had to have a certain training behind her and her work had to be viewed as skilled since she was now responsible for the eternal salvation, not only of new-born infants, but also even the smallest embryos deep inside the womb. The high number of new-borns christened during birth at the end of the eighteenth century, and the reports of abortions to be found in the archives of the time, are strong evidence for the diffusion of this preoccupation with, and fear for, the soul of the child. As often as not, it turns out to be the midwife herself who insists on the child being taken – even precociously – to the baptismal font.[45]

State intervention

Up until the mid-eighteenth century, interference by State institutions in the activities of midwives was rather limited and, when it did occur, it was intimately bound up with the aims and finalities of the Church. Directives issued in the name of the State in most instances built on decrees already formulated by the ecclesiastical institutions, or they entirely conformed with them, since their aims were fundamentally the same. The attempts made by historians to draw a clear line between Church and secular jurisdictional spheres ultimately remain contrived for this period, given that the two institutions generally interacted very closely. With a policy that was in perfect harmony with that of the Church, the secular authorities initially aimed to identify and to keep a close check on all midwifery practitioners. Access to the profession was regulated by norms which, in many instances, formalized and gave an official status to traditional forms of apprenticeship and, at the same time, they acknowledged the role of the parish priest.

In Venice, a state particularly advanced in respect to health measures, the *Magistratura di Sanità* ordered as early as 1624 that women aspiring to become midwives should come before a committee in order to obtain an official licence and to be entered on the midwives roll. Amongst her references, she was required to present a testimonial from the parish priest, confirming her capacity to administer baptism, and one from a midwife declaring that the woman had completed an apprenticeship of at least two years under her supervision.[46] In 1719, the Republic made attendance at anatomy sessions obligatory as part of the training of a midwife. However, as we can see from the midwives' heated assertions of never having time to attend anatomy sessions, and as evidenced by the fact that they were allowed to practise all the same, it was apprenticeship and parish approval that won the day.[47] The committee's examination was no more than a *pro forma*, as a Verona proclamation of 1755 insisting on its gratuitous nature suggests. None of the women who took the examination was failed, even if she lacked other paper qualifications.[48] The civic authorities tended to delegate responsibility for approving midwives to the parish priest with a clear recognition that this was his role.

In the mid-eighteenth century, however, there was a decided change in some states (the Duchy of Milan, the Grand Duchy of Tuscany and the Serene Republic of Venice). The main impulse derived from deep changes in the politics of 'Enlightened governments' (influenced by Enlightenment philosophical and political views), especially a growing and increasingly direct interest in the people, itself due to the princes' perception of the needs of their subjects and of the duties of rulers. This conviction was adopted as being at the very roots of government and the support of the State. Demographic expansion, therefore, became important for political affirmation and, concerned about expansion, the civil authorities turned to the doctors for assistance in bettering, qualitatively and quantitatively, the lot of the population. This new State *Polizia medica* (medical police), aimed at bringing mortality rates down and combating disease, was applied in the spirit of 'good government', as Panseri has put it 'a strategy for the elimination of the causes, moral and physical, of de-population'.[49] The first preoccupation of Enlightened government was to reduce infant mortality which had reached alarming proportions. As a Treviso doctor declared in 1777 in a letter to the Venetian *Magistratura della Sanità*, infant mortality was decimating 'that class which is most useful to the State'.[50]

Measures were taken to care for poor pregnant women and to ensure that the poorest quarters of the towns had the services of a midwife, as was implemented in Florence and Turin.[51] With respect to training, a new midwife was created, but with a reduced area of competence. The Enlightenment governments, then, together with the demands, public and private, of the doctors, provided new objectives for regulating the midwife. High infant mortality was unthinkingly attributed to the ignorance and inability of those who delivered children, and this, logically, gave rise to a whole battery of new laws on midwifery training and practice and an official fight against illegal practitioners. As it happened, the accusations against midwives could not be proven, but they created a climate where all hopes were founded on 'science' and its prospects and development.[52] In this climate of scientific development and reform in public education, many Italian states opened schools of obstetrics for both surgeons and midwives. The states also recognized some of the private schools set up by doctors to train midwives and surgeons.

Between 1757 and 1779, for the most part in Venice and the Duchies, thirteen midwifery schools were founded.[53] In the neighbourhood of either a hospital or an anatomy theatre, with accommodation for trainee midwives from the rural areas, these schools were all run by surgeons, who taught using various '*suppelletix obstetrica*', such as drawings and models of the body in glass, wood or wax. Manzolini Brothers in Bologna became specialists in manufacturing such teaching aids.

Those who wanted to become midwives had to show that they could read and write, that they could memorize theoretical ideas, and give proof of attendance at anatomy classes but, above all, that they could understand what they had been taught.[54] The examination was a true test of what these would-be midwives had learnt on the course; they were the 'new' or 'modern' midwives, very much acclaimed and à la mode at a time when modernity meant science.

The break with tradition was clear and profound. No older or illiterate women became midwives. This eliminated the majority of ordinary working-class or rural women from practice. The unquestionable authority of male doctors meant that it was no longer the midwife who gave access to the profession, choosing her own apprentices; her social autonomy and professional standing in the community diminished.

Enlightened governments also set about codifying, in detail, all the therapeutic tasks involved in obstetrics, assigning some to the surgeon, some to the physician and some to the midwife. Medicines taken by mouth could not be given by the midwife, the midwife could not apply leeches, nor could she use any instrument 'useful though it be in the obstetric art'.[55] This meant that the midwife was only authorized to carry out normal deliveries.

The break with tradition and new conflicts

The new Enlightened policy of governments had a very different impact in the various Italian states with regard to the role and function accredited to the midwife. In the Papal States and the Two Sicilies, training did not stray very far from the old ways, and new laws actually enabled the midwife to use instruments where deemed necessary. 'Scholarship' as a condition for access to the profession was something that was imposed in the 'Enlightened' states in the north of the country. Here the midwife's duties were drastically reduced, while the role of the obstetric surgeon and his authority during births was upheld. This had a double effect. First, the old harmony between Church and midwife was destroyed and, second, conflict developed among the midwives themselves, especially during the last three decades of the eighteenth century.

The Church authorities saw their traditional hold on the midwife evaporating. They looked on both the new figure of the doctor and the scientific approach to female sexuality with suspicion, as being outside their direct control. The reaction of the priesthood at the time was also twofold. Some theologians entered into the new debate, taking up research and experimentation, which they directed at interpreting and upholding the priority of the spiritual life of the foetus in the womb. But the majority of the clergy, above all its lower echelons, took up the cause of those who greeted this new debate with incomprehension, and it was they who led the opposition. Many cases are recorded of parish priests turning in protest to the authorities to ask that the law admit exceptions, to plead the cause of aged midwives in no position to go to school, and to assure the magistracy of their ability and devotion.[56]

The strongest opposition arose in the rural areas. The parish priests related their parishioners' refusal to send their daughters to school in the town. Married women were in no position to go, not only because of family commitments and heavy work-loads, but also because of the diffidence and moral suspicion aroused by uprooting a woman from her family and exposing her to the dangers of the town. The schools did not find pupils easily, especially from the countryside. In Milan, in 1791, the school's first year, only ten pupils enrolled. Again only ten attended the Padua school in 1776.[57] In Venice the average attendance in 1794 was five.[58] Even among those who attended, the results were not always positive, and did not necessarily lead to the re-establishment of a 'state registered midwife' in her home environment. In many cases she was simply rejected either on grounds of moral suspicion or because, as a result of the knowledge and skills that she had obtained, a cultural gulf had opened up between her and her own people. In the countryside surrounding Milan, some parish priests refused outright to have anything to do with midwives from the city's midwifery school.

> Some parish priests refuse to publicly proclaim the names of mid-wives, from the altar, even though these are qualified to practise their art by the Faculty of Medicine. It seems that it is claimed, with undue presumption, that it is the priest who still has the right to sanction this activity.[59]

Empress Maria Theresa of Austria found herself constrained from inter-vening directly with the Archiepiscopal Curia in very firm terms, but in December 1770 she revindicated the State's rights in this matter, citing the relevant laws, and demanding that the clergy be called to order. A power struggle ensued, resulting in numerous regulations, suggestions and requests. One example of this was the question of the veto on the use of instruments. While some states prohibited their use to the midwife, the Church, as we have already seen, more preoccupied with the spiritual than the material welfare of the child, even in the womb, actually obliged her to do a caesarean section post-mortem in cases of necessity. J.P. Frank, speaking out against the fanaticism of some parish priests,[60] was very explicit on this point. In 1794 a midwife was put on trial in the Duchy of Milan for carrying out a caesarean section, following the priest's instructions.[61] Similar dissension between Church and State developed out of the question of excessively precocious baptism, which often implied a lengthy journey and exposure of the infant which might itself lead to its death. With regard to the abandonment of children to the hospices, late in the eighteenth century when the State was trying to reduce this practice, the parish priests were pushing in the other direction, approving the consignment of illegitimate children to the institutions to keep scandal out of the parish. And indeed the rate of abandonment did rise early in the nineteenth century.[62] The Austrian government finally intervened, publishing a circular in 1832 'On the obligation of parish priests not to suggest that mothers put their illegitimate babies into hospices'.[63]

The new regulations created splits within the body of midwives them-selves, at times developing into open conflict. Various strategies were employed by these women when dealing with the law. Some openly ignored it, and went on working as they had always done. Others recog-nized it, but did not follow it. For some this was impossible (for example, for those who were illiterate or who could not leave their villages); others wished to avoid the law for reasons of expediency, pleading exceptional circumstances with the magistrates. There were also those who followed the law to the letter often in the hope of acquiring a steadier income, 'to establish themselves in their work' or to overcome competition.[64]

The earliest result, then, of these new laws was schism and the beginnings of differentiation between literate and illiterate midwives, between countryside and town, where there was the opportunity to attend school, and between the more and the less educated, with the creation of the new institutional midwives, the teacher-midwife (in the midwifery schools that had been founded in a number of hospitals), and the municipal midwives, nominated to assist poor women in some northern cities in the 1780s.[65] Out of this arose profound incomprehension, reciprocal suspicion and open professional conflict. The new graduates from the schools all too often saw their hopes of secure employment dashed. The innovation that they represented to the community was often rejected, especially in the countryside. At Abbiate Guzzone, a village near Milan, the inhabitants refused to pay a graduate what the old midwives received, being 'disgusted at the new midwife because she had been to the hospital and seen anatomical demonstrations when she was at school there'.[66] The new graduates who were at the forefront in the battle against illegality, turned to the magistrates to resolve their difficulties. The volume of 'appeals' made by the 'authorized' midwives against the 'unauthorized' ones, is large enough to demonstrate a split in the profession that drew in all the forces of the law. The old midwives upheld tradition, unwritten law and their own work. Their advocates were the parish priest and the people. The new, 'state registered' midwives called on the support of civil law and the necessity of education and authorization. They were proud of their diplomas and the name of the professor who had taught them. The basic aim of both groups, however, was the same – a steady job; their methods of going about this were different, but they were also proud of the differences.

What is interesting in this whole picture of schism is the position taken by some of the better-educated midwives who tried to mediate in the conflict. They did not underestimate the value of tradition, yet, at the same time, saw the importance of education in the sciences associated with midwifery, which they regarded as the means of sustaining this traditionally female province.

One of these figures was Teresa Ployant, a French midwife working as a *maestra* in the Incurabili in Naples during the last thirty years of the century. In the foreword to her midwifery manual, the *Breve Compendio dell' Arte Ostetricia* (1787), the only manual to be written by a woman in Italy in the eighteenth century, she set out her reasons for taking such a task in hand, declaring that she has written the book to encourage women to study 'not as the occasion demands but methodically and according to the principles proper to an art so necessary to the people',[67] in order to conserve this art for women. Teresa Ployant's cause, which became that of many other midwives, such as Benedetta Trevisan in Venice in 1800 and

Maddalena De Marinis in Naples in 1838, was simple: to participate in what they called the 'bettering' of the art, improving the midwives' practice through scientific knowledge, accepting the professional nature of their craft, and winning back a monopoly in the field from the male doctors who were invading it. So Ployant urged women to go to midwifery school, while recognizing the fact that the midwives' knowledge is rooted in their being women or, as Benedetta Trevisan wrote in 1800, 'not of a different sex'.[68] For women like these, the risks to the profession were not those connected to schismatic conflict, but rather those of losing their role in childbirth altogether with the advent of the obstetrician and his 'horrible instruments of cruelty'. They were turning their eyes to the northern European situation, where 'they already leave the pregnant woman in the hands of men',[69] a threat, as they saw it, incumbent on Italy. Ployant concluded with a heartfelt appeal to women in the name of women:

> Let us then be quick to stem this fatal turn of events and through untiring study make the public realize that we are the ones that can bring births to a happy outcome and at the same time save women's modesty.[70]

Surgeons and '*mammane*'

Teresa Ployant and Benedetta Trevisan were writing about their work around the end of the eighteenth century. The picture they give is of an Italy where births were still very much the province of the midwife. The man-midwife's appearances were still sporadic, not to say exceptional, and masculine competition in the profession was felt more as a threat than reality. In their eyes, Italy was privileged in Europe as a whole.

This difference is worthy of note because it is characteristic of Italy: throughout the century, the presence of the man-midwife at a birth was rare to say the least, a fact recognized by the Colleges of Surgeons themselves.[71] Surgeons who took up obstetrics – the *chirurghi-ostetricanti* – were few up until the end of the eighteenth century. The more precise and formal definition of the figure of the obstetrician, as a surgeon specializing in difficult births, was only reached in the early nineteenth century. The law obliged the midwife to call for a surgeon in difficult births, and in many states only the surgeon had the right to use obstetrical instruments. Yet instruments were used in only a few cases; on the rare occasions when it did happen, it was exceptional enough to be published in the scientific press.

Forceps, for example, were known in Italy from the middle of the eighteenth century, but their use was very limited. They were successfully used for the first time in Venice in 1766. Benedetto Maja, who applied them, lost no time in informing the College of Surgeons and the most illustrious professors of the neighbouring universities.[72] However, they were employed by only a small number of surgeons, such as Giuseppe Vespa, a pupil of the French man-midwife Levret, and holder of the chair in obstetrics founded at the Hospital Santa Maria Nuova in Florence in 1761, and another of Levret's pupils, Lorenzo Nannoni, a demonstrator in surgery and obstetrics in the Innocenti Hospital in Florence since 1794. Cangiamila knew only of the '*speculum matricis*', and says that it was rarely used in Sicily.[73]

The first caesarean section on a living patient was carried out in the small Istrian village of Pirano in 1780. The surgeon who conducted the operation published an article on the subject, but his work brought him so little fame that he died in poverty in Venice. By the end of the century, his example had been followed by only two other surgeons.[74] The first symphyseotomy was carried out in Genoa in 1781 by the surgeon Antonio Lavagnino. It aroused the wrath of the whole city to the point that the funeral of the woman, who died after the operation, had to take place at night 'to avoid any scandalous consequences'.[75] One, albeit indirect, confirmation of the paucity of activity on the part of surgeons is provided in the nominations to university posts in obstetrics and to the midwifery schools. Posts were awarded on the grounds of competence, but most candidates had only a theoretical background and a history of articles and studies.[76] The only field in which claims were made for practical experience was that of caesarean section post-mortem, something which could hardly be considered as obstetric experience.

Men-midwives at the end of the eighteenth century, then, were theoreticians rather than practitioners, but it must be said that, given the dearth of maternity homes in Italy at the time, in contrast to many larger cities in Northern Europe, that they had precious little chance of gaining practical experience.[77] The defamation campaign launched against the midwife in Italy thus took on a quite different character from the rest of Europe. It aimed at control of them and the services they rendered rather than engaging in professional conflict and competition. This is confirmed by the great effort that was put into training midwives, an effort that brought together urban and rural doctors, and which produced huge numbers of manuals intended for midwives. There were no less than twenty-four manuals published between the 1760s and the close of the century.[78]

Italy stands out from other European countries in the eighteenth century for many reasons – the opposition of the Catholic Church to the involvement of doctors in obstetrics, the climate of public opinion which was opposed to change, the strong aversion on the part of childbearing women to the presence of a male practitioner and, finally, the prestige of the midwife amongst women.

168

> The demureness of women and their absolutely unreasonable
> blushing at exposing themselves to who could be of help to them
> [says a doctor in 1774] lies at the root of the midwife practising this
> very important art of obstetrics.[79]

Blushing and shame, along with other basic aspects of the culture of the
time, was also bound up with confidence in the art of the midwife and the
credit she enjoyed in the community. 'Confidence' was a frequently used
word in the writings of those days. 'In our Italy', said the famous Bolognese
surgeon Gian Antonio Galli, 'women giving birth are used to claiming her
help alone and having confidence in only the skill of the midwife.'[80] The
Milan Medical Commission, enquiring into midwives' activities in the area,
reported to the government that women will 'confide' only 'in persons of
their own sex'.[81] In other words, it is to the midwife, the 'other mamma',
that women were sure they could turn. Even if she could not read or write,
her charges were 'very glad' that she was there. Cringing, real diffidence,
even horror and repulsion might well be the words to describe how they
felt about the attentions of the surgeon. The College of Surgeons in Venice
recognized that 'women giving birth like to be assisted by women, and it is
rare to find one who does not shudder with fear at being handled by one
of the men who practise the art'.[82] When one reads accounts of the time,
and learns of the ham-handedness and truculence with which doctors
operated, one is left in no doubt of why women reacted as they did.

The better-educated midwives, gathering in their own defence the
notion of protecting female modesty, their competence in dealing with
their own sex and rejection of surgeons in the field, not only took up the
cudgels on the part of their sister-midwives, but also appealed more widely
to the sensibilities of all women. Public opinion was on their side as far as
the assumption of the art by male surgeons was concerned.

Even one so much informed by the spirit of the Enlightenment as
Ludovico Antonio Muratori, author of *Della Pubblica Felicità* (1749), found
it 'more decent' that the art should be practised by women and underlined
the fact that the important thing, as far as public welfare was concerned,
was to educate them. This was a thought shared by many a doctor and even
a few famous surgeons, Bertrandi, Malacarne and Valota. The latter were
also in favour of women learning to use surgical instruments, since they not
only had considerable manual skill, but also because in some remote
country areas there was next to no chance of finding a surgeon for difficult
births. The profound roots that the midwife with all her dexterity had in
the community led these doctors to believe that the midwife could still be
useful. Certain functions and competence should not have been taken out
of their hands; indeed new instruments could be given to them. Even
among doctors, then, there were differences of opinion.

In the end, however, at least in principle, the midwife's practice and her role was to be cut down. French influence was to be a determining factor with the Napoleonic armies spreading – apart from revolutionary politics – the social welfare structures and new approaches that were widespread in their own country. The creation of maternity hospitals and clinics, launched by the French and continued by many Italian governments, was decisive in strengthening the man-midwife.

A further turning point in Italian obstetrical history was the development of the obstetrician, from being only a practitioner of instrumental surgery, into a practitioner of what was classified as 'minor' or manual surgery at the turn of the nineteenth century, leaving the midwife as a '*raccoglitrice del bambino*', a kind of nurse.[83]

But contradictions would not die out for a very long time. There was conflict between law and reality and, throughout the nineteenth century, the unauthorized midwife dominated, especially in country areas outside the control of doctors. Law and reality were to run a parallel race for a long time yet, and, when they did meet it could result in either compromise or conflict. For the most part, however, they remained strangers to each other.[84] The changing status of the midwife and the takeover of the man-midwife was a longer and more complex process than what the eighteenth century itself, with all its Enlightened ideals in medicine and politics, had promised.

Acknowledgements

I am grateful to Hilary Marland for her generous support and to Dr Lidia Sciama and Dr Maria Balboni for their advice regarding translation.

Notes

1. A. Corradi, *Dell' Ostetricia in Italia dalla metà del secolo scorso fino al presente* (Bologna, 1874), 49.

2. There are two main lines of research on the midwife and obstetric practice in Italy. Medical historical studies of the eighteenth century are often eulogistic in tone and carried out by doctors. For example, Corradi, *Dell' Ostetricia in Italia*; A. Guzzoni degli Ancarani, *L'Italia Ostetrica* (Catania, 1902); O. Viana and F. Vozza, *L'Ostetricia e la Ginecologia in Italia* (Milano, 1933); E. Curatolo, *L'Arte di Juno Lucina in Roma. Storia dell' Ostetricia dalle sue origini sino al secolo XX* (Roma, 1901); G.M. Nardi, *Il Pensiero Ostetrico-Ginecologico nei secoli* (Milano, 1954); L. Premuda, *Personaggi e vicende dell' ostetricia e della ginecologia nello studio di Padova* (Padova, 1958); L. Belloni, *La Scuola Ostetrica milanese dai Moscati ai Porro. Cenni storici* (Milano, 1960). A more recent and specialized line of research is within the field of gender history, usually undertaken by women scholars, which flourished during the 1980s. See L. Accati, V. Maher and G. Pomata (eds) *Parto e Maternità: momenti della autobiografia femminile*, *Quaderni Storici*, 44 (1980); G. Pomata, 'Barbieri e

comari', in *Medicina, erbe e magia* (Milano, 1981); F. Pizzini (ed.) *Sulla scena del parto: luoghi, figure e pratiche* (Milano, 1981); D. Pillon, 'La comare istruita nel suo ufficio. Alcune notizie sulle levatrici fra il '600 e il '700', *Atti dell' Istituto Veneto di Scienze, Lettere e Arti*, 140 (1981), 65–78; *idem*, 'Medici e mammane nel '700. La scuola ostetrica di Padova', *Schema*, 5 (1982), 159–65; G. Calvi, 'Manuali delle levatrici (sec. XVII–XVIII)', *Memoria. Rivista di Storia delle Donne*, 3 (1983), 108–13; G. Fiocca, 'Mammane e medici a Roma tra sette e ottocento', in A. Lazzarini (ed.) *Economia e società nella storia dell' Italia Contemporanea. Fonti e metodi di ricerca* (Roma, 1983), 143–53; C. Pancino, 'La comare levatrice. Crisi di un mestiere nel XVIII secolo', *Società e Storia*, 13 (1981), 593–638; *idem*, *Il Bambino e l'acqua sporca. Storia dell' assistenza al parto dalle mammane alle ostetriche (secoli XVI–XIX)* (Milano, 1984); A. Parma, 'Didattica e pratica ostetrica in Lombardia (1765–1791)', *Sanità, Scienza e Storia*, 2 (1984), 101–55; N.M. Filippini, 'Con le mani disarmate: la vicenda di una levatrice-chirurgo veneziana (1800–1802)', *Sanità, Scienza e Storia*, 2 (1984), 156–72; *idem*, 'Levatrici e ostetricanti a Venezia tra sette e ottocento', *Quaderni Storici*, 58 (1985), 149–80; A. Lonni, 'Il mestiere di ostetrica al confine tra il lecito e l'illecito', *Società e Storia*, 25 (1984), 563–90; A. Oakley *et al.*, *Le Culture del parto* (Milano, 1985); L. Chinosi (ed.) *Nascere a Venezia. Dalla Serenissima alla Prima Guerra Mondiale* (Torino, 1985); L. Guidi, 'Parto e maternità a Napoli nell' ottocento: carità e solidarietà spontanee, beneficenza istituzionale (1840–1880)', *Sanità, Scienza e Storia*, 1 (1986), 111–48. Much of this research is local in character and confined to northern Italy.

3. G. Grevembroch, *Gli Abiti dei Veneziani di quasi ogni età con diligenza raccolti e dipinti nel secolo XVIII* (Museo Correr, Venezia, n.d., presumed 1754).

4. In 1760 the city of Venice had a population of 149,476 and births in that year totalled 4,996. The average number of births per midwife per annum, as reported by Beltrami, was fifty. These data should be treated with great caution, as there are differences in the figures for civil and ecclesiastical registration. A. Beltrami, *Storia della popolazione di Venezia dalla fine del secolo XVI alla caduta della Repubblica* (Padova, 1954).

5. This is how widowed and unmarried midwives were registered. Social standing can often be gauged by the trade of the husband, as indicated in apprenticeship listings in the midwives roll for Venice in 1790. The husbands were employed in the poorest and least reliable trades, as waiters, cooks, tailors, shoemakers, boatmen, masons, porters, etc. State Archives of Venezia (hereafter ASV), Provveditori alla Sanità, b.584.

6. M. Scipione, *La Comare o Ricoglitrice* (Venezia, 1596), 72.

7. Parma, 'Didattica e pratica ostetrica', 117.

8. The Verona midwives roll covers the years 1755 to 1821 and includes examination results. State Archives of Verona (hereafter ASVR), Ufficio Sanità, Registri 31. In Venice there are rolls for the years 1786 and 1790; the names of apprentices are listed alongside the name of the midwife.

9. ASV, Provveditori alla Sanità, b.589.

10. A 1774 law of the Provveditori alla Sanità in Venice complained of 'certain midwives . . . using in such a craft, as jealously guarded as it is inexpert, those who usually are their serving-wenches'. ASV, Compilazione leggi, b.277. The information comes from Grevembroch, *Gli Abiti de Veneziani*.

11. For the role of midwife as expert witness in England and Germany, see chs 2, 3 and 4 in this volume by David Harley, Ann Giardina Hess and Merry Wiesner.

12. Processo per deflorazione e successiva infezione gallica di Antonia Elisabetta Brighenti, 23 marzo 1795. ASV, Esecutori contro la Bestemmia, b.47. For such trials, see M. Gambié, 'La donna e la giustizia penale veneziana nel XVIII

secolo', in G. Cozzi (ed.) *Stato, Giustizia e Società nella Repubblica Veneta (Sec. XV–XVIII)* (Roma, 1980), 529–70.

13. Processo per deflorazione con promessa di matrimonio di Anna Perina Galvan, 1 agosto 1794. ASV, Esecutori contro la Bestemmia, b.47.

14. Terminazione, 24 febbraio 1624. ASV, Provveditori alla Sanità, Notatorio 739.

15. F. E. Cangiamila, *Embriologia Sacra. Ovvero dell' Ufficio de' Sacerdoti, Medici e Superiori circa l'Eterna Salute de' Bambini racchiusi nell' utero* (Palermo, 1745), 168.

16. J. Panzani, 'Un parto difficile', *Giornale di Medicina*, 12 (1774), 253.

17. Pancino, *Il Bambino e l'acqua sporca*, 38.

18. Pillon, 'Medici e mammane nel '700', 67.

19. Panzani, 'Un parto difficile', 253.

20. Pomata, 'Barbieri e comari'.

21. The Dean of the Venice College of Surgeons wrote in 1800, 'At this moment, midwives make use of leeches and manual operations, illicitly.' Letter of 13 Dec. 1800. Cited in Filippini, 'Levatrici e ostetricanti', 179, n. 70.

22. Parma, 'Didattica e pratica ostetrica', 103.

23. F. Della Peruta, 'Infanzia e famiglia nella prima metà dell' ottocento', *Studi Storici*, 3 (1979), 487.

24. Grevembroch, *Gli Abiti dei Veneziani*, III, 154.

25. Ibid.

26. Pillon, 'La comare istruita nel suo ufficio', 75.

27. My research was carried out in the parish of San Giacomo dell' Orio, in Sante Croce, Venice for the year 1786. Cross-referencing the names of midwives in the baptismal rolls and midwives rolls, it was possible to confirm that 84 per cent of the births in the parish were attended by four of the midwives resident in the quarter. The remaining 16 per cent of births was distributed amongst eleven other midwives from rather more distant parishes. Parish Archives of San Giacomo dell' Orio (Venezia), Libro Battezzi 1785–92. For repeat practice in seventeenth-century London, see ch. 1 in this volume by Doreen Evenden.

28. N.M. Filippini, 'L'assistenza al parto nel primo ottocento: appunti sull' intervento istituzionale', in Oakley *et al.*, *Le Culture del parto*, 64; Guidi, 'Parto e maternità a Napoli nell' ottocento', 115.

29. See G. Cappelletto, 'Infanzia abbandonata e ruoli di mediazione sociale nella Verona del settecento', *Quaderni Storici*, 53 (1983), 421–44; and V. Hunecke, *I Trovatelli di Milano. Bambini esposti e famiglie espositrici dal XVII al XIX Secolo* (Bologna, 1989), 125–30.

30. Processo per deflorazione con promessa di matrimonio di Anna Perina Galvan, 1 agosto 1794.

31. N.M. Filippini, *Noi, quelle dei campi. Identità e rappresentazione di sé delle contadine veronesi del primo novecento* (Torino, 1983), 76–84.

32. The 1832 report can be found in a bulky enquiry into midwives' activities, undertaken by the civil authorities on the request of the clergy. ASVR, Sanità, b.219.

33. J. Gélis, *La sage femme ou le médecin. Une nouvelle conception de la vie* (Paris, 1988).

34. L. Accati, 'Il padre naturale. Tra simboli dominanti e categorie scientifiche', *Memoria. Rivista di Storia delle Donne*, 21 (1987), 79–106; *idem*, 'Matrimony and chastity', *International Journal of Moral and Social Studies*, 1 (1990), 23–33.

35. See C. Ginzburg, *I Benandanti. Stregoneria e culti agrari tra cinquecento e seicento* (Torino, 1966). Taking a stillborn child to church in the hopes of a

momentary revival so that he might be baptized was widespread in northern Italy, in Trentino and Friuli in particular. This rite was carried out by women. The Holy Office definitively condemned these practices in 1729. See S. Cavazza, 'La doppia morte: resurrezione e battesimo in un rito del seicento', *Quaderni Storici*, 50 (1982), 551–82; J. Gélis, *L'Arbre et le Fruit. La naissance dans l'occident moderne XVIe–XIXe siècle* (Paris, 1984), 509–20.

36. Pancino, *Il Bambino e l'acqua sporca.*

37. For the involvement of the Church in midwife regulation in England and Spain, see chs 1, 2 and 5 in this volume, and for the midwife's role in baptism in early modern Germany, ch. 4 by Merry Wiesner.

38. Parma, 'Didattica e pratica ostetrica', 102.

39. Fiocca, 'Mammane e medici a Roma', 147.

40. P. Darmon, *Le mythe de la procréation à l'âge baroque* (Paris, 1977).

41. I am completing a doctoral thesis on this question and that of caesarean section for the École des Hautes Études en Sciences Sociales in Paris, 'La naissance extraordinaire. Transformations culturelles et sociales dans la pratique de la césarienne, entre dix-huitième et dix-neuvième siècle' (forthcoming 1993).

42. Pancino, *Il Bambino e l'acqua sporca*, 77 (Filippini's emphasis).

43. E. Brambilla, 'La medicina del settecento: dal monopolio dogmatico alla professione scientifica', in F. Della Peruta (ed.) *Malattia e Medicina. Annali 7* (Torino, 1984), 5–147.

44. G. Baruffaldi, *La Mammana istruita per validamente amministrare il Santo Sacramento del Battesimo in caso di necessità alle creature nascenti* (Verona, 1746), 8.

45. Here too I consulted the baptismal rolls for San Giacomo (see note 27) for 1786 with the following results: 20 per cent of new-born infants were baptized by the parish priest at home for fear they should die, 35.7 per cent were taken to be baptized in church the day of their birth or the following day, 33 per cent on the second or third day after their birth. Thus more than half the children born in the parish were christened on the day of their birth or the following day.

46. Filippini, 'Levatrici e ostetricanti'.

47. In Venice, for example, an apprentice midwife, Bortola Marchesini, hotly affirmed 'not having time' to go to anatomy demonstrations but to know all there is to know about 'all that the above-mentioned demonstration can show'. Bortola Marchesini was not alone in making declarations of this kind. ASV, Provveditori alla Sanità, b.589.

48. This proclamation is dated 16 Sept. 1755. ASVR, Ufficio Sanità, b. XLV. Similar regulations, with analogous formality, also were in force in the Papal States. See Fiocca, 'Mammane e medici a Roma'.

49. G. Panseri, 'La nascita della polizia medica: l'organizzazione sanitaria nei vari stati italiani', in G. Micheli (ed.) *Scienza e tecnica nella cultura e nella società dal rinascimento a oggi, Storia d'Italia. Annali 3* (Torino, 1980), 192.

50. The Treviso doctor was Giuseppe Zara. See Filippini, 'Levatrici e ostetricanti', 158–9. J.P. Frank, who was government councillor for medical issues in the Duchy of Milan, dedicated a chapter of his *System einer Vollstandigen Medizinischen Polizei* (Mannheim, 1779–88) to this problem. Frank's work was translated into Italian, with the title *Sistema Completo di Polizia Medica* (Milan, 1807). The relevant chapter is 'Della cura che in ogni Repubblica aver si deve delle partorienti e delle puerpere', in vol. II.

51. M.T. Caffaratto, *L'Ospedale Maggiore di San Giovanni Battista e della città di Torino. Sette secoli di assistenza socio-sanitaria* (Torino, 1984); Pancino, *Il Bambino e l'acqua sporca.*

52. Infant mortality rates, as elaborated by Beltrami, *Storia della Popolazione,*

161–70, belie this theory. In fact infant mortality rates (from birth to 1 year of age) were rising at this time. The rate was 30 per cent in the early years of the seventeenth century, increasing to 40 per cent by the end of 1797. The institution of a midwifery school in 1770 made no difference to these rates, which yield other information if broken down into months. For example, in 1760 6.2 per cent of infant deaths occurred at birth, 62.4 per cent within the first 3 months, and 31 per cent between 3 months and 1 year. The greatest number of infant deaths, then, were not at the moment of birth but rather within the first 3 months of life. Causes included exposure to the cold (also for precocious baptism), and poor feeding and infant care practices, exacerbated, as Beltrami has pointed out, by a progressive deterioration in living conditions for the poorer classes throughout the century.

53.   Pancino, *Il Bambino e l'acqua sporca*, 92–121.

54.   This echoes traditions outlined in ch. 6 in this volume by Helen King. For more structured forms of midwife training in Spain, France and Holland, see chs 5, 7 and 10 in this volume.

55.   Filippini, 'Levatrici e ostetricanti', 154.

56.   Pancino, *Il Bambino e l'acqua sporca*, 136–9; Pillon, 'La comare istruita nel suo ufficio', 74–5.

57.   Parma, 'Didattica e pratica ostetrica', 153; Pillon, 'Medici e mammane nel '700', 162.

58.   Filippini, 'Levatrici e ostetricanti', 176.

59.   Parma, 'Didattica e pratica ostetrica', 136.

60.   Frank, *Sistema Completo di Polizia Medica*.

61.   Pancino, *Il Bambino e l'acqua sporca*, 150–9.

62.   The rate doubled between the 1780s and the decade 1810–19. Some 1,938 foundlings were abandoned in the city of Milan alone, compared with 359 in the years 1780–89. Hunecke, *I Trovatelli di Milano*, Table 1.

63.   N.M. Filippini, 'Il bambino prezioso: maternità e infanzia negli interventi istituzionali del primo ottocento', in Chinosi, *Nascere a Venezia*, 37.

64.   Domenica Fadiga, a midwife working in what is now Porec (then in Istria), chose to go to school in Venice in 1781, to have 'such an important title' solely to overcome competition from others in her trade. ASV, Provveditori alla Sanità, b.589. The pupils' point of view has tended to be overlooked in recent research.

65.   M.T. Caffaratto, 'L'assistenza ostetrica in Piemonte dalle origini ai nostri tempi', *Giornale di Batteriologia, Virologia ed Immunologia*, 1: 6 (1970), 176–209.

66.   Pancino, *Il Bambino e l'acqua sporca*, 130–1.

67.   T. Ployant, *Breve Compendio dell' Arte Ostetricia* (Napoli, 1787). Quote taken from 3rd edn (Bologna, 1803), 4.

68.   Filippini, 'Con le mani disarmate', 170.

69.   Ployant, *Breve Compendio dell' Arte Ostetricia*, 6.

70.   Ibid.

71.   Filippini, 'Levatrici e ostetricanti'. See chs 2, 5, 9 and 10 in this volume for the challenge to midwives presented by male practitioners in England, Spain, Germany and Holland.

72.   Filippini, 'Levatrici e ostetricanti'.

73.   Cangiamila, *Embriologia Sacra*, 168.

74.   N.M. Filippini, 'Il corpo violato. La pratica del taglio cesareo nell' Italia del primo ottocento', *Società e Storia*, 40 (1988), 295–333.

75.   Nardi, *Il Pensiero Ostetrico-Ginecologico nei Secoli*, 296.

76.   Filippini, 'Levatrici e ostetricanti', 160.

77.   N.M. Filippini, 'Gli ospizi per partorienti e i reparti di maternità tra sette

e ottocento', in M.L. Berti and M. Bressan (eds) *Gli Ospedali in Area Padana tra settecento e novecento, Sanità, Scienza e Storia* (Milano, 1992), 395–411.

78. Pancino, *Il Bambino e l'acqua sporca*, 59–61; Calvi, 'Manuali delle levatrici'.
79. Panzani, 'Un parto difficile', 249.
80. Pancino, *Il Bambino e l'acqua sporca*, 99.
81. Ibid., 52.
82. Filippini, 'Levatrici e ostetricanti', 165.
83. Filippini, 'Il bambino prezioso', 164.
84. Lonni, 'Il mestiere di ostetrica'.

9

Professionals? Sisters? Rivals?
Midwives in Braunschweig, 1750–1800

Mary Lindemann

Q

→

Time and historical indifference have obscured the lives of most midwives in the past. Few enjoyed more than the local esteem of contemporaries and posterity celebrates a mere handful, among them Justine Siegemund, Louise Bourgeois and now, of course, Mme du Coudray.[1] Yet this long-standing and almost institutionalized neglect has not quite rendered their biographies either inaccessible or historically irrelevant.[2] Their lives, their struggles, their ambitions, their frustrations and their successes can be recovered, and these experiences reveal much about the social construction of life in early modern Europe.

Midwifery has been studied most extensively in England and, for a later period, the United States. These emphases have to some extent imposed the tyranny of an Anglo-Saxon model on the history of midwifery. According to this model, the crucial issue is the mortal combat that raged between midwife and *accoucheur* (or between women and male-dominated science in general) for hegemony. But what has emerged as a central issue of debate in Anglo-Saxon arenas may be of limited importance, perhaps even irrelevant, to the experiences of midwives elsewhere. In the German states and cities, the history of midwifery was shaped by different issues as the example of the city of Braunschweig in the eighteenth century demonstrates.[3]

→

Eighteenth-century Braunschweig served as *Residenz* to the court of a very modest territory, Braunschweig-Wolfenbüttel, which quietly nestled between more puissant Hanoverian and Prussian neighbours. Braunschweig was the duchy's most populous city with about 27,000 inhabitants in 1793. No midwife in Braunschweig amassed the international reputation or exerted the political and politico-medical influence of a Bourgeois, a Siegemund or a du Coudray, although two had authored midwifery manuals.[4] But I am not principally concerned here with these twin anomalies. It is rather the everyday and the ordinary that form the substance of this investigation; that is, the careers of that relatively small number of women who comprised the corps of licensed midwives and their assistants – the evocatively named warming-women (*Wärme-Frauen*) – during the last half of the eighteenth century.

Historians have often cast the discussion of midwives and midwifery into one of two broader models: professionalization or medicalization. These models have spawned a rich debate on how the relationships between medicine, state, society and gender evolved. Most discussions of medical professionalism in the nineteenth and twentieth centuries implicitly or explicitly accept as paradigmatic the model constructed by sociologists such as Ernst Greenwood, Morris L. Cogan and Talcott Parsons. Paul Starr in his *The Social Transformation of American Medicine* defined a profession as 'an occupation that regulates itself through systematic, required training and collegial discipline; that has a base in technical, specialized knowledge; and that has a service rather than profit orientation, enshrined in its code of ethics'.[5] Thus most studies of the professions have focused on formal education, the coalescence of professional organizations, and the maturation of professional hegemony, and regard these places as the sites where professional identities unfolded. But these standards proved less useful when historians began to consider 'professionalism' in the early modern period and 'professions' dominated by females. If we accept the criteria that seem to typify professionalism in the nineteenth and twentieth centuries, then early modern historians, like scholars working on the history of women in medicine, must relegate medical practitioners before the late eighteenth century to a catch-all category of 'non-professional' or to an unsatisfactorily defined intermediate state of 'semi-professionalism'. Alternatively, they may scratch around trying to unearth the roots from which a lusher professionalism eventually sprouted. Another solution is to alter the meaning of professional so that the term may be applied to early modern medical practitioners without sounding hopelessly anachronistic or, worse, Whiggish. Some suggest we simply expand the classification: 'professionals' are then defined as those people who at particular moments in their lives identified themselves as engaged in medical practice, or who were consulted as healers in their communities, and who practised medicine outside the setting of the family.[6]

I remain somewhat sceptical as to whether it is profitable to cast the discussion of early modern midwifery *primarily* into the arena of professionalization (and to a lesser degree, medicalization) debates. It makes good sense, on the one hand, to ignore the more rigorous standards attributed to nineteenth- and twentieth-century professions when discussing early modern practitioners, or, for that matter, when discussing female practitioners of any era (such as the lay midwives of the late twentieth century), and to rely on the looser definitions suggested above. On the other hand, it remains unclear to what extent midwives understood themselves as professionals (by any definition) or, in contrast, viewed themselves as 'sisters'.[7] Moreover, is the often discussed tension between 'professional' and 'sister' in fact anachronistic when applied to the early modern world in that *neither* label characterized midwives' conceptions of themselves and their job? It seems more likely that their lives and their *métier* were moulded by quotidian circumstances, to which, of course, they alone were not subject. The 'defining events' which determined the norms and shaped the daily experience of midwifery occurred not only in the midwives' dealings with physicians, with government agencies and with ecclesiastical authorities, but also, perhaps even principally, in their assocations with other midwives, with their apprentices and, ultimately, with their patients. And yet retaining some sense of how midwives and early modern medical practitioners in general compare to our more modern standards of professionalism helps us understand their world by focusing our eyes on the inevitable points of similarity and difference. By trying to understand these issues and by grappling with the incongruities, we can unearth the basic features of early modern midwifery that scholars have only cursorily considered or dismissed as unimportant or irrelevant.

One articulate insider was Anne Horenburg, who served as a midwife in Braunschweig at the end of the seventeenth century. In 1700, she published a midwifery text presenting the art of midwifery in the conventional form of a conversation between two sisters. Although Fasbender's magisterial history of obstetrics[8] dismisses the book as 'insignificant', it is nonetheless an important source, for in the preface Frau Horenburg described her life.[9]

She was born the daughter of a regimental surgeon named Güldapffel in Wolfenbüttel (at that time the ducal *Residenz*). As a child she was taught to sew and knit, and as a young woman entered the ducal household as a seamstress. There she fell under the influence of the reigning duchess, who, 'animated by a great desire to succour her fellow human beings in illness', maintained a free apothecary for the poor, providing them, according to Horenburg, with 'sage advice' in illness. Horenburg relates how she began 'to think more about such things . . . and as Her Highness the Duchess possessed several books on midwifery in her library . . . I studied them and pondered these matters whenever I had time and thus gradually acquired a certain modest perception and knowledge'.

Later, Anne married Hans Christoph Horenburg, a corporal in the cavalry, 'and together we travelled the wide world'. The first birth she assisted was that of her landlady in Westphalia which

> turned out so happily that I thereafter no longer felt misgivings about being called to such work and during the war helped deliver many children. It also occurred that occasionally when the midwife made mistakes, I warned her and showed her the right way to proceed, and because of this [the midwives] were often sour with me and told me that it was not fitting for me, a young woman, [to presume] to correct her elders.

After her husband was discharged from the army, they settled in Eisleben, bought a house, and lived there for fifteen years. During this time, she frequently attended neighbours in childbirth. After she successfully delivered the niece of a certain Dr Keulings, he suggested to her that she consider becoming a midwife. At first she declined, arguing that 'I am still in my fruitful years, having already borne eight children.' Later, however, she reconsidered and became midwife to the towns of Eisleben and Mansfeld, receiving *ex officio* free lodging and allowances of firewood and grain. After her husband died, she returned to Braunschweig where her family still resided. On her mother's urging, she became a midwife there by submitting documentation attesting to her previous work in Eisleben and Mansfeld to the city authorities, and after the city's Physicus declared her 'competent'.

Clearly Horenburg enjoyed no regular instruction in midwifery: she had neither attended a school for midwives, nor listened to lectures on female anatomy, nor assisted a mistress-midwife as apprentice. Much of her learning, at least initially, came from reading books. It cannot be claimed, of course, that Horenburg's experience was typical, but it serves as a useful template and as a measure of contrast and comparison with the life stories of those women who served as midwives in Braunschweig during the last half of the eighteenth century.

Between 1750 and the end of the century, the number of licensed midwives, that is, midwives who had been examined by the duchy's *Collegium medicum* (board of health) and sworn-in by the city magistrates, rose from five to eight. In 1797, for example, eight were active.[10] I have clearly identified twenty-six women who filled these positions and for all of these, as well as for many of their warming-women, the archives yielded up information on their careers as midwives, as well as on their socio-economic position, their marital status, their ages and their husbands' occupations. The amount of evidence varied from individual to individual, of course.[11] Yet these materials permit a short (and somewhat tentative) analysis of the characteristic features of midwifery in eighteenth-century Braunschweig, and one that probes, moreover, beyond statistical profiles by concentrating on *mentalité*, illustrating how midwives conceived of their practice and interpreted their role.

Their composite life-history might well begin with the process of becoming a midwife. The Midwifery Ordinance of 1757 laid out a course of theoretical and practical instruction, making compulsory a formal training in female anatomy and physiology by the professor of obstetrics and gynaecology at the Anatomical-Surgical Institute (*Das Anatomisch-Chirurgische Institut*)[12] in Braunschweig. In addition, prospective midwives were to complete a rather loosely structured apprenticeship as warming-women. After the construction of a lying-in facility (*Accouchir-Haus*) in 1767, on-going students honed their skills by delivering babies under the watchful eye of a male supervisor.[13] This apparently often amounted to little more than extra, unpaid toil for the midwife-to-be. Despite the provision for structured theoretical training, throughout the eighteenth century the education of a midwife continued to be largely that of learning-by-doing. It approximated the artisan's training: an older midwife passed her knowledge on to an apprentice-like assistant. Most instruction was transmitted orally, although the Midwifery Ordinance of 1757 required that midwives must be able to read and write and, judging from Braunschweig's archival evidence, all could sign their names. Some were quite literate, possessing and apparently consulting texts on midwifery; at least one, Clara Catrina von der Mühle, annotated her copy of *Siphra und Pua* (a commonly-used midwifery manual).[14]

Until the middle of the eighteenth century, neither the *Collegium medicum* nor the city prescribed any regular procedure for the selection, training and appointment of warming-women: the midwife and her prospective helper apparently struck a mutually satisfying agreement. It appears that midwives were not legally entitled to any reimbursement for taking on apprentices, although it is possible they nevertheless received payment. No law, except custom, compelled a midwife to engage a helper, although many did. In 1755, in an explicit attempt to supervise more closely the education of midwives and to alleviate what was viewed as a scarcity of trained midwives in the city (and, for that matter, throughout the duchy), the *Collegium medicum* ordered 'that each midwife in the city of Braunschweig be appointed a helper, under the name of a warming-woman'. City magistrates were to identify suitable subjects and then report their names to the *Collegium medicum* for further scrutiny.[15] The selection of these warming-women, their position in the hierarchy of midwifery, and their activities (legal and otherwise), created moments of intense conflict between the *Collegium medicum* and the midwives, on the one hand, and between the midwives and their helpers, on the other. The documents generated in the course of these confrontations supply the historian with richly detailed information from which may be pieced together the daily reality of midwifery in eighteenth-century Germany.

The city of Braunschweig promised warming-women that 'although at first there are no *emolumenta*' – no salaries – connected with their job they were nominated *in spe succedendi*, that is, they took a place in line for a midwife's post in the future. Strictly worded regulations forbade warming-women to deliver babies, except in emergencies; neither were they permitted to carry children to the church to be christened ('*zum Taufe tragen*').[16] These were not uncommon arrangements in early modern cities. The privileges warming-women savoured during their apprenticeship were few; work was hard, hours long, wages uncertain, prestige non-existent. Not until 1767 did the government guarantee midwives an annual wage of 50 thaler. But this commitment took effect only slowly and as late as 1806 only five of the city's nine practising midwives actually received 50 thaler annually.[17] In addition, of course, midwives collected fees for the specific services they rendered. The Midwifery Ordinance of 1757 published detailed tables, which calibrated payments according to the difficulty of the birth, the hours of attendance and the social status of the mother. Fee tables alone, however, provide only a very shaky basis on which to calculate what midwives or warming-women actually earned. In order to estimate even crudely the 'typical' midwife's income, one would also need to know – at the very least – how many women each midwife delivered in a year.[18] What data exist are scanty and widely strewn. For example, the *Collegium medicum* reported that 685 women had given birth in Braunschweig during 1789. As there were at that time nine licensed midwives, this averages out to approximately seventy-six births for each midwife.[19] Yet this is a worthless statistic: some midwives had more extensive practices than others;[20] older women possibly attended fewer births in a year than did younger, more active women; personalities and reputations played conspicuous roles in a midwife's popularity with the public.[21] Thus the historian cannot compute the earnings of the 'average' midwife in Braunschweig, unless she or he is satisfied with rather meaningless numbers that reflect reality only imperfectly. The 50-thaler salary four or five midwives drew regularly after 1767, along with the freedom from some property taxes they traditionally enjoyed,[22] must have compared favourably to what many artisan families lived on. But a haze of reciprocal arrangements, family circumstances and property ownership that is from the distance of two centuries hard to penetrate, continues to obscure their true economic circumstances from the historian's gaze. Some owned property, some did not; some had inheritances, some had none; some laboured alone for their families, some contributed extras to family economies. Socially, judging by the known occupations of their husbands (among them we find lathe-turners, tailors, basket makers, peddlers, wheelwrights, textile weavers, barber-surgeons, journeymen and apprentices, soldiers and the like),[23] they came from the artisan milieu, although they usually were found at the lower end of this occupational category, among the poorer and more congested trades, such as tailoring and weaving.[24]

What reverberates throughout this documentation is the sense of need, the sense of misfortune, and the sense of frustration that almost all midwives and prospective midwives wove into the fabric of their petitions and protests. Of course, they were obviously concerned about displaying their cases in the best possible light and in stressing their 'deservedness' over the claims of rivals; thus, they constructed 'tales' they felt would be believed.[25] Yet there is little reason to doubt the general veracity of the facts provided, especially as they are so often corroborated by other evidence. Women usually chose midwifery (probably as they chose other work) because they had to support themselves or their families. Because the midwifery ordinanccs and custom dictated that they be past childbearing age themselves (and had already borne children), few midwives or warming-women were under 40. In 1751, Christina Maria Altvater, 44 years of age, related that she had given birth to thirteen children, of whom eight were still young and uneducated. Moreover, she had assisted many 'reputable women in travail . . . whereby I acquired the skills necessary to a midwife'. Her 60-year-old husband was a citizen of Braunschweig who eked out a pitiful living as a dancing master (*Tanzmeister*). But, she continued, 'the [price] of food rises from day to day . . . [and thus] I solicit [*sollicitire*] most humbly the office' of midwife. She was appointed in 1752.[26] While the *Collegium medicum* and the city magistrates never named women they regarded as 'unqualified' to be midwives, they were frequently swayed by economic arguments to appoint a poorer woman over one even slightly better-off. Furthermore, they often scaled wages to need.[27] This was not sheer humanitarianism on their part: poor women, especially widows with children, counted among the most frequent recipients of poor relief in early modern cities.

Compared to the licensed midwife, however, the anticipated earnings – in wages, tips and gifts – of a warming-woman were negligible. One midwife, Antoinette Elisabeth Becker, reported that despite her best efforts she had failed to locate any woman eager to take on the job 'because they can expect to earn nothing, and they are scared away by the fact that they must pay Professor Wagler thirty thaler pro informatione [for their instruction in midwifery]'. She herself had laboured as a warming-woman for fourteen years and during that time had earned no more than 2 or 3 thaler in total. Two other midwives, likewise unable to locate candidates for warming-women, pointed out that a warming-woman's anticipated income was so miserable that 'a woman could do far better as a seamstress'. Another midwife, Dorothea Elisabeth Seehausen, agreed, adding that 'the lying-in women do not want the warming-women around'. Not only did mothers fret about the extra costs involved (warming-women were allowed a small fee for their assistance at a birth and it was probably more or less customary to tip them and offer them some refreshment during their wait), they also resented the intrusion of strangers into a ritual to which their best friends were summoned and where an invitation to a birthing (or the lack of one) carried significant social messages.[28] None of this made midwifery seem a particularly attractive option for women. Of the four women the *Collegium medicum* interviewed in 1764 only one exhibited much enthusiasm about taking on the job of warming-woman. The one exception was Anna Magdalena Schrader, the wife of a barber-surgeon. Yet she would accept the post only if the city paid for her training 'in that I am almost destitute, and burdened by a husband who has suffered a stroke, and [am] bereft of all income'.[29] Thus, a woman could envision little profit and even less social prestige accruing from her service as a warming-woman. Moreover, instructional costs were substantial even though the *Collegium medicum* had decided in 1765 that warming-women need pay only one-third of the specified amount, and public funds would cover the other two-thirds. Still, this was a benefit enjoyed only briefly: in 1772, the *Collegium medicum* reversed its decision, maintaining that 'as midwives in Braunschweig now receive a generous salary and [furthermore] can expect good earnings; the thirty thaler instructional fee is for them a sound investment and they can no longer demand that the government subsidize their education'.[30]

What quickly becomes evident here is that warming-women had both motive and opportunity to overstep the boundaries marking the limits of their position. They often waited years for a midwifery post to open up, usually until the death of the previous occupant. Frau Becker, perhaps atypically, waited fourteen years, but other warming-women narrated similar tales of trial and tribulation. In 1776, when Frau Heidorn applied for a position that had just fallen vacant, she stressed that,

> for over five-and-a-half years I have faithfully attended the instruction in the *Accouchir-Haus*, and have shied away from neither the costs . . . nor the need to neglect my home and family to be present whenever required; all in the expectation eventually to be able to nourish myself and my children by the exercise of this craft, [which I must do] because my husband, a tailor, is almost blind and can work no more.[31]

The road to a midwife's licence could be a long and rocky one. Securing the desired prize necessitated patience, perseverance and a good deal of luck. In 1774, Dorothea Margaretha Nußbaum renewed her application for the position her deceased mother-in-law had once held. When she had first applied, in 1772, the *Collegium medicum* denied her appeal, advising her '[to] first acquire a thorough grounding in midwifery', and that once she had obtained a certificate attesting to her proficiency from Professor Sommer, she 'would be helped'. In this hope, she maintained that 'I spared myself neither expense nor effort in achieving the requisite [level of] skill . . . in midwifery'. Moreover, she explained how 'in the two years that I was constantly in attendance at the *Accouchir-Haus*, I earned nothing although I often had to hold myself in readiness two or three days at a time, while totally ignoring my household duties'. Furthermore, she insisted that 'I will [soon] be ruined if I continue "breadless" much longer.'[32] This petition, as well as ones she subsequently filed each year from 1775–78 were all rejected. It was not until 1785 that the *Collegium medicum* finally selected her to fill a vacancy.[33]

Once a position was available, the *Collegium medicum* consulted its roster of warming-women and of women who had already passed the midwifery examination for a suitable replacement. Seniority usually determined the choice, although a candidate was also required to produce on demand a pastor's attestation of the propriety of her conduct, her good morals and her Christian life-style.[34] Especially after mid-century (and perhaps heart-ened by the prospect of a 50-thaler salary), warming-women habitually took the midwifery examination once they had completed the theoretical and practical phases of their training. Success in the examination, however, did not bestow on them the right to act as midwives. On the contrary, they were expressly forbidden to do so. This inevitably resulted in a surplus of trained women for whom no legitimate practice existed. In some instances, the *Collegium medicum* and the city government agreed to the naming of 'supernumeraries' again *in spe succedendi*. They authorized these supernumerary or 'extraordinary' midwives to assist women in child-birth but allowed them no salary; they could (and did), however, demand the regular fees for their services.[35] It is not hard to imagine that in these circumstances the relations between licensed midwives, their warming-women, and the supernumeraries were tense, quarrelsome and even combative.

The friction to a large degree resulted from economic pressures. Warming-women and supernumeraries repeatedly agitated for greater incomes, while midwives reacted belligerently to those who poached on their territory. Complaints about the professional misconduct of warming-women, supernumeraries and others arose almost routinely.[36] A fat dossier of grievances signed by all the licensed midwives in Braunschweig in the years 1795–96, and directed against Margaretha Elisabeth Krüger, reveals the complex and consequential issues involved in such accusations:

> We see ourselves forced to denounce those midwives from outside Braunschweig as well as some [midwife] candidates, who clan-destinely attend women in childbed; such [actions] greatly damage our incomes, [and] to speak more plainly, steal the very bread from our mouths.[37]

Here we find ourselves catapulted into the realm of what was deemed 'quackery' in early modern Europe. 'Quackery', as paradoxical as the argument may sound, was the nucleus around which many early modern professionals defined the prerogatives of their professions and the mirror in which they perceived their own professional identities. Throughout the century, as earlier, the preferred word for such 'encroachment', for such 'quackery', was *Pfuscherey*. A *Pfuscher* was the guild's expression of scorn for an unprivileged, non-guilded worker who was an interloper but not necessarily or even usually an incompetent. Special proficiency was to be feared far more. To the modern definition of the word 'quack' cling connotations of tricksterism, ignorance and deceit. But the traditional meaning of 'quack' was different and far richer. In the eighteenth century a quack might be unskilled, but she or he was invariably seen as a 'disturber' (*Störer*) of communal tranquillity or as a 'thief' (*Dieb*) who preyed on the protected and legally defined 'livelihood' (*Nahrung*) of others.[38]

Frau Krüger personified the early modern quack. She resided in the small town of Holzminden and was, in Holzminden, an officially installed midwife who had passed the standard midwifery examination with the grade of '*sehr gut*'. That gave her *no* right to practise in the city of Braunschweig, however. But she did. She was, her detractors asserted, so 'cheeky . . . that she peddles her services to people unbidden'. When called upon to justify her actions, Frau Krüger conceded that she had in truth delivered several babies in Braunschweig. She offered as her defence that 'I have only assisted very poor women, from whom the midwives could hardly have anticipated much compensation.' Furthermore, she claimed that she had been dispatched as a midwife to Holzminden 'in a way completely contrary to my own wishes'. The move forced her to sell her house in Braunschweig at a loss. Her husband, a cobbler, had to pay substantial entrance fees to join the shoemakers' guild in Holzminden. She had only gone to Holzminden in the first place because Professor Sommer assured her that, as the only midwife there, her earnings would be more than ample. Holzminden, however, turned out to be less than a paradise: in a period of six months, she maintained that she had only delivered seven infants there and thus saw herself compelled to cast around for additional employment in Braunschweig.[39] It is crucial to note that nowhere in the midwives' denunciation of Krüger emerged any indication that she was unskilled, irresponsible or a menace. In this context, their opposition to her practice was solely economic and occupational: it involved in equal measure considerations of money and livelihood.[40] Similarly, midwives objected to warming-women who performed the emergency baptism (*Noth-Taufe*) 'quite unnecessarily', robbing them of the perquisites they 'rightfully enjoyed' from their participation in the festive christening ceremony.[41]

The concept of livelihood provides the essential key to understanding how people constructed and perceived professional identities in eighteenth-century Europe. Granting the right to exercise a livelihood within the community was a process of entitlement as well as a judgment of competency. Most conflicts between midwives and the *Collegium medicum* crystallized around those issues of economic survival and social status firmly encased within the early modern concept of livelihood. To assure a living for each midwife, it was felt necessary to divide the market equally (or relatively so) between them and to shield them from the unfair and injurious activities of interlopers, to protect them from such 'quacks' as Frau Krüger.[42]

The principle was almost universally accepted: the quotidian execution of it was hotly contested. The midwives, the city government, the warming-women and the *Collegium medicum* often harboured quite contradictory notions of what a 'sufficient' and a 'superfluous' number of midwives might be. Warming-women and supernumeraries, who desperately sought appointments as midwives, insisted that the number of midwives in the city was too small to provide adequate care for the entire female population of childbearing age. The *Collegium medicum*, calculating on the basis of population size, repeatedly denied appeals to increase the number of midwives to more than eight, arguing that eight was 'quite enough for a city of 30,000 inhabitants'.[43] Midwives, not surprisingly, countered that too many licensed midwives were already practising in Braunschweig, and this over-crowded situation had effectively denied each one of them an adequate living.

The small earnings of the warming-women and their long, sometimes futile wait for a position as a licensed midwife often propelled them into quackery. But economic distress was an argument the *Collegium medicum*, as well as the midwives themselves, would not countenance as a legitimate excuse for quackery. The midwives pointed out that they, too, had served equally protracted and equally penurious apprenticeships. Leaping to the offensive, they charged that many warming-women seemed far more pre-occupied with lining their pockets than with mastering the essentials of their craft. Dr Martini, dean of the *Collegium medicum*, also refused to listen to such 'nonsense'. He contended that, like the medical student at a university, warming-women should not be reluctant to invest time and money in their future.[44] Thus although such 'trespassing' (which was what quackery amounted to, after all) was expressly forbidden, and occasionally even punished (if mildly; most offenders got off with a warning), it remained – and had to remain – more or less accepted, to some extent tolerated, and certainly expected in this historical context. Quackery formed an integral part of almost every midwife's life and was perhaps her earliest 'professional' experience. Frequently, even regularly, the entire corps of midwives collectively denounced the quackery of one or another warming-woman or supernumerary. Yet these same interlopers almost always (if they lived long enough or did not leave the city in the interim) became midwives who were as alacritous and as vehement in protesting the quackery of *their* warming-women and as zealous in defence of *their* livelihood as their erstwhile critics had been. Their experiences in first attaining and then protecting their livelihoods largely defined their profession and their professional identities.

Is it possible then to describe a professional identity, as done here, almost solely on the basis of discord and competition? Had no sense of professional solidarity emerged? It might be argued that the conflict por-trayed here is overstated or illusory, an epiphenomenon of the sources rather than a true state of affairs. This criticism cannot be dismissed out of hand. Harmony tends to spawn little documentation whereas the medi-ation of disputes (like the investigation of criminal charges) generates much. Another explanation is that while the conflict between midwives and warming-women certainly existed, perhaps we should view it as a common life-experience uniting them more than an embittered battle dividing them. After all, almost all the warming-women eventually *did* become midwives, as did even the much persecuted Frau Krüger. No matter what their stance – aggrieved or defiant – they all spoke the same language of 'livelihood' and 'privileges', of 'rights' and 'commitments', and it is this discourse, these points of agreement that defined them as medical practitioners and members of a professional group.

Common language

Notes

1. Siegemund, Bourgeois and du Coudray were all authors: J. Siegemund, *Die König. Preußische und Chur-Brandenb. Hof-Wehe-Mutter, Das ist: Ein höchst nöthiger Unterricht von schweren und unrecht-stehenden Geburthen, In einem Gespräch vorgestellt,* ... (Berlin, 1752); L. Bourgeois, *Observations Diverses sur la Stérilité, Perte de Fruict, Foecondité, Accouchement et Maladies des Femmes et Enfants Nouveaux Naiz, amplement Traiteés et Heursement Pratiquées* (Paris, 1609, 1626); A.M. Le Bousier du Coudray, *Abrégé de l'Art des Accouchements* (Paris, 1778). See W. Perkins, 'Midwives versus doctors: the case of Louise Bourgeois', *The Seventeenth Century*, 3 (1988), 135–57; *idem*, 'The relationship between midwife and client in the works of Louise Bourgeois', *Seventeenth-Century French Studies*, 11 (1989), 28–45; and ch. 7 in this volume by Nina Gelbart.

2. It is, of course, impossible to review here the extensive historical literature dealing with midwives. Of the works on midwives in early modern Germany, one should mention E. Haberling, *Beiträge zur Geschichte des Hebammenstandes* (Berlin, 1940); G. Buckhard, *Die deutschen Hebammenordnungen von ihren ersten Anfängen bis auf die Neuzeit* (Leipzig, 1912); F. C. Wille, *Über Stand und Ausbildung der Hebammen im 17. und 18. Jahrhundert in Chur-Brandenburg* (Berlin, 1934); W. Gubalke, *Die Hebamme im Wandel der Zeiten: Ein Beitrag zur Geschichte des Hebammenwesens* (Hanover, 1964); D. Tutzke, 'Über statistische Untersuchungen als Beitrag zur Geschichte des Hebammenwesens im ausgehenden 18. Jahrhundert', *Centaurus*, 4 (1956), 351–9; *idem*, 'Zur materiellen Lage der Niederlausitzer Hebammen im 18. Jahrhundert', *Sudhoffs Archiv*, 45 (1961), 334–40; *idem*, 'Die Entwicklung des Hebammenwesens in der Oberlausitz bis zum Beginn des 19. Jahrhunderts', *Oberlausitzer Forschung* (1961), 284–306; B. Menssen and A.-M. Taube, 'Hebammen und Hebammenwesen in Oldenburg in der zweiten Hälfte des 18. und zu Beginn des 19. Jahrhunderts', in E. Hinrichs and W. Norden (eds) *Regionalgeschichte: Probleme und Beispiele* (Hildesheim, 1980), 165–224; M.E. Wiesner, 'Early modern midwifery: a case study', *International Journal of Women's Studies*, 6 (1983), 26–43, and ch. 4 in this volume by Merry Wiesner. On midwives in Braunschweig, there is some important older literature. See esp. A.F. Nolde, *Notizen zur Kultur-Geschichte der Geburtshülfe in dem Herzogthum Braunschweig* (Erfurt, 1807). See also the very useful section on 'Das Collegium Anatomico-Chirurgicum und die Accouchir-Anstalt in Braunschweig', in *Zum Aufbau der Hebammenschulen in Niedersachsen im 18. und 19. Jahrhundert*, exhibition catalogue (Hanover, 1981), 17–21. More generally, the (not always reliable) K.-R. Döhnel, *Das Anatomisch-Chirurgische Institut in Braunschweig* (Braunschweig, 1957) and Walter Artelt's pioneering article, 'Das medizinische Braunschweig um 1770', *Medizinhistorisches Journal*, 1 (1966), 240–60.

The major ordinances concerning medical practice in Braunschweig are collected in A. Hinze, *Lexikon aller herzoglichen braunschweigischen Verordnungen, welche die medizinische Polizei betreffen* (Stendal, 1793).

3. For example, the conflict between men and women midwives never developed in Germany. For the most part, midwives continued to deliver women throughout the eighteenth and nineteenth centuries. Physicians did try to gain control of the education of midwives in attempts to 'improve' their training, but never really tried to muscle them out of the business entirely. There were, of course, male physicians and surgeons who delivered babies. For relationships between midwives and medical practitioners in eighteenth-century Holland, see ch. 10 in this volume by Hilary Marland.

4. A. Horenburg, *Wohlgemeynender und Nöhtiger Unterricht der Heeb-Amme* (Hanover and Wolfenbüttel, 1700). Christian Franz Paullini refers to the work as 'a useful little book, that I recommend to all midwives . . . ' in *Das Hoch- und Wohl-gelahrte Teutsche Frauen-Zimmer Nochmals mit mercklichen Zusatz vorgestellet* (Frankfurt and Leipzig, 1705), 74. The midwifery manual written by Elisabeth Margarethe von Keil (also Reil), who died in 1699, is also favourably mentioned by Paullini in *Das Hoch- und Wohl-gelahrte*, 81. Keil's husband was a physician who practised in Celle in the late seventeenth century.

5. P. Starr, *The Social Transformation of American Medicine: The Rise of a Sovereign Profession and the Making of a Vast Industry* (New York, 1982), 15; E. Friedson, *Profession of Medicine* (New York, 1970); and *idem, Professional Dominance: The Social Structure of Medical Care* (New York, 1970). For Germany, see C. Huerkamp, *Der Aufstieg der Ärzte im 19. Jahrhundert. Vom gelehrten Stand zum professionellen Experten: Das Beispiel Preußens* (Göttingen, 1985), esp. 14–21. Although the pre-history of the professions can be traced to the Middle Ages, 'according to the sociological canon', the professions 'attained a nearly recognizable form in the late eighteenth and nineteenth centuries and "took off" at that time, eventually becoming, . . . one of the hallmarks of modernity in the West'. J. Goldstein, 'Foucault among the sociologists: the "disciplines" and the history of the professions', *History and Theory*, 23 (1984), 174.

6. M. Pelling, 'Medical practice in early modern England: trade or profession?' in W. Prest (ed.) *The Professions in Early Modern England* (London, 1987), 90–128; M.H. Green, 'Women's medical practice and health care in Medieval Europe: review essay', *Signs: Journal of Women in Culture and Society*, 14 (1989), 438–9.

7. For a discussion of these issues in a late twentieth-century setting, see M. Reid, 'Sisterhood and professionalization: a case study of the American lay midwife', in C. S. McClain (ed.) *Women as Healers: Cross-Cultural Perspectives* (New Brunswick and London, 1989), 219–38. I would like to thank Hilary Marland for calling my attention to this article.

8. H. Fasbender, *Geschichte der Geburtshülfe* (Jena, 1906), 143.

9. Horenburg, *Wohlgemeynender und Nöhtiger Unterricht der Heeb-Amme*. All details of Horenburg's life are taken from the preface.

10. There were five midwives in 1755, six in 1759, and five in 1764. Stadtarchiv Braunschweig (hereafter StadtB) C VII S20 vol. VII, 238, 281, 293.

11. From the following sources: StadtB C VII S20 vol. VII; Niedersächsisches Staatsarchiv-Wolfenbüttel (hereafter StAWf) 2 Alt 11416–11420, esp. 11419–11420; StAWf 111 Neu 1757, 111 Neu 1762, 111 Neu 1764, 111 Neu 1768, and 111 Neu 1797.

12. For its history, see Döhnel, *Das Anatomisch-Chirugisches Institut in Braunschweig.*

13. *Serenissimi gnädigste Verordnung, das Hebammenwesen betreffend. De Dato Braunschweig, von 18. Febr, 1757* (hereafter MO 1757), pars 3–4; and StAWf 40 Slg 11250, 16 March 1771. The Anatomisch-Chirurgische Institut was established in

1750. Döhnel, *Das Anatomisch-Chirurgische Institut in Braunschweig*, 25–8, 34–6. See also the section on 'Das Collegium Anatomico-Chirurgicum und die Accouchir-Anstalt in Braunschweig', in *Zum Aufbau der Hebammenschulen in Niedersachsen im 18. und 19. Jahrhundert*, 17–21; *s.v.* 'Das Gebährhaus in Braunschweig', in Hinze, *Lexicon.* Lectures for midwives were often advertised in the town's newspaper.

14. Von Mühle was appointed a midwife in Braunschweig in 1739, as she recorded in her own hand in the back of her copy of Johan von Hoorn, *Die zwo um ihrer Gottesfrucht und Treue willen von GOTT wohlbelohnte Weh-Mütter Siphra und Pua*, ..., 2nd edn (Stockholm, 1737), which can be found in the Herzog August Bibliothek (Wolfenbüttel) under accession number Mr143.

15. Procedures for choosing and appointing warming-women are described in StadtB C VII S20 vol. VII, 289. The appointment of warming-women became standard practice for the entire duchy in the MO 1757, pars 3 and 19; see also StAWf 111 Neu 1727. Among medical reformers, there was almost universal agreement that midwifery was in a miserable state in the eighteenth century. Bernhard Christoph Faust, in his influential and widely-read *Gedanken über Hebammen und Hebammenschulen auf dem Lande* (Frankfurt, 1784), maintained that 'midwives are *certainly* among those most responsible for the destruction of the health and the vitality and therefore also [among the principal causes of] the misery and decay of the human race' (p. 5). See, in addition, J.G. Krünitz, *D. Johann Georg Krünitz's ökonomischtechnologische Encyklopädie oder allgemeines System der Staats-, Stadt-, Haus-, und Landwirthschaft und der Kunstgeschichte in alphabetischer Ordnung* (Berlin, 1782–1858), *s.v.* 'Heb-Amme'; J.D.F. Brunner, *Entdeckung der Irrthümer und Bosheiten der Hebammen* (Solingen, 1740); E. Ettner, *Unvorsichtige Hebamme* (Leipzig, 1715); J.P. Frank, *System einer medicinischen Polizey* (Mannheim, 1779), vol. 1, 609–78; A. Hinze, 'Vorschläge zur Verbesserung des Hebammenwesens, insonderheit der Hebammen des platten Landes', *Braunschweigisches Magazin*, 16 April 1791; and A. Fischer, *Geschichte des deutschen Gesundheitswesens* (Berlin, 1933), vol. 1, 233–4. One result of all this bad publicity was an attempt to improve midwifery standards, partially through increased education and partially through stricter supervision and control. These dual initiatives led to a new series of midwifery ordinances passed in quick succession in the mid-eighteenth century. Among other places, we find new midwifery ordinances in Augsburg (1750), Basel (1770), Holstein (1767), Nuremberg (1755) and Strasburg (1757). Fischer, *Geschichte des deutschen Gesundheitswesens*, vol. 1, 234–5.

16. MO 1757, par. 1 forbade anyone 'other than [properly] appointed and sworn-in midwives, except in emergencies, to assume the duties of a midwife'. This was repeated many times. See especially the order of 7 May 1772 which grounded the prohibition on the need to protect the livelihoods and incomes of official midwives. StadtB C VII S20 vol. VII, 219.

17. An edict of 24 June 1767, StAWf 111 Neu 1757, 164, provided an annual salary of 50 thaler out of city funds for each midwife appointed *in the future.* Salaries were introduced gradually. For example, in 1777, the *Collegium medicum* distributed 'salary improvements' to two midwives, raising one woman's salary to the stipulated 50 thaler, while the other received 25 thaler. StAWf 111 Neu 1764. Nolde, *Notizen zur Kultur-Geschichte*, 103–4, noted that in 1765, each midwife received 5 thaler 29 mariengulden in salary plus limited tax advantages. By 1806, of the nine midwives in the city, the five senior practitioners each received 50 thaler, the next two 25 thaler, the eighth 8 mariengulden, and the ninth, a supernumerary, no payment.

18. MO 1757, pars 21–2.

19. 'Summarischer Auszug aus den Listen der Gebohrenen, Gestorbenen und

Copulirten de 1789 a) Von den Städten b) vom platten Lande', in StAWf 2 Alt 11417, 30.

20. The extent of each practice is impossible to calculate as we have no case books nor even (with scattered exceptions) the monthly lists registering births attended by each midwife which she was supposed to forward to the *Collegium medicum*. However, in spring 1797, the *Collegium medicum* and city magistrates requested midwives to send in lists of babies they had recently delivered. The authorities were searching for a suspected infanticide. These reports, which must be very like the monthly reports midwives filed (at least occasionally!), are mere slips of paper. But from them I have put together a very rough calculation of the relative size of each midwife's practice.

Table 9.1 Relative sizes of midwifery practices in Braunschweig, 1797

Midwife	No. of deliveries	Time period (in weeks)	Births per year (approx.)
Voges	4	3	69
Becker	2	5	21
Bollmann	6	10	31
Goetze	13	12	56
Zobebier	10	7	74
Niederhütter	18	8	117
Nußbaum	16	11	76

Source: StadtB C VII S20 vol. VII, 51–72.

21. For midwives' repeat practices in seventeenth-century London, see ch. 1 in this volume by Doreen Evenden.

22. Nolde, *Notizen zur Kultur-Geschichte*, 104; StadtB CVII S20 vol. VII, 347, 383.

23. List of husbands' occupations compiled from the files noted in note 11.

24. Compare the similar findings of Menssen and Taube, 'Hebammen und Hebammenwesen in Oldenburg', and of Tutzke, 'Über statistische Untersuchungen'.

25. Natalie Z. Davis explored elements of 'fiction' in analysing how people of sixteenth-century France composed pardon tales to save their skins. According to Davis, they selected incidents, language, and forms of argumentation that would influence their audiences. As she points out, she makes

> the 'fictional' elements of these documents . . . the center of analysis. I do not mean their feigned elements, but rather using the other and broader sense of the word *fingere*, their forming, shaping, and molding elements: the crafting of a narrative . . . . I think we can agree with Roland Barthes, Paul Ricoeur, and Lionel Grossman that shaping choices of language, detail, and order are needed to present an account that seems to both writer and reader true, real, meaningful, and/or explanatory.

N.Z. Davis, *Fiction in the Archives: Pardon Tales and their Tellers in Sixteenth-Century France* (Stanford, 1987), 3.

26. Altvater's petition from 8 Nov. 1751 in StAWf 111 Neu 1757, 19–20.

27. See, for example, a decision reached in 1777 in StAWf 111 Neu 1764.

28. StadtB C VII S20 vol. VII, 235, 238, 246; StAWf 2 Alt 11420, 2.

29. StadtB C VII S20 vol. VII, 239–41.
30. Cited in Nolde, *Notizen zur Kultur-Geschichte*, 99, 103.
31. StadtB C VII S20 vol. VII, 216.
32. StadtB C VII S20 vol. VII, 137–8.
33. On Nußbaum, see StadtB C VII S20 vol. VII, 136–60; also StAWf 111 Neu 1797 and 111 Neu 1757.
34. I have reconstructed the sequence of events from the files listed in note 11. For examples of cases decided between 1750 and 1800, see StadtB C VII S20 vol. VII and StAWF 111 Neu 1757.
35. Dorothea Elisabeth Seehausen petitioned to be allowed the status of a supernumerary in 1755, an appointment she received in October of that year. In 1756, an official midwife post opened up and she was selected to fill it. StAWf 111 Neu 1757, 34–6, 40. Similarly, Christiane Henriette Margaretha Backhaus was appointed 'extraordinnaire' in 1784. StAWf 111 Neu 1757, 255.
36. See, for example, 'Acta die Hebammen-Pfuscherey der Peitschen, Heidorn, Leitloffen und Nußbaum hieselbst betref. 1773', in StAWf 111 Neu 1797, 2. Renewed complaints about these women appear in StAWf 111 Neu 1797, 13–14.
37. 'Acta die Beschwerde der hiesigen Heb-Ammen gegen die Hebammen Candidata Krügern betrf.', StadtB C VII S20 vol. VII, various complaints from 1795–1800.
38. *S.v.* 'Pfuscherey' and 'Nahrung' in J.H. Zedler, *Großes vollständiges Universal-Lexikon, aller Wissenschaften und Künste . . .* (Halle, 1732–50), and *s.v.* 'Pfuscherey', 'Quacksalberey', and 'Marktschreyer' in *Krünitzs Encyklopädie.* By the middle of the nineteenth century the term 'Pfuscherey' had undergone a gradual, although never complete, metamorphosis and had come to approximate the modern meaning of 'unskilled' or 'incompetent'.
39. StadtB C VII S20 vol. VII, 79–86.
40. A complaint about Krüger's 'irresponsibility' (a complaint that was close to what we would today term 'professional negligence') was, however, raised by a gardener, Georg Heinrich Billing. He testified that Krüger, after 'offering her aid' to his pregnant wife, then refused to attend to her when she went into labour. It was in the middle of the night and Krüger had given him the 'flimsy excuse' that she was ill. But the next day Billing saw her on the streets doing her shopping, apparently in perfect health. From 7 Nov. 1799, in StadtB C VII S20 vol. VII, 29.
41. Complaint submitted on 12 June 1798, in StadtB C VII S20 vol. VII, 33–6.
42. MO 1757, par. 20.
43. See, for example, the decision of the *Collegium medicum* dated 10 April 1779 in StadtB C VII S20 vol. VII, 133.
44. Note dated 20 Nov. 1773 in StAWf 111 Neu 1797, 7.

10

The *'burgerlijke'* midwife: the *stadsvroedvrouw* of eighteenth-century Holland

Hilary Marland

On 18 June 1763 Sara van der Wegh, wife of Wijnand Reuseveld, then midwife in Rijswijk, following the departure of Margaretha Perks, was appointed midwife to the small harbour town of Delfshaven, 'to serve the women folk, who in their need looked to her'. She was to reside in Delfshaven and help poor and indigent women as well as the rich 'with all friendliness and care, and further to follow herself the rules and ordinances that existed'. Her salary was to be 60 guilders per annum, and for this sum she was, together with the other town midwife in Delfshaven, to deliver women and to care for infants in their first days of life.[1]

By the eighteenth century a distinct group of midwives had evolved in the Netherlands, the *stadsvroedvrouwen* (town or municipal midwives), who were authorized and paid by local councils to deliver poor women residing within the town walls.[2] The *burgerlijke*[3] figures appointed to such posts had usually followed a recognized training with a local midwife and lessons given under the auspices of local medical corporations, had taken an examination and sworn an oath, and had been issued with a licence to practise. Arrangements for teaching and regulating midwives dated back to the mid-seventeenth century; by the eighteenth they had been adopted by a large number of towns, and in a number of ways the position of the *stadsvroedvrouw* was becoming more formalized and her role more important. Towards the end of the century, *stadsvroedmeesters* (town men-midwives) were also being appointed, but the midwife was still expected to attend normal deliveries.

At a time when the midwife was reputed to be in decline in Europe, in terms of practice and status,[4] a corps of trained and licensed midwives, with recognized functions, was being built up in the Netherlands. The *stadsvroed-vrouw* demonstrates the possibilities of change and the formalization of the midwife's role in a positive direction, and of regulation associated not with squeezing the midwife out of practice but with consolidating her position, albeit in a way dictated largely by local hierarchies and the medical community.

The *stadsvroedvrouw* coexisted with licensed midwives without municipal appointments, and the 'unofficial' midwives, who continued to practise in the Netherlands throughout the eighteenth century. The coexistence of these groups was not acceptable to the town authorities and medical corporations (or often to the licensed midwives) – the situation in the countryside, where uncontrolled practice was rife, was a particular cause of concern – but little could be done to bring the unlicensed midwife into line. Unlicensed rural practice was still being cited as a major problem in the early decades of the twentieth century.[5] The coexistence of formally trained, licensed midwives practising alongside the untrained and un-recognized was not unique to the Netherlands,[6] but the carefully regulated and very visible *stadsvroedvrouw* system[7] brings the dichotomy of midwifery practice into especially sharp focus. It was a division based largely on towns and rural areas; by the eighteenth century most Dutch towns had taken steps to supervise midwifery practice, while in the countryside the un-regulated midwife remained the norm.

This dichotomy, however, tells us little about the competence of the two groups. Although the *stadsvroedvrouw* had generally undergone a lengthy period of apprenticeship with a recognized midwife, together with a brief grounding in obstetrics in lessons given by members of the local medical hierarchy, perhaps also witnessing a couple of dissections, this was no guarantee of practical skills. Formal recognition and a licence by no means ensured that the *stadsvroedvrouw* was fully equipped to deliver babies, especially at a time when there was often a shortage of women to fill these posts. The unlicensed midwife, with her skills acquired through word of mouth and hands-on practical experience, sometimes also accompanied by a period of informal apprenticeship with a competent midwife, may have been equally if not better fitted for her task. Vrouw Catharina Schrader is an outstanding example of a midwife who, working without a formal training and without a licence, with knowledge picked up from her hus-band's practice as a rural surgeon, probably supported by book-learning, achieved fame and credit for her work in the harbour town of Dokkum in Friesland in the early years of the eighteenth century.[8] Working as the town's midwife, she attended the births of many prominent members of the Dokkum community, the wives of local doctors and surgeons, town officials and ministers, as well as assisting many poor inhabitants.[9]

One of the strongest points in favour of the town midwife was that she practised regularly, attending a large number of deliveries each year, often several a week. There is no doubt that she was kept busy, and in some cases was over-pressured, as in Gouda during the 80 Years' War when the town authorities struggled to keep three *stadsvroedvrouwen* in service for a popu-lation of 12,000.[10] Though not a guarantee of skill, regular practice could confirm it. Yet many rural midwives also had flourishing practices.

Vrouw Schrader, while based in the small town of Dokkum, attended many rural births, often having to travel long and difficult distances. An acknowledged local expert in complicated deliveries, with a considerable repeat business, she delivered some 3,060 children during her 50 years in practice, in her peak years over one hundred per annum.[11] While praising some of her colleagues, Schrader also was quick to point to the low standards of many midwives, who she referred to as 'torturers', 'dreadful know-nothings' or 'messy bunglers'.[12] Schrader's case records demonstrate some of the problems of assessing midwifery in this period, referring to a mix of urban and rural practice, good and bad midwives, and skilled and incompetent rural surgeons and men-midwives.

1711 on 10 February I was fetched to Nijkerk to Wattse Jennema, whose wife was called Alltie Jouwkes. She wanted me to attend her, but didn't call for me. And fetched a midwife from Morra, *who tortured her for three days.* She turned it over to the man-midwife, doctor Van den Berrg. He said, he must cut off the child's arms and legs. He took her for dead. *And he said, the child was already dead.* Then I was fetched in secret. When I came there her husband and friends were weeping a great deal. I examined the case, suspected that I had a chance to deliver [her]. The woman was very worn out. I laid her in a warm bed, gave her a cup of caudle, also gave her something in it; sent the neighbours home, so that they would let her rest a bit. An hour after her strength awakened again somewhat. And I had the neighbours fetched again. And after I had positioned the woman in labour, [I] heard that the doctor came then to sit by my side. I pulled the child to the birth canal and in half of a quarter of an hour I got a living daughter. *And I said to the doctor, here is your dead child, to his shame. He expected to earn a hundred guilders there.* The friends and neighbours were very surprised. The mother and child were in a very good state.[13]

Early initiatives in the municipal regulation of midwives

What then was the background to the development of the *stadsvroedvrouw* system? In a number of large towns midwives acting in the service of the community can be traced back to the early seventeenth century; account books record payments to midwives for delivering the poor, and some towns kept lists of midwives who were to re-register at regular periods. In Dordrecht several '*stadsvroedvrouwen*' were recorded in the account books for 1602.[14] In Rotterdam the first midwife to be named in the town records was Janne Danielsr, the wife of Pieter Huybregtse Kuyper, who in February 1611 was described as midwife in the town's service 'on the condition that she be examined beforehand before the town doctors to demonstrate her knowledge'.[15] It was made compulsory for midwives to register with the surgeons' guild annually and to pay a fee to practise, yet one hundred years passed before a closely regulated system of controlling and examining midwives and appointing *stadsvroedvrouwen* was established in Rotterdam.

It was as the Dutch Republic reached its heyday in the mid-seventeenth century[16] that town councils and local medical corporations began to make more rigorous attempts to outline and control the work of the midwife. The practices of instituting lessons, licences and oaths and of appointing *stadsvroedvrouwen* often went hand in hand. At a time when Church and State were becoming separate entities in Holland, the *stadsvroedvrouw*, while maintaining a number of 'moral' functions – the right to perform emergency baptisms, the role of expert witness, and extractor of the names of the fathers of illegitimate children – became an example of the secularization of Dutch society and the concentration of power in local authorities.[17] Towns flourished in this period. It was almost as if Holland was made up of a collection of small nation states, self-contained, self-important municipal powerhouses, with active civic leaderships: 'To *be* Dutch was to be local, parochial, traditional and customary. It meant insisting that power ascended from the local community to higher authorities only on specific terms and conditions . . . .'[18] During this period, the town authorities also became increasingly concerned with indigency and regulating the poor. Efforts to control midwife practice and formalize midwives' status and tasks fitted into the wider trends of organizing all aspects of civic life and offsetting problems associated with need. The midwife came to be seen as an important figure in securing safe (and orderly) childbirth and enabling the population to increase. Yet although the bustling civic activity associated with the seventeenth century saw the introduction of midwife regulation, it was only in the eighteenth century, in a period of rising poverty and economic decline, that most towns followed these precedents, appointing *stadsvroedvrouwen* as one means of relieving the situation of the poor. What began as a '*burgerlijk*' initiative, a sign of municipal strength and concern for the less fortunate, came to be perceived as a necessity.

Several of the more important Dutch towns introduced statutes to control local midwives, and set up lessons and examinations to test their competence to practise in the seventeenth century. The midwives of Delft, the first to be systematically regulated in the Netherlands, were brought under the supervision of the surgeons' guild and town council as early as 1656. Midwives working in the town were to submit to the rules and provisions of the guild, whose members would also be responsible for examining them and teaching them anatomy.[19] Those passing the examination would receive protection from the guild against women attempting to practise without authorization. This deal for the midwife, which could be interpreted as an attempt to ensure good standards and security for the licensed midwife, or as a consolation in return for loss of independence, was to be struck in other communities.

Although Delft was the first known town to regulate midwives closely, Amsterdam provided the model that was largely taken up and followed. Amsterdam made the examination of midwives compulsory in 1668, something held by many to be a good thing, for as the *Willekeur* declared in March of that year, there were many midwives who practised their profession 'without acquiring enough knowledge and expertise for it', so that 'out of her mishandling, many heavy ailments and disasters [occur]'.[20] From 1668 all women wishing to practise as midwives in Amsterdam were to take an examination before the *Collegium Obstetricum*[21] and the lector in anatomy. In the same year, enactments intended to improve the quality of midwives' work were introduced: midwives were instructed to teach apprentices for two years, the official 'learning period' for midwives was fixed at four years, and midwives were ordered not to undertake 'heavy' operations or to give medicine without advice.

Theoretical teaching was given to the Amsterdam midwives by Hendrik van Roonhuysen (1622–1672), surgeon and *stadsvroedmeester*, followed by Frederick Ruysch (1638–1731), lector in anatomy. After 1679 attendance was made compulsory for midwives wishing to work in the town. It could be argued that such lessons were of no use to midwives, for these men were poorly equipped in practical midwifery skills, with little experience of normal deliveries. Practical midwifery, however, was not what they intended to teach. The courses supplemented apprenticeship with an experienced midwife, and their aim was to provide a theoretical background and to fill the midwives in on more complicated, 'unnatural' cases of childbirth. Men of high calibre, certainly amongst the most learned of obstetric doctors, the Amsterdam medical hierarchy were probably better equipped than most to do this, though this was not necessarily the case in all the towns which set up courses. Ruysch was particularly keen to improve anatomical knowledge, and in 1674 suggested to the town council that once every three months 'a recently dead Body be brought in the quiet of the evening from the hospital, and afterwards brought back to the place where it had come from' for demonstrating to midwives and their pupils.[22] One of the primary intentions of the teachers, however, was to train midwives to recognize cases which required the intervention of men-midwives and obstetric doctors, and to instil into them the idea of deferring in complicated deliveries to these higher authorities. So motives were mixed. How helpful this knowledge eventually was to the midwife is questionable, but it is of no little importance that she was believed capable of acquiring it.

The stepping up of regulation in the eighteenth century

Other towns followed Amsterdam, though not with any great urgency. Regulation of midwives generally took place in two phases; rules were implemented to control apprenticeship and personal requirements, followed by the institution of theoretical training by the town's medical hierarchy, the *stadsvroedmeester*, the lector in anatomy or members of the medical corporations. Rotterdam drew up regulations for midwives in 1717, Leiden set up an examination in 1719, but other communities were slower to act, Zwolle in 1757, Groningen in 1766 and Utrecht in 1778.[23] In towns with midwife ordinances expectations concerning the midwife's ability and fitness to practise were similar; they were looking for marks of citizenship, marital status, good character and education. Some communities – in spite of their dissociation from the Church in regulating midwives – superimposed religious qualifications. In Enkhuizen no woman was admitted to the examination unless she was a member of the Protestant Reformed Church (*Gereformeerde*).[24] In Zwolle there was resistance to the appointment of Roman Catholic midwives around 1750, but on 19 July 1778 the town council resolved that 'the Jewess Sibilla Markus be given permission to practise midwifery for Jewish women and other minority folk, who chose her . . .'.[25]

Before taking an examination before the surgeons' guild, *Collegium Medicum* or *Collegium Obstetricum*, candidates of a minimum age of around 25 to 30 were expected to have trained for several years under an established midwife, and to have attended ten to sixteen deliveries. In Haarlem, where examinations for midwives were instituted in 1694, those admitted to the examination had to be at least 30 years old, citizens of Haarlem, of good reputation, to have borne children and be able to read and write well. They had to have worked for three consecutive years under a midwife, who had practised for at least ten years, and under her supervision have delivered at least sixteen women.[26] In 's-Hertogenbosch

> No woman shall be admitted to the afore-mentioned examination, unless she herself is of good name and reputation; legally married, or [a] Widow; have or have had children from a legal marriage; can read and write well; healthy and strong in body; and have learned the skill (*konst*) a long time and have had several children herself.[27]

In Haarlem the second phase of the process of regulation was implemented in 1744 with the setting up of a *Collegie van de vroetkunde* (college of midwifery), the appointment of a *Praelector* in midwifery and the revision of earlier regulations. The Haarlem *stadsvroedmeester* and *stadschirugijn* (town surgeon) Pieter Sannie was to give lessons to midwives; for this and other duties he received a salary of 300 guilders per annum. The college was made up of Sannie, the two *stadsdoctoren* (town doctors) and two other doctors. Pupil midwives were to follow the courses for two years. The lessons were to be given on the first Thursday of each month, and those taking them were to pay the yearly fee of 50 guilders.[28]

In Rotterdam the *Ordannantie op de Anatomie* of 1705 instituted special demonstrations in anatomy to be given by the town's lector in anatomy, Philippus Mazimiliaan Helvetius (*c.* 1660–1708). In cases where 'a subject of the female sex would be dissected' the lector was to give a 'special demonstration . . . of the parts necessary for the skill of midwifery'.[29] It was compulsory for the town's aspirant and practising midwives to attend. Helvetius also wrote a special booklet to be used in conjunction with the lessons to prepare midwives for the examination, based on the formula of short questions and answers.[30] Helvetius's successor Willem Vink (*c.* 1680–1763) put the teaching and licensing of Rotterdam midwives on a firmer basis when he introduced his *Pligt van de Vroed-vrouwen* in 1717.[31] This set out in detail the requirements and duties for midwives practising in the town, a 3-year training, followed by an examination before the lector in anatomy, *stadsdoctoren* and representatives of the surgeons' guild.[32] Vink had worked intensively with midwives prior to 1717, had written a thesis on difficult childbirth (*De partu difficili,* 1703) and was a close contact of Hendrik van Deventer. The timing of the introduction of regulations, lessons and examinations in particular towns was often related to the appointment of men with a special interest in obstetrics to municipal posts.

On passing the examination, and swearing an oath of office, midwives were entitled to hang up a board advertising their profession[33] and, under given conditions, to practise independently. Many towns put together whole pamphlets outlining their role, duties and limitations. The small town of Enkhuizen on the Zuiderzee published a twenty-four-page booklet in 1786 with regulations for midwives working within the town boundaries.[34] Frequently separate lists of rules were drawn up for licensed midwives, *stadsvroedvrouwen* and *stadsvroedmeesters.* The brief of the *stadsvroedvrouw* was to attend at births taking place within the town walls, at the cost of the town authorities, but wealthier inhabitants were to remunerate the midwife out of their own pockets for her time and trouble. It was to avoid the midwife being tempted by the lure of attending richer women that the ordinances rigorously stipulated that the *stadsvroedvrouw* was on no condition to leave a poor woman in the throes of childbirth to attend at the home of a richer neighbour. The regulations drawn up by Willem Vink in Rotterdam in 1717 were typical, instructing midwives not to make the labouring woman frightened, but to calm and comfort her, not to rush or abandon a delivery in order to attend on a richer woman, and ordering midwives to call for the assistance of a surgeon or man-midwife in difficult labours.[35] Some regulations forbade *stadsvroedvrouwen* from leaving the town without giving notice; others warned against drinking, insisted on cleanliness and neatness, and enjoined midwives not to gossip:

> in her reason she must be gentle, patient and not miserable, in the work not too hasty, comfort the labouring women, to abstain herself from strong drink, and to rid herself of all superstitious things.[36]

The regulations stipulated with great force that in difficult cases of child-birth, the midwife was to call in a man-midwife, obstetric doctor or surgeon to take over, limiting her work to normal deliveries. Midwives were not permitted to use instruments – except for the catheter and enema syringe, with softening oils. The regulations drawn up in Dordrecht in 1720 stated that

> no midwife shall be capable of attending unnatural births where the fruit may be dead, or carry out other heavy operations on the body of the woman or force the fruit in any way with the use of any instruments or other means . . . and are not permitted to speed up any extraordinary delivery with or without instruments . . .[37]

Yet there was ambivalence concerning such rulings, and midwives clearly did employ instruments on occasion. Regulations could be vague, interpretations no doubt vaguer. Vrouw Schrader had her own instrument collection, including a crochet, which she used sparingly in emergency deliveries.[38]

The formula for and means of regulating midwives varied from town to town, with responsibility usually being shared by the medical corporations and the town council. In one variation on the general theme, Delft's midwives were regulated by the surgeons' guild, town council and governors and doctors of the *Gasthuis*, the town's hospital, working in close co-operation. By the 1730s the day-to-day regulation and appointment of Delft's *stadsvroedvrouwen* had been turned over to the *stadsdoctoren*, who also functioned as doctors to the *Gasthuis*.[39] By this time, the *Gasthuis* had become a centralized organization with responsibility for the town's medical services, particularly the relief of the sick poor. The town council's role was largely confined to rubber-stamping the recommendations of the *Gasthuis* doctors.

Women wishing to practise in Delft or nearby Delfshaven[40] as midwives were to take their examination before the surgeons' guild, and to swear the oath of office dating back to 1656. The midwife was to call in a doctor in difficult cases, and was to take great care to ensure that the afterbirth was delivered whole. The midwife was not to give the women she delivered alcohol or 'anything else of consequence' – only 'oil of sweet almonds between mother and child a spoonful of cinnamon water, camomile beer, or something similar of little consequence'. She was not to work 'beyond her knowledge'.[41]

Delft had the longest history of midwife regulation in Holland, dating back to 1656, but it was in a period of crisis that efforts were made to step up medical care for the poor and the supervision of the town's midwives. For the town of Delft, its economy based on earthenware, brewing and distilling, and textiles, was experiencing serious economic decline and falling population and birth rates in the late seventeenth and eighteenth centuries.[42] With its population of around 15,000 in the 1730s, Delft was divided up into five areas and a midwife appointed to each of them; Delfshaven, with around 2,100 inhabitants, into two districts.[43] It was stipulated that the midwife was to live in the area where she worked. This rule was applied firmly, and in 1783 Jannetje Buijsterling, who had replaced Geertruij Dorpman as *stadsvroedvrouw* ten years previously, was dismissed when she moved to nearby Schipluiden.[44]

The division of the town paralleled that made for the *stadsdoctoren*, with the most senior midwife being appointed to the same area as the senior *stadsdoctor*.[45] If, when called to a delivery, the *stadsvroedvrouw* of the district was already occupied, another would be called to fill her place and, if all the *stadsvroedvrouwen* were busy, then another licensed midwife would be called in. The salaries paid to the *stadsvroedvrouwen* in Delft were fixed at around 60 to 80 guilders per annum, and we can be fairly sure that they were paid promptly twice a year, together with the *stadsdoctoren* and other *Gasthuis* appointees.

The aims of the regulators/the status of the midwife

In all towns, despite small local differences, the aims were the same – by means of regulation, to make the midwife answerable to the town authorities and local medical hierarchy, to control her qualifications and practice. If the midwife broke the regulations, she was liable to punitive action – a fine, dismissal as town midwife, or the removal of her board, the symbol of her craft and her authorization to practise. In 's-Hertogenbosch the punishment for using instruments was a ban on practice for six weeks for a first offence, six months for a second, and a life ban for the third offence.[46] Despite their often punitive nature, however, the regulations were presented neither as being overly restrictive of the midwife's practice nor as a form of protection of the practices of men-midwives and obstetric doctors, but rather as a safeguard for the regulated midwife herself against her unqualified competitors.

As the midwife became more closely regulated during the late seventeenth and eighteenth centuries, the costs of training and taking an examination also rose rapidly. Midwives were compensated for taking on apprentices, but the rewards were small, and many experienced midwives were reluctant to co-operate in training pupils. Arrangements between midwife and pupil were worked out privately, but towns often imposed guidelines; by the mid-eighteenth century pupils in 's-Hertogenbosch were to pay a maximum of 10 guilders a year, plus half a guilder for a delivery over and above the first six,[47] in Haarlem the maximum was 30 guilders a year, plus 1 guilder for each delivery above the first ten.[48] Theoretical lessons had to be paid for, and an examination fee was usually demanded. In Haarlem after 1744 the lessons cost 100 guilders for a two-year period, plus 15 guilders for the examination fee,[49] in Rotterdam by 1773 41 guilders and 10 stuivers was demanded by the surgeons' guild from candidates wishing to take their examination in midwifery.[50] Payment for a licence was additional, 25 guilders in Amsterdam in 1703 and 100 guilders from 1786, a considerable proportion of a *stadsvroedvrouw's* annual salary.[51] While apprenticeship fees remained low, the impositions of the medical corporations meant that, all in all, training was an expensive business, which presumably excluded many from qualifying (though not from practising midwifery). This system served to confirm the distinction between those working within town regulations, who were likely to gain employment as *stadsvroedvrouwen*, from those working outside the town boundaries or unofficially within the town. It also reinforced the divide between urban and rural practice.

Though complaints were heard of the generally low level of knowledge of midwives, much was demanded of them in terms of examination knowledge, so much so that it is hard to give credence to the idea that, following a handful of theoretical lessons, the candidate midwives suddenly became equipped to fulfil what was required of them. A reasonable standard of general knowledge, literacy and practical experience can be assumed, much perhaps picked up during apprenticeship. In 1700 the Amsterdam *Collegium Medicum et Obstetricum's Promotieboek der Vroedvrouwen* listed amongst the aspects of midwifery that candidates were expected to understand – knowledge of the uterus, how to induce labour, how to 'lay, place and handle' the woman in labour, what to do if the child is not properly turned, what to do if the waters have broken but the woman has no contractions, to recognize if the 'fruit' is living or dead, or if it is a 'mola' or misformed. The midwife was also to have a complete understanding of how to deliver the afterbirth, how to care for the mother and child, and what to do if the baby was born dead.[52] Most midwives working in the towns appear to have been literate – they could sign their names, while some, such as Anna Hensbeek of Gouda, became active petitioners[53] – and a few were very learned.

The sisters Van Putten who worked in Rotterdam in the closing decades of the eighteenth century and early years of the nineteenth were at the very least unusual, but perhaps unique, in that they both acquired, in addition to their midwifery diplomas, licences to practise as *vroedmeesters* (men-midwives).[54] Elisabeth van Putten (1755–1848) registered as a pupil midwife with the Rotterdam surgeons' guild in 1769, and in 1773 (in the same year that her father, the Rotterdam surgeon Hendrik van Putten was elected headman of the guild), took her examination.[55] This was no ordinary examination for midwives, however, for Elisabeth was also examined in operative midwifery. On the basis of her knowledge, the guild qualified her as '*vroedmeesteres*'

201

—7   (female man-midwife!) 'with permission to use the forceps or the secret of Roonhuysen if circumstances require this'.[56]

Neeltje van Putten (1761–1828), following in her older sister's footsteps, registered with the surgeons' guild as a pupil in 1778, took her midwives' examination in 1781[57] and, as Elisabeth had done, followed the theoretical lessons in obstetrics given by the town's lector Hendrik Vink. Neeltje followed her apprenticeship not with one of the *stadsvroedvrouwen,* but with the *stadsvroedmeester,* Cornelius Imchoor (in a more general response of the guild to the shortage of *stadsvroedvrouwen* in Rotterdam and consequent lack of placings for apprentices). In 1783 Neeltje also qualified as *vroedmeesteres.*[58] Both sisters lacked the usual requirements demanded of midwives. Although Elisabeth married a wealthy Rotterdam merchant in 1779, the marriage producing some fourteen children (including two sets of twins), at the time she took her diploma in 1773, she was single and only 18 years of age. Neeltje, aged 22 when she qualified as *vroedmeesteres,* never married.[59] In terms of social cachet, however, they ranked higher than most midwives.

After some three decades in practice, Neeltje published two articles in the medical journal *Hippocrates,* in 1814 and 1816.[60] The articles, illustrated with cases of difficult births that she had attended, argued against too liberal instrumental intervention; even in difficult cases of childbirth, nature should be allowed, if possible, to take its course. Neeltje van Putten did use forceps, but stressed the need to employ them in conjunction with and not in opposition to nature, to observe carefully, particularly to note at an early stage the position of the child in the womb. Van Putten cited a number of midwifery works, especially from the French school, indicating a respectable (though far from exhaustive) working knowledge of obstetric texts.[61] Indirectly, the articles vindicated women as the traditional midwifery practitioners, employing skills acquired through experience and patient observation, as did the Van Putten sisters directly through their practices. No doubt many other midwives worked in a similar way, employing instruments, including the forceps, on a limited basis,[62] but what is unusual about the Van Puttens is that they were licensed by the Rotterdam surgeons' guild to do so, to work legitimately as 'men-midwives'. They attempted to straddle the boundary between man-midwife and midwife, combining the policy of allowing nature to take its course with the judicious use of instruments.[63]

The case of the Van Putten sisters is clearly special, and closely related to the Rotterdam situation, where efforts were being made to reform surgical and obstetric practice not via the academic branch of medicine, but by the surgeons themselves.[64] There seems to have been no opposition within the guild to this highly unusual development, though it is unclear whether the town's surgeons considered the awarding of diplomas in man-midwifery to the Van Puttens as isolated initiatives, or as a viable method of attracting more women of a higher calibre to midwifery.

In general, while midwife regulations protected and reinforced the power of the medical corporations who were to oversee training and licensing, during this period of municipal control medical men were concerned primarily with supervising the midwife, rather than seeking to replace her. Occasionally this was simply not feasible – some towns had only a small number of men-midwives and obstetric doctors – but the reverse was more often the case, many communities having too few midwives.[65] Rotterdam, Delft and Gouda all recorded shortages of *stadsvroedvrouwen* during the eighteenth century and anxiety about recruiting suitable women. This was not constant; at times in Delft there were too many candidates and a waiting list,[66] but often there was a dearth. There were frequent vacancies for the posts in Delfshaven, and in February 1780 it was predicted that around fifty women would have to be delivered by one *stadsvroedvrouw* before the end of March! Despite placing newspaper advertisements, one year passed before Maria Bosschieten was appointed second midwife to the harbour town.[67]

Regulation was closely associated with efforts to increase the number of licensed midwives, and not the diminishment of their role. While *stadsvroedmeesters* were employed in increasing numbers towards the end of the century, their task was to take over difficult cases, primarily those requiring instrumental intervention. The fact that their positions were less demanding was reflected by their low salaries, which compared poorly with those of *stadsvroedvrouwen*. The amount paid by town authorities varied greatly, as did work-loads. In Gouda, Anna Puyt was employed as town midwife to the fourth quarter of the town in 1739 at a salary of 30 guilders per annum. Upon the death of another midwife, she moved to the third quarter in 1746 and her salary consequently increased to 60 guilders. Ten years later, in 1756, she became midwife to the second quarter receiving 70 guilders per annum, and in 1762 she took over the first quarter and a salary of 98 guilders.[68] By 1799 salaries in Gouda were much higher, 300 guilders for the most senior midwife to 200 guilders for the fourth, a response to a shortage of candidates for the posts and the repeated petitioning of midwives for better remuneration. Gouda's *stadsvroedmeester* received 100 guilders, a reflection of his comparatively light work-load.[69] A *stadsvroedmeester* was first appointed in Delft in 1739, with a salary of 50 guilders, again lower than that of the *stadsvroedvrouwen*, but he was only to attend emergency deliveries.[70] His salary was a third of that paid to the *Gasthuis* doctors, who were receiving 150 guilders per annum in 1737; surgeons' salaries were fixed at 350 guilders in 1756.[71] Like the *stadsvroedvrouw*, the *stadsvroedmeester* was a municipal employee, subject to a long list of regulations, and accountable to the *Gasthuis* doctors.

In the eighteenth century *vroedmeesters* and obstetric doctors were generally only present in the birthing chamber to assist in obstructed deliveries, cases of placenta praevia, multiple births or other obstetric emergencies.

Employing their instruments, the task of delivering a dead infant or, more rarely, performing a caesarean section, fell usually to them; in theory they were to be called in by the midwife once she encountered difficulties delivering the child.[72] Resistance to the figure of the doctor in the birthing chamber on the grounds of tradition and modesty took similar forms to elsewhere in Europe,[73] but the lack of initiatives on the part of medical men to push the midwife out of practice seems to account in part at least for her continuing importance.[74]

Yet initiatives were taken to raise standards amongst midwives. Supplementing the training courses set up in towns, the eighteenth century saw the large-scale production of books, by Dutch authors or translations from French, English and German,[75] intended largely to improve the midwife's knowledge, and not at persuading the public and medical men that the midwife was redundant.[76] Van Deventer's publications, *Dageraet der Vroedvrouwen* (1696) and *Manuale Operatien Zijnde een Nieuw Ligt voor Vroedmeesters en Vroedvrouwen* (1701), though containing some fierce criticisms of midwives, embodied the understanding that they were to remain the normal childbirth attendants. Married to a practising midwife, Van Deventer realized that the profession was not about to disappear, but urged that the midwife's training be improved, her knowledge (though not her competence) extended. He also emphasized that a good midwife was one who did not hesitate to call in a man-midwife in difficult cases.[77]

Though rhetoric was used against midwives throughout the eighteenth century – they were criticized for everything from a lack of skill to an absence of social graces – no determined effort was made to put them out of business. Jacob Denys, the *stadsvroedmeester* for Leiden, railed against the midwife early in the eighteenth century – 'no art is practised in a more slovenly, reckless and stupid way' than obstetrics by midwives.[78] Yet he was talking about the poorly trained, the unlicensed, and both Denys and his successor, Cornelius Terne, believed the solution to lie in instruction, separating the wheat from the chaff, the ignorant, uneducated midwife from those who had followed their lessons and sworn an oath of practice.[79]

Conflicts between midwives and medical men chiefly centred around disputes over teaching, minutiae of regulation, individual charges of malpractice or salaries, and not around the broader division of labour. Midwives themselves were silent (or their comments unrecorded) on the larger issues of midwifery practice, which may indicate that such issues were simply not being discussed. The conflicts that are recorded often tell us more about the assertive and independent character of the midwife than indicating subjugation to medical authority. In all towns midwives petitioned regularly for salary increases – they did not always receive them, but the shortage of *stadsvroedvrouwen* strengthened their hand. In Leiden it was the midwives, led by Anna van Abcoude, who complained about the *stadsvroedmeester* Terne, his lessons and deportment in cases of childbirth.

The midwives' complaints were 'heard and taken seriously' by the *Collegium Obstetricum*, and frequently resolved in their favour.[80] In Gouda the *stadsvroedvrouw* Anna Hensbeek came before the town authorities in 1796 when she failed to ask a woman she had attended in labour to declare the name of the father of her illegitimate child. She refused to pay a fine of 25 guilders and was dismissed but, after a petition was drawn up by the other midwives in the town, she was quickly reinstated.[81] More serious accusations of malpractice could end badly for the midwife. One of the very few disputes recorded between the town authorities and midwives in eighteenth-century Delft, but one resulting in severe retribution, occurred in 1773 when the *stadsvroedvrouw* Martijntje Kneijne was packed off to the house of correction for two years for her poor behaviour and drunken debauchery. Kneijne was accused of attending a delivery whilst drunk, and extracting the baby with such force that shortly after it died.[82]

Conclusion

It is difficult to make an assessment of the effects of local regulations on midwife practice, or to judge whether standards were higher in the towns with their *stadsvroedvrouwen* than the countryside. Apprenticeship remained the key to training. Many midwives were unable (or unwilling) to take advantage of the lessons and anatomy demonstrations given in the towns and, for those that did, this made little impact on their practical skills. Even in the nineteenth century, after schools were established for midwifery training, practical teaching with a qualified midwife remained one of the most important features of the courses offered to both midwives and men-midwives. Many midwives remained outside the reach of the examination and licensing systems set up by the towns; simply by living beyond the town boundaries, they were exempt from their ordinances.

The examined and licensed *stadsvroedvrouw* shared many features with members of other trades in eighteenth-century Holland. Controlled by a guild or corporation – albeit not one they could be member of or which they had elected – they were subject to a series of rules of admission and a strict definition of their role. Upon qualification, they were entitled to hang up a board, usually adorned with symbols of their trade, the enema spout, a birthing stool or cherubic infant.[83] They could be reprimanded and sanctions imposed for failing to provide a satisfactory service or for breaking guild rules. Yet the *stadsvroedvrouwen* were also salaried employees, expected to be loyal to the town councils, working in effect as a combination of early community midwife and civil servant.

Though critics of the midwife were to be found, the medical corporations and town authorities were interested in preserving them (and perhaps encouraging their contributions to the guild coffers through their payments for lessons and licences), although in a closely controlled form which suited their needs. Only in the nineteenth century was this system upturned, with the collapse of the guilds and decline in the power of the towns, following the invasion of the French into the Netherlands in 1795. What came to replace the authority of the guilds and town councils was a nationally regulated system of control, whereby the midwife was legislated for together with other medical practitioners, with distinct duties and limitations on her work. Yet the system of midwife regulation imposed after 1818 for the country as a whole shared many features with the schemes set up by individual towns since the mid-seventeenth century.[84]

The story of the Dutch midwife is not one of decline from the eighteenth century.[85] Emphasis remained on reform, not replacement. Midwives were seen as being essential in the eighteenth century, all the better if they were *burgerlijke*, respectable, well-trained, and a close eye kept on their activities. The functions of the midwife were curtailed during the eighteenth century – regulations forbidding her from using instruments were strengthened, her role in gynaecology and minor surgery undermined, her competence confined to normal births, falling under the supervision of the doctors. Yet her position as attendant in normal cases of childbirth was guaranteed, something not assured in other European countries. The eighteenth century laid the groundwork of a confirmation of the midwife's role in the nineteenth, with the *stadsvroedvrouwen* system forming a basis for the future organization of midwife practice. In the nineteenth century emphasis remained on supervising the midwife's work and restricting her activities, rather than on excluding her from practice.[86]

Today, the Dutch midwife occupies a unique position of professional and workplace autonomy, including attendance at large numbers of domiciliary births.[87] Already, the roots of later developments in Holland, which were to set its obstetric services apart from those of other countries, were discernible in the eighteenth century. Though it is to the nineteenth and twentieth centuries that we must look to trace the legislative and professional developments which confirmed the midwife's position and the different path taken in the organization of obstetric care in Holland compared with other European countries, the predecessors of modern Dutch midwives are to be found in the eighteenth-century women who worked in the service of the community.

Acknowledgements

I would like to acknowledge the help of the Gemeente Archieven in Delft and Rotterdam, and to thank Lara Marks and Mart van Lieburg for commenting upon an earlier version of this article.

Notes

1. Gemeente Archief Delft (hereafter GAD), Archief van het Oude en Nieuwe Gasthuis te Delft (hereafter ONGD), Register houdende opgave van aanstelling, ontslag en bezoldiging van, alsmede instructies voor de stads- en gasthuisdoctoren, chirurgijns, pestmeester, apotheker en vroedvrouwen, *c.* 1725–*c.* 1765, f. 95.

2. For midwives in the early modern period, see, for example, E. van der Borg, 'Beeldvorming over vroedvrouwen in de Noordelijke Nederlanden (1600–1900)', *Verzorging*, 3 (1988), 2–17; *idem*, 'Wijze volksvrouwen. Beroepsvorming van vroedvrouwen in Nederland tot 1865', *Focaal. Tijdschrift voor Antropologie*, 14 (1990), 13–34; H.A. van der Borg, *Vroedvrouwen: Beeld en Beroep. Ontwikkelingen in het Vroedvrouwschap in Leiden, Arnhem, 's-Hertogenbosch en Leeuwarden, 1650–1865* (Wageningen, 1992); W. Frijhoff, 'Non satis dignitatis . . . Over de maatschappelijke status van geneeskundigen tijdens de Republiek', *Tijdschrift voor Geschiedenis*, 96 (1983), 379–406; *idem*, 'Medische beroepen en verzorgingspatroon in de Franse Tijd: een dwarsdoorsnede', *Tijdschrift voor de Geschiedenis der Geneeskunde, Natuurwetenschappen, Wiskunde en Techniek*, 8 (1985), 92–122; H.M. Dupuis *et al.*, *Een Kind Onder het Hart. Verloskunde, Volksgeloof, Gezin, Seksualiteit en Moraal Vroeger en Nu* (Amsterdam, 1987), esp. ch. 1; F.W. van der Waals, 'Doorbraken in de verloskunde'; M.J. van Lieburg and H. Marland, 'Elisabeth en Neeltje van Putten: twee 18e-eeuwse grensgangers tussen de beroepsvelden van vroedvrouw en vroedmeester', *Tijdschrift voor de Geschiedenis der Geneeskunde, Natuurwetenschappen, Wiskunde en Techniek*, 12 (1989), 181–97; A. Hallema, 'Vroedvrouwen in stad en dorp in het westen van Noord-Brabant', *Nederlands Tijdschrift voor Geneeskunde*, 99:III (1955), 2660–7; C.R. Post, 'De Amsterdamse vroedvrouw uit de 18de eeuw', *Bijdragen tot de Geschiedenis der Geneeskunde*, 36 (1985), 1–8; A.J. van Reeuwijk, *Vroedkunde en Vroedvrouwen in de Nederlanden in de 17e en 18e Eeuw* (Amsterdam, 1941).

3. The dictionary gives a wide definition of '*burgerlijke*' – middle class, bourgeois, conventional, civilian, smug. The word here is taken as representing a mix of these elements, the midwife as a self-assured municipal employee, a 'good citizen', an important (and perhaps also self-important) figure in the community. *Van Dale Grootwoordenboek Nederlands-Engels.*

4. As Mary Lindemann has pointed out in ch. 9 in this volume, our reliance on Anglo-Saxon studies has affected our vision of the place of the midwife in the eighteenth century. For studies of decline in England and North America, see, for example, J. Donnison, *Midwives and Medical Men. A History of Inter-Professional Rivalries and Women's Rights* (London, 1977); J.B. Donegan, *Women and Men Midwives. Medicine, Morality, and Misogyny in Early America* (Westport, CT and London, 1978). Mary Lindemann also outlines some of the dangers of calling even trained and recognized groups of midwives 'professionals' in this period. See also chs 5, 7 and 8 in this volume for the enduring role of the midwife in eighteenth-century Spain, France and Italy.

5. H. Marland, 'The medicalization of motherhood: doctors and infant welfare in the Netherlands, 1901–1930', in V. Fildes, L. Marks and H. Marland (eds) *Women and Children First. International Maternal and Infant Welfare 1870–1945* (London and New York, 1992), and for a regional analysis, M. Pruijt, 'Roeien, baren en in de arbeid zijn. Vroedvrouwen in Noord-Brabant, 1880–1960', in M. Grever and A. van der Veen (eds) *Bij ons Moeder en ons Jet. Brabantse Vrouwen in de 19de en 20ste Eeuw* (Zutphen, 1989), 122–42.

6.   See chs 5 and 8 in this volume by Teresa Ortiz and Nadia Filippini, for the parallel existence of the 'modern' trained midwife and her 'traditional' counterpart in Italy and Spain.

7.   And generally well-documented in town archives and the records of the medical corporations, in the form of ordinances, regulations and details of appointments. This is in contrast to non-licensed midwives who, as elsewhere in Europe, are thinly documented.

8.   H. Marland, M.J. van Lieburg and G.J. Kloosterman, *'Mother and Child were Saved'. The Memoirs (1693–1740) of the Frisian Midwife Catharina Schrader* (Amsterdam, 1987). For a brief summary of Schrader's life and work, see H. Marland, 'All well for mother and child. The notebook and practice of Vrouw Catharina Schrader, 1693–1745', *Nursing Times,* 83 (7 Oct. 1987), 49–51, and S. Schama, *The Embarrassment of Riches. An Interpretation of Dutch Culture in the Golden Age* (London, 1987), 525–35. See also the fuller transcription of Vrouw Schrader's notebook with introductory essays, M.J. van Lieburg (ed.) *C.G. Schrader's Memoryboeck van de Vrouwens. Het Notitieboek van een Friese Vroedvrouw 1693–1745* (with an obstetric commentary by G.J. Kloosterman) (Amsterdam, 1984); B.W.Th. Nuyens, 'Het dagboek van Vrouw Schraders', *Nederlands Tijdschrift voor Geneeskunde,* 70:II (1926), 1790–801, and, for a commentary on the Dutch edition of the notebook, W. Frijhoff, 'Vrouw Schrader's beroepsjournal: overwegingen bij een publikatie over arbeidspraktijk in het verleden', *Tijdschrift voor de Geschiedenis der Geneeskunde, Natuurwetenschappen, Wiskunde en Techniek,* 8 (1985), 27–38. See chs 2 and 3 in this volume by David Harley and Ann Giardina Hess for the rural midwife in England.

9.   Marland, Van Lieburg and Kloosterman, *'Mother and Child were Saved',* 14.

10.   J.G.W.F. Bik, *Vijf Eeuwen Medisch Leven in een Hollandse Stad,* MD thesis, University of Amsterdam (Assen, 1955), 348.

11.   See Marland, Van Lieburg and Kloosterman, *'Mother and Child were Saved',* 9–13, for the extent and range of Vrouw Schrader's practice. For repeat practice in seventeenth-century London, see ch. 1 in this volume by Doreen Evenden.

12.   Marland, Van Lieburg and Kloosterman, *'Mother and Child were Saved',* 19.

13.   Ibid., 63–4 (Marland's emphasis).

14.   A.C. Drogendijk, *De Verloskundige Voorziening in Dordrecht van 1500 tot Heden,* MD thesis, University of Amsterdam (Amsterdam, 1935), 44.

15.   M.J. van Lieburg, 'Het verloskundig onderwijs te Rotterdam vóór 1828', in E. Scholte, M.J. van Lieburg and R.O. Aalbersberg, *Rijkskweekschool voor Vroedvrouwen te Rotterdam* (Leidschendam, 1982), 6.

16.   Schama, *The Embarrassment of Riches;* J. Huizinga, *Dutch Civilization in the 17th Century* (London and New York, 1968); J.L. Price, *Culture and Society in the Dutch Republic During the 17th Century* (London, 1974).

17.   See H. Schilling, 'Religion und Gesellschaft in der calvinistischen Republik der Vereinigten Niederlande – "Öffentlichkeitskirche" und Säkularisation; Ehe und Hebammenwesen; Presbyterien und politische Partizipation', in F. Petri (ed.) *Kirche und gesellschaftlicher Wandel in deutschen und niederländischen Städten der werdenden Neuzeit* (Köln, 1980), 197–250. Schilling uses the case of Dutch midwives to support Talcott Parsons's thesis that the development of modern society dates back to the seventeenth century. T. Parsons, *The System of Modern Societies* (Englewood Cliffs, NJ, 1971). The secularization of midwives' tasks signalled a break with the Middle Ages and a profound change in mentality, a shift in concentration from the 'soul' to the mother and baby, and a move towards 'professionalization'. A link was forged between midwife practice and local authority supervision, which in the nineteenth century became State control. As

Eva Abraham has pointed out, this establishment of midwives as a (semi-) 'professional' group did not necessarily imply high standards of practice, nor a steady advance through the centuries. E. Abraham-Van der Mark, 'Dutch midwifery in the past and present', unpub. paper, Amsterdam, 1990. For the battle between the Catholic Church and State in eighteenth-century Italy, see ch. 8 in this volume by Nadia Filippini.

18. Schama, *The Embarrassment of Riches,* 62 (Schama's emphasis).

19. GAD, Stadsarchief, Chirurgijnsgildeboeke, 1584–1749, accession no. 1981, Resolution of 11 Sept. 1656; H.L. Houtzager, *Medicyns, Vroedwyfs en Chirurgyns. Schets van de Gezondheidszorg in Delft in Beschrijving van het Theatrum Anatomicum Aldaar in de 16e en 17e Eeuw* (Amsterdam, 1979), 45–6; D.P. Oosterbaan, *Zeven Eeuwen Geschiedenis van het Oude en Nieuwe Gasthuis te Delft* (Delft, 1954), 201–5.

20. Dossier Vroedvrouwen, Gemeente Archief Amsterdam. Cited Post, 'De Amsterdamse vroedvrouw uit de 18de eeuw', 1.

21. The *Collegium Obstetricum,* a branch of the *Collegium Medicum,* was established in only a few of the larger towns, including Amsterdam and Leiden. Obstetric doctors (*obstetriae doctoren*), who had followed a university training, were few in number and concentrated in larger centres; they had the same tasks, primarily to undertake complicated deliveries, as their non-university educated man-midwife (*vroedmeester*) colleagues.

22. Cited R.E. Kistemaker, 'De praktijk van de Amsterdamse vroedvrouw in de 17de en 18de eeuw', *Ons Amsterdam,* 39 (1987), 179.

23. See, for local studies of midwife practice, Van der Borg, 'Wijze volks-vrouwen', and *idem,* Vroedvrouwen (for Leeuwarden, Arnhem, 's-Hertogenbosch and Leiden), and Bik, *Vijf Eeuwen Medisch Leven in een Hollandse Stad,* esp. 347–74 (for Gouda).

24. *Reglement Bij die van den Geregte der Stad Enkhuizen, Gemaakt, Verbeeterd en Vermeerderd, Rakende het Vroedwerk, Binnen dezelve Stadt* (Enkhuizen, 1786), 5.

25. Resolutieboek van Raad en Schepenen der Stad Zwolle. Cited J.H. Hagenbeek, *Het Moederschap in Overijssel. Een Onderzoek naar de Verloskundige Voorziening en de Zuigelingenzorg in de Provincie Overijssel* (Zwolle, 1936), 46.

26. H. Bitter, 'Vroedvrouwen en leerling-vroedvrouwen te Haarlem in de 17de en 18de eeuw', *Nederlands Tijdschrift voor Geneeskunde,* 59:IB (1915), 2197, 2199.

27. Regelement en ordonnantie voor de vroedvrouwen, binnen de stadt 's-Hertogenbosch, 1761. Cited P.E.G. van der Heijden, *De Zorg voor Moeder en Kind in Noord-Brabant,* MD thesis, University of Amsterdam, 1934, 39.

28. Bitter, 'Vroedvrouwen en leerling-vroedvrouwen te Haarlem', 2203.

29. *Ordannantie op de Anatomie,* 1705, art. 20. Gemeente Archief Rotterdam (hereafter GAR), Oud Stadsarchief, accession no. 37, ff. 224–5, 6 June 1705. Cited Van Lieburg, 'Het verloskundig onderwijs te Rotterdam vóór 1828', 8.

30. P.M. Helvetius, *Teel-Thuin van 't Menschelijk Geslagt* (Leiden, 1698).

31. *Ordannantie op de Chirurgie, Pligt van de Vroed-vrouwen, ende Saken tot de Chirurgie Behoordende* (Rotterdam, 1717).

32. See Van Lieburg, 'Het verloskundig onderwijs te Rotterdam vóór 1828', 6–11.

33. M.A. van Andel, 'Vroedvrouwenbordjes', *Nederlands Tijdschrift voor Genees-kunde,* 72:II (1928), 2665–9.

34. *Reglement Bij die van den Geregte der Stad Enkhuizen.*

35. *Ordannantie op de Chirurgie, Pligt van de Vroed-vrowen, ende Saken tot de Chirurgie Behoordende.*

36. *Reglement Bij die van den Geregte der Stad Enkhuizen,* 5. Vrouw Schrader was able to combine a deep and driving faith, a true religious vocation, with 'matter-

of-fact' superstitions, sharing a belief with many of her clients in the influence of maternal imagination and maternal behaviour on the foetus ('*verzien*'), a baby born with a 'pig's head' because its mother had spent too much time working with pigs, a malformed child born to a 'dishonoured' innkeeper's daughter, who had sworn that she would not get pregnant, a child born with a growth on its head, to a woman who preferred curly-haired children: 'How careful the pregnant woman must be to conduct herself well in all she says and thinks.' Marland, Van Lieburg and Kloosterman, '*Mother and Child were Saved*', 61–2, 67.

37. Ordonnantie en reglement voor de vroedvrouwen, 1720. Cited Drogendijk, *De Verloskundige Voorziening in Dordrecht*, 39.

38. Marland, Van Lieburg and Kloosterman, '*Mother and Child were Saved*', 20, 37.

39. GAD, Stadsarchief, Memoriaal Burgemeesteren, 23 Dec. 1730, and for Delfshaven 21 Nov. 1739. Cited Oosterbaan, *Zeven Eeuwen Geschiedenis van het Oude en Nieuwe Gasthuis te Delft*, 204.

40. Delfshaven, Delft's harbour town, was a dependency of the Delft town council until 1885, when jurisdiction shifted to Rotterdam.

41. GAD, Stadsarchief, Chirurgijnsgildeboeke, 1584–1749, Resolution of 11 Sept. 1656.

42. T. Wijsenbeek-Olthuis, *Achter de Gevels van Delft* (Hilversum, 1987), chs 1 and 2.

43. Ibid., 27; GAD, ONGD, Register houdende opgave van aanstelling, ontslag en bezoldiging van . . . de stads- en gasthuisdoctoren, chirurgijns, pestmeester, apotheker en vroedvrouwen, *c.* 1725–*c.* 1765, Extract uit het register van de officianten der stad Delft, 5 Sept. 1734, Extract uit de resolutien van de Heeren Burgermeesteren der stad Delft, 21 Nov. 1739, f. 6.

44. GAD, ONGD, Des ouden Gasthuis journaal. Van instructiën, contracten en commissiën van rentmeesters, predikanten, doctoren, chirurgijns, apothecars, vroedvrouwen, binnenvaders en moeders, *c.* 1765–*c.* 1850, f. 71

45. Oosterbaan, *Zeven Eeuwen Geschiedenis van het Oude en Nieuwe Gasthuis te Delft*, 205.

46. Regelement en ordannantie voor de vroedvrouwen, binnen de stadt 's-Hertogenbosch, 1761. Cited Van der Heijden, *De Zorg voor Moeder en Kind in Noord-Brabant*, 41.

47. Ibid., 40.

48. Bitter, 'Vroedvrouwen en leerling-vroedvrouwen te Haarlem', 2204.

49. Ibid., 2203–4.

50. GAR, Arch. Gilden, inv. no. 30, Rekenboek van het chirurgijnsgilde, 13 Oct. 1773.

51. Post, 'De Amsterdamse vroedvrouw uit de 18de eeuw', 1.

52. Archief van *Collegium Medicum et Obstetricum Amstelaed*, no. 13, Gemeente Archief Amsterdam. See ch. 4 in this volume by Merry Wiesner for similar requirements in Germany.

53. Bik, *Vijf Eeuwen Medisch Leven in een Hollandse Stad*, 367–74.

54. Van Lieburg and Marland, 'Elisabeth en Neeltje van Putten'.

55. GAR, Arch. Gilden, inv. no. 30, 12 Jan. 1769; Rekenboek van het chirurgijnsgilde, 13 Oct. 1773.

56. GAR, Oud Stadsarchief, inv. no. 325, ff. 264–6.

57. GAR, Arch. Gilden, inv. no. 30, 19 Jan. 1778, May 1781.

58. 'Lijsten van erkende geneeskunstoefenaren', supp. to *Provinciale Bladen*, and listings in Archief Plaatselijke Commissie voor Geneeskundig Toevoorzigt, GAR, inv. no. 4, items 22 and 25. Neither of the Van Putten sisters are listed in the registers of midwives, GAR, Oud Stadsarchief, inv. nos 2845, 2846, 2851.

59. Van Lieburg and Marland, 'Elisabeth en Neeltje van Putten', 183.

60. N. van Putten, 'Eenige aanmerkingen en waarnemingen als bijdragen tot de verloskunde', *Hippocrates*, 1 (1814), 389–412; *idem*, 'Bijdrage tot de verloskunde', *Hippocrates*, 2 (1816), 433–51.

61. Van Lieburg and Marland, 'Elisabeth en Neeltje van Putten', 193–4.

62. For the use of forceps by Italian midwives, see ch. 8 in this volume by Nadia Filippini.

63. Van Lieburg and Marland, 'Elisabeth en Neeltje van Putten', 196.

64. M.J. van Lieburg, 'De geneeskunde en natuurwetenschappen binnen de Rotterdamse genootschappen uit de 18e eeuw', *Tijdschrift voor de Geschiedenis der Geneeskunde, Natuurwetenschappen, Wiskunde en Techniek*, 1 (1978), 14–22; *idem*, *Het Medisch Onderwijs te Rotterdam 1467–1967. Een Kort Historisch Overzicht* (Amsterdam, 1978); *idem*, 'Het verloskundig onderwijs te Rotterdam vóór 1828'.

65. For the relationship between the number of medical personnel and population in the early nineteenth century, see Frijhoff, 'Medische beroepen en verzorgingspatroon in de Franse Tijd'.

66. In 1749 Margaretha Perks was appointed *stadsvroedvrouw* in Delft, without payment, on the condition that she would receive her first salary on the death or departure of one of the other *stadsvroedvrouwen*. She waited some six years before being awarded her first salary of 60 guilders per annum for a post in Delfshaven. GAD, ONGD, Register houdende opgave van aanstelling, ontslag en bezoldiging van . . . de stads- en gasthuisdoctoren, chirurgijns, pestmeester, apotheker en vroedvrouwen, *c.* 1725–*c.* 1765, 28 June 1755, f. 86.

67. GAD, ONGD, Register van resoluties van het college van regenten, 1756–85, 26 Feb. 1780, 25 Feb. 1781.

68. Bik, *Vijf Eeuwen Medisch Leven in een Hollandse Stad*, 357.

69. Ibid., 373.

70. GAD, ONGD, Register houdende opgave van aanstelling, ontslag en bezoldiging van . . . de stads- en gasthuisdoctoren, chirurgijns, pestmeester, apotheker en vroedvrouwen, *c.* 1725–*c.* 1765, Extract uit de resolutien van de Heeren Burgermeesteren der stad Delft, 21 Nov. 1739, f. 6.

71. Oosterbaan, *Seven Eeuwen Geschiedenis van het Oude en Nieuwe Gasthuis te Delft*, 180, 189

72. On 15 October 1713 a tailor's wife in the Dronkermanssteeg in Rotterdam went into labour. A midwife was called who observed 'that the child came with his bottom first and that the birth could not proceed, but stayed unmovingly stuck'. After five days, the midwife summoned Dr Willem Vink who also saw no means of delivering the child. Hendrik van Deventer was then brought in, but was unable to save the woman. The head of the child was 'on the right side of the mother with its chin wedged fast on its breast', the child was dead and 'rotting fast'. The woman died the day after. Van Deventer was so influenced by this grim saga that he cited it in his book *Manuale Operatien Zijnde een Nieuw Ligt voor Vroedmeesters en Vroedvrouwen*, published in 1701. M.J. van Lieburg, 'Uit de medische stadsgeschiedenis van Rotterdam. Vroedvrouwen, verlosmeesters en doctoren', *Monitor*, 4 (1975), 77.

73. For Italy, see ch. 8 in this volume by Nadia Filippini.

74. The case notes of Catharina Schrader indicate that we should not place too much credence on a strict division of labour – midwives normal, men-midwives difficult births. Schrader took over difficult cases from other midwives or doctors, or co-operated closely with them at a delivery, or *vroedmeesters* were called in to attend normal births. Other factors, such as availability, the need to attend other pressing cases, and problems of transport, must also have played a part in rural

areas with a thin covering of medical personnel. Marland, Van Lieburg and Kloosterman, *'Mother and Child were Saved'*.

75. G.J. Kloosterman, 'Verloskundige kanttekeningen bij Vrouw Schraders "Memoryboeck"', in Van Lieburg, *C.G. Schrader's Memoryboeck van de Vrouwens*, 47–56. Popular midwifery manuals included translations of E. Roesslin's *Der Schwanngeren Frawen und Hebammen Rosengarten* (Frankfurt, 1513) (*Den Roseghaert van den Bevruchten Vrouwen*, 1516), J. Rueff's *De Conceptu et Generatione Hominis* (Frankfurt, 1580) (*'t Boeck van de Vroet-wijfs*, 1591), F. Mauriceau's *Traité des Maladies des Femmes Grosses* (Paris, 1668) (*Tractaet van de Siekten der Zwangere Vrouwen*, 1683), and the works of H. van Deventer.

76. For a comparison with Spain, see ch. 5 in this volume by Teresa Ortiz.

77. Van der Waals, 'Doorbraken in de verloskunde', in Dupuis *et al.*, *Een Kind Onder het Hart*, 27–31; A.J.M. Lamers, *Hendrik van Deventer Medicinae Doctor 1651–1724. Leven en Werken* (Assen, 1946).

78. J. Denys, *Verhandelingen over het Ampt der Vroed-vrouwen en Vroedmeesters* (Leiden, 1733), 1. Cited Van der Borg, 'Beeldvorming over vroedvrouwen', 6.

79. C. Terne, *Lucina. Ontdekkende de Waare Oorzaken* (Leiden, 1784).

80. E. van der Borg, 'Het ontslag van de stadsvroedmeester Cornelius Terne. Wedijverende beroepsgroepen te Leiden in de achttiende eeuw', *Holland*, 2 (1990), 109–20.

81. Bik, *Vijf Eeuwen Medisch Leven in een Hollandse Stad*, 369.

82. GAD, ONGD, Register van resoluties van het college van regenten, 1756–85, 28 March 1772, 9 Oct. 1773.

83. Van Andel, 'Vroedvrouwenbordjes'.

84. See M.J. van Lieburg and Hilary Marland, 'Midwife regulation, education, and practice in the Netherlands during the nineteenth century', *Medical History*, 33 (1989), 296–317.

85. More sombre interpretations of the decline of the midwife owe much to an over-reliance on Anglo-American sources when, clearly, the division of labour between midwives and medical men took a very different course in Holland, as reflected in midwives' working situations today. The negative image of eighteenth-century midwives is based largely on the writings of nineteenth-century and early twentieth-century 'midwife opponents', particularly A. Geyl (1853–1914), surgeon, gynaecologist and would-be medical historian, who published a series of articles attacking midwives in the *Medisch Weekblad* in 1897 and 1911. His polemical articles, coinciding closely with the publication of reports on the state of midwife practice at the turn of the twentieth century, discussed the status of midwives in the fifteenth to eighteenth centuries, concluding that they were generally unskilled, brutal, careless and lacking in integrity. A. Geyl, 'Over de opleiding en maatschappelijke positie der vroedvrouwen in de 17de en 18de eeuw', *Medisch Weekblad*, 4 (1897–98), 6–10, 18–26, 35–41, 53–62, 67–73, 86–90, 115–7, and *idem*, 'Beschouwingen en mededeelingen over vroedvrouwen uit de 15de tot en met de 18de eeuw', *Medisch Weekblad*, 18 (1911–12), 227–31, 266–70, 279–83, 318–22, 341–5, 353–7, 368–9, 377–81, 401–6, 414–17, 425–30. Yet Geyl's pronouncements seem untypical of both medical opinion in the eighteenth century or at the turn of the twentieth. For the relationship between doctors and midwives in the nineteenth and early twentieth centuries, see H. Marland, 'The guardians of normal birth: the debate on the standard and status of the midwife in the Netherlands around 1900', in E. Abraham-van der Mark (ed.) *Successful Home Birth and Midwifery: The Dutch Obstetric Model* (Amherst, MA, forthcoming).

86. See Van Lieburg and Marland, 'Midwife regulation, education, and practice'; Marland, 'The guardians of normal birth'.

87.   See the essays in Abraham-van der Mark (ed.) *Successful Home Birth and Midwifery,* J.J. Klinkert, *Verloskundigen en Artsen Verleden en Heden van Enkele Professionele Beroepen in de Gezondheidzorg* (Alphen aan den Rijn and Brussels, 1980); J.M.L. Phaff, 'De Nederlandse verloskunde in Europees perspectief', in P.E. Treffers *et al.* (eds) *Voortgang en Visie. 25 Jaar Verloskunde en Gynaecologie* (Utrecht, Antwerp and Bohn, 1983); L.A.M. van der Hulst (ed.) *De Vroedvrouw, de Spil van de Verloskunde* (Bilthoven, 1991).

Select bibliography

This select bibliography is intended to serve as an introductory guide to further reading. It deals primarily with the history of midwives in the early modern period, and not the associated topics of women's medical practice, the medical professions, obstetrics and gynaecology, women's health, maternal and infant mortality and welfare, the family, or the history of child-rearing. It is far from exhaustive and for a more detailed literature the reader should refer to *Current Work in the History of Medicine*. Short sections have been included here on topics not covered in this volume, namely the 'United States' and 'Medieval and Renaissance midwifery'.

Britain

Aveling, J.H. (1872) *English Midwives. Their History and Prospects*, London, repr. New York, 1977.

Burnby, J.G.L. (1991) 'The apothecary and developments in the practice of midwifery', *Medical Historian – Bulletin of the Liverpool Medical History Society* 4: 10–19.

Chamberlain, M. (1981) *Old Wives' Tales. Their History, Remedies and Spells*, London.

Clark, A. (1919) *Working Life of Women in the Seventeenth Century*, London, repr. 1968, 1991.

Donnison, J. (1977) *Midwives and Medical Men. A History of Inter-Professional Rivalries and Women's Rights*, London, 2nd edn 1988.

Eccles, A. (1977) 'The early use of English for midwiferies 1500–1700', *Neuphilologische Mitteilungen* 78: 377–85.

—— (1982) *Obstetrics and Gynaecology in Tudor and Stuart England*, London.

Erickson, R.A. (1982) '"The books of generation": some observations on the style of the British midwife books, 1671–1764', in P.-G. Boucé (ed.) *Sexuality in Eighteenth-Century Britain*, Manchester, 74–94.

Evenden-Nagy, D. (1991) 'Seventeenth-century London midwives: their training, licensing and social profile', unpub. PhD diss., McMaster University.

Fildes, V. (ed.) *Women as Mothers in Pre-Industrial England*, London and New York.

Forbes, T.R. (1964) 'The regulation of English midwives in the sixteenth and seventeenth centuries', *Medical History* 8: 235–44.

—— (1971) 'The regulation of English midwives in the eighteenth and nineteenth centuries', *Medical History* 15: 352–62.

—— (1988) 'A jury of matrons', *Medical History* 32: 22–33.

214

Giardina Hess, A. (1994) 'Social aspects of local midwifery practice in latter seventeenth-century England and New England', unpub. PhD thesis, University of Cambridge.

Gordon, J.E. (1975) 'Mrs Elizabeth Cellier – the "Popish Midwife" of the Restoration', *Midwife, Health Visitor and Community Nurse* 11(5): 139–42.

Guy, J.R. (1982) 'The episcopal licensing of physicians, surgeons and midwives', *Bulletin of the History of Medicine* 56: 528–42.

Harley, D.N. (1981) 'Ignorant midwives – a persistent stereotype', *Bulletin of the Society for the Social History of Medicine* 28: 6–9.

—— (1993) 'Ethics and dispute behaviour in the career of Henry Bracken of Lancaster, surgeon, physician and manmidwife', in R. Baker, D. Porter and R. Porter (eds) *The Codification of Medical Morality in the Eighteenth and Nineteenth Centuries*, Dordrecht, 47–71.

—— (forthcoming) 'Providence and the problem of cunning folk in England', in J. Barry (ed.) *Essays on Witchcraft.*

King, H. (1986) 'Agnodike and the profession of medicine', *Proceedings of the Cambridge Philological Society* 32: 53–77.

Lane, J. (1987) 'A provincial surgeon and his obstetric practice: Thomas W. Jones of Henley-in-Arden, 1764–1846', *Medical History* 31: 333–48.

Lewis, J.S. (1986) *In the Family Way. Childbearing in the British Aristocracy, 1760–1860*, New Brunswick, NJ.

Loudon, I. (1986) 'Deaths in childbed from the eighteenth century to 1935', *Medical History* 30: 1–41.

—— (1986) *Medical Care and the General Practitioner 1750–1850*, Oxford.

Pelling, M. (1987) 'Medical practice in early modern England: trade or profession?', in W. Prest (ed.) *The Professions in Early Modern England*, London, 90–128.

Pelling, M. and Webster, C. (1979) 'Medical practitioners', in C. Webster (ed.) *Health, Medicine and Mortality in the Sixteenth Century*, Cambridge, 165–235.

Porter, R. (1987) 'A touch of danger: the man-midwife as sexual predator', in G.S. Rousseau and R. Porter (eds) *Sexual Underworlds of the Enlightenment*, Manchester, 206–32.

Schnorrenberg, B.B. (1981) 'Is childbirth any place for a woman? The decline of midwifery in eighteenth-century England', *Studies in Eighteenth-Century Culture* 10: 393–408.

Shorter, E. (1985) 'The management of normal deliveries and the generation of William Hunter', in W.F. Bynum and R. Porter (eds) *William Hunter and the Eighteenth-Century Medical World*, Cambridge, 371–83.

Smith, H. (1976) 'Gynaecology and ideology in seventeenth-century England', in B. Carroll (ed.) *Liberating Women's History*, Urbana, IL, 97–114.

Spencer, H.R. (1927) *The History of British Midwifery from 1650 to 1800*, London, repr. New York, 1978.

Towler, J. and Bramall, J. (1986) *Midwives in History and Society*, London.

Versluysen, M.C. (1980) 'Old wives' tales? Women healers in English history', in C. Davies (ed.) *Rewriting Nursing History*, London, 189–97.

—— (1981) 'Midwives, medical men and "poor women labouring of child": lying-in hospitals in eighteenth century London', in H. Roberts (ed.) *Women, Health and Reproduction*, London, 18–49.

Wilson, A. (1982) 'Childbirth in seventeenth- and eighteenth-century England', unpub. PhD thesis, University of Sussex.

—— (1983) 'Ignorant midwives – a rejoinder', *Bulletin of the Society for the Social History of Medicine* 32: 46–9.

—— (1985) 'William Hunter and the varieties of man-midwifery', in W.F. Bynum and R. Porter (eds) *William Hunter and the Eighteenth-Century Medical World*, Cambridge, 343–69.

—— (1985) 'Participant or patient? Seventeenth-century childbirth from the mother's point of view', in R. Porter (ed.) *Patients and Practitioners. Lay Perceptions of Medicine in Pre-Industrial Society*, Cambridge, 129–44.

—— (1990) 'The ceremony of childbirth and its interpretation', in V. Fildes (ed.) *Women as Mothers in Pre-Industrial England*, London and New York, 68–107.

—— (forthcoming) *A Safe Deliverance: Ritual and Conflict in English Childbirth, 1600–1750*, Cambridge.

France

Darmon, P. (1977) *Le mythe de la procréation à l'âge baroque*, Paris, repr. 1986.

Dumont, M. and Morel, P. (1968) *Histoire de l'obstétrique et de la gynécologie*, Lyon.

Gelbart, N. (1989) 'Mme du Coudray's manual for midwives: the politics of Enlightenment obstetrics', *Proceedings of the Annual Meeting of the Western Society for French History* 16: 389–96.

—— (forthcoming) 'Delivering the goods: patriotism, property and the midwife mission of Mme du Coudray', in J. Brewer and S. Staves (eds) *Changing Conceptions of Property in Early Modern Europe.*

—— (forthcoming) *Delivering the Goods: The Midwife Mission of Mme du Coudray in 18th Century France.*

Gélis, J. (1976) 'L'accouchement au XVIIIe siècle. Pratiques traditionnelles et contrôle médical', *Ethnologie Française* 6: 325–40.

—— (1977) 'Sage-femmes et accoucheurs: l'obstétrique populaire aux XVIIe et XVIIIe siècles', *Annales E.S.C.* 32: 927–57.

—— (1977) 'La formation des accoucheurs et des sage-femmes aux XVIIe et XVIIIe siècles: evolution d'un matériel et d'une pédagogie', *Annales de Démographie Historique*, 153–80.

—— (1980) 'L'Enquête de 1786 sur les "Sage-femmes du Royaume"', *Annales de Démographie Historique*, 299–343.

—— (1980) 'Regard sur l'Europe médicale des Lumières: la collaboration internationale des accoucheurs et la formation des sages-femmes au XVIIIe siècle', in A.E. Imhof (ed.) *Mensch und Gesundheit in der Geschichte*, Husum, 279–99.

—— (1984) *L'Arbre et le Fruit. La naissance dans l'occident moderne (XVIe–XIXe siècle)*, Paris.

—— (1985) 'Les villes et la diffusion de la conscience moderne du corps: le révalateur de l'obstétrique (XVIe–XVIIIe siècles)', *Annales de Démographie Historique* 45: 2–13.

—— (1988) *La sage femme ou le médecin. Une nouvelle conception de la vie*, Paris.

Gélis, J., Laget, M. and Morel, M.-F. (1978) *Entrer dan la vie: Naissances et enfances dan la France traditionelle*, Paris.

Gibson, W. (1989) *Women in Seventeenth-Century France*, Basingstoke.

Kalisch, P.A., Scobey, M. and Kalisch, B.J. (1981) 'Louyse Bourgeois and the emergence of modern midwifery', *Journal of Nurse Midwifery* 26 (4): 3–17.

Kniebiehler, Y. and Fouquet, C. (1983) *La femme et les médecins. Analyse historique*, Paris.

Laget, M. (1977) 'La naissance aux siècles classiques. Pratique des accouchements et attitudes collectives en France aux XVIIème et XVIIIème siècles', *Annales E.S.C.*, vol. 32: 958–93.

—— (1980) 'Childbirth in seventeenth- and eighteenth-century France: obstetrical practices and collective attitudes', in R. Forster and O. Ranum (eds) *Medicine and Society in France. Selections from the Annales*, vol. 6, Baltimore, 137–76.

—— (1982) *Naissances: L'accouchement avant l'âge de la clinique*, Paris.

Perkins, W. (1988) 'Midwives versus doctors: the case of Louise Bourgeois', *The Seventeenth Century* 3: 135–57.

—— (1989) 'The relationship between midwife and client in the works of Louise Bourgeois', *Seventeenth-Century French Studies* 11: 28–45.

Petrelli, R.L. (1971) 'The regulation of French midwifery during the *ancien régime*', *Journal of the History of Medicine* 26: 276–92.

Germany

Birkelbach, D., Eifert, C. and Leuken, S. (1981) 'Zur Entwicklung des Hebammenwesens vom 14. bis zum 16. Jahrhundert am Beispiel der Regensburger Hebammenordnungen', in *Frauengeschichte: Dokumentation des 3. Historikerinnentreffens in Bielefeld, April 1981*, Munich.

Buckhard, G. (1912) *Die deutschen Hebammenordnungen von ihren ersten Anfängen bis auf die Neuzeit*, Leipzig.

Elmeer, G.P. (1964) 'The regulation of German midwifery in the 14th, 15th and 16th centuries', unpub. MD thesis, Yale University School of Medicine.

Gubalke, W. (1964) *Die Hebamme im Wandel der Zeiten: Ein Beitrag zur Geschichte des Hebammenwesens*, Hanover.

Haberling, E. (1940) *Beiträge zur Geschichte des Hebammenstandes*, Berlin.

Hanke, G. (1989) 'Die Dachauer Hebammen vom 17. bis zum Beginn des 20. Jahrhunderts', *Amperland* 25 (1,2): 192–202, 237–43.

Horsley, R.J. and Horsley, R.A. (1987) 'On the trial of the "witches": wise women, midwives and the European witch hunts', in M. Burkhard and E. Waldstein (eds) *Women in German Yearbook 3: Feminist Studies and German Culture*, Washington, DC, 1–28.

Labouvie, E. (1992) 'Selbstverwaltete Geburt. Landhebammen zwischen Macht und Reglementierung (17.–19. Jahrhundert)', *Geschichte und Gesellschaft* 18: 477–506.

Lefftz, J.-P. (1985) *L'art des accouchements à Strasbourg et son rayonnement européen de la Renaissance au Siècle des Lumières*, Strasbourg.

Menssen, B. and Taube, A.-M. (1980) 'Hebammen und Hebammenwesen in Oldenburg in der zweiten Hälfte des 18. und zu Beginn des 19. Jahrhunderts', in E. Hinrichs and W. Norden (eds) *Regionalgeschichte: Probleme und Beispiele*, Hildesheim, 165–224.

Meyer, K. (1985) *Zur Geschichte des Hebammenwesens im Kanton Bern*, Berner Beiträge zur Geschichte der Medizin und der Naturwissenschaften, Neue Folge, 11, Bern.

Tatlock, L. (1992) 'Speculum feminarum: gendered perspectives on obstetrics and gynaecology in early modern Germany', *Signs: Journal of Women in Culture and Society* 17: 725–60.

Tutzke, D. (1956) 'Über statistische Untersuchungen als Beitrag zur Geschichte des Hebammenwesens im ausgehenden 18. Jahrhundert', *Centaurus* 4: 351–9.

—— (1961) 'Zur materiellen Lage der Niederlausitzer Hebammen im 18. Jahrhundert', *Sudhoffs Archiv* 45: 334–40.

—— (1961) 'Die Entwicklung des Hebammenwesens in der Oberlausitz bis zum Beginn des 19. Jahrhunderts', *Oberlausitzer Forschung*: 284–306.

Wiesner, M.E. (1983) 'Early modern midwifery: a case study', *International Journal of Women's Studies* 6: 26–43.

—— (1986) 'Hospitals, healing, and health care', in M.E. Wiesner (ed.) *Working Women in Renaissance Germany*, New Brunswick, NJ, 37–73.

Select bibliography

Wille, F.C. (1934) *Über Stand und Ausbildung der Hebammen im 17. und 18. Jahrhundert in Chur-Brandenburg*, Berlin.

Italy

✝ Accati, L., Maher, V. and Pomata, G. (eds) (1980) *Parto e Maternità: momenti della autobiografia femminile, Quaderni Storici*, 44.

Caffaratto, M.T. (1970) 'L'assistenza ostetrica in Piemonte dalle origini ai nostri tempi', *Giornale di Batteriologia, Virologia ed Immunologia* 1 (6): 176–209.

Calvi, G. (1983) 'Manuali delle levatrici (sec. XVII–XVIII)', *Memoria. Rivista di Storia delle Donne* 3: 108–13.

Chinosi, L. (ed.) (1985) *Nascere a Venezia. Dalla Serenissima alla Prima Guerra Mondiale*, Torino.

Filippini, N.M. (1983) *Noi, quelle dei campi. Identità e rappresentazione di sé delle contadine veronesi del primo novecento*, Torino.

—— (1984) 'Con le mani disarmate: la vicenda di una levatrice-chirurgo veneziana (1800–1802)', *Sanità, Scienza e Storia* 2: 156–72.

—— (1985) 'Levatrici e ostetricanti a Venezia tra sette e ottocento', *Quaderni Storici* 58: 149–80.

—— (1985) 'Il bambino prezioso: maternità e infanzia negli interventi istituzionali del primo ottocento', in L. Chinosi (ed.) *Nascere a Venezia. Dalla Serenissima alla Prima Guerra Mondiale*, Torino, 28–40.

—— (1985) 'L'assistenza al parto nel primo ottocento: appunti sull' intervento istituzionale', in A. Oakley *et al.*, *Le Culture del parto*, Milano, 63–73.

—— (1992) 'Gli ospizi per partorienti e i reparti di maternità tra sette e ottocento', in M.L. Berti and M. Bressan (eds) *Gli Ospedali in Area Padana tra settecento e novecento, Sanità, Scienza e Storia*, Milano, 395–411.

—— (1993) 'La naissance extraordinaire. Transformations culturelles et sociales dans la pratique de la césarienne, entre dix-huitième et dix-neuvième siècle', thesis Doctorat en Histoire, École des Hautes Études en Sciences Sociales, Paris.

Fiocca, G. (1983) 'Mammane e medici a Roma tra sette e ottocento', in A. Lazzarini (ed.) *Economia e società nella storia dell' Italia Contemporanea. Fonti e metodi di ricerca*, Roma, 143–53.

Lonni, A. (1984) 'Il mestiere di ostetrica al confine tra il lecito e l'illecito', *Società e Storia* 25: 563–90.

Nardi, G.M. (1954) *Il Pensiero Ostetrico-Ginecologico nei secoli*, Milano.

Oakley, A. *et al.* (1985) *Le Culture del parto*, Milano.

Pancino, C. (1981) 'La comare levatrice. Crisi di un mestiere nel XVIII secolo', *Società e Storia* 13: 593–638.

—— (1984) *Il Bambino e l'acqua sporca. Storia dell' assistenza al parto dalle mammane alle ostetriche (secoli XVI–XIX)*, Milano.

Parma, A. (1984) 'Didattica e pratica ostetrica in Lombardia (1765–1791)', *Sanità, Scienza e Storia* 2: 101–55.

Pillon, D. (1981) 'La comare istruita nel suo ufficio. Alcune notizie sulle levatrici fra il '600 e il '700', *Atti dell' Istituto Veneto di Scienze, Lettere e Arti* 140: 65–78.

—— (1982) 'Medici e mammane nel '700. La scuola ostetrica di Padova', *Schema* 5: 159–65.

Pizzini, F. (ed.) (1981) *Sulla scena del parto: luoghi, figure e pratiche*, Milano.

Pomata, G. (1981) 'Barbieri e comari', in *Medicina, erbe e magia*, Milano.

Premuda, L. (1958) *Personaggi e vicende dell' ostetricia e della ginecologia nello studio di Padova*, Padova.

Viana, O. and Vozza, F. (1933) *L'Ostetricia e la Ginecologia in Italia*, Milano.

The Netherlands

Abraham-van der Mark, E. (1990) 'Dutch midwifery in the past and present', unpub. paper, Amsterdam.

Bik, J.G.W.F. (1955) *Vijf Eeuwen Medisch Leven in een Hollandse Stad*, MD thesis, University of Amsterdam.

Borg, E. van der (1988) 'Beeldvorming over vroedvrouwen in de Noordelijke Nederlanden (1600–1900)', *Verzorging* 3: 2–17.

—— (1990) 'Wijze volksvrouwen. Beroepsvorming van vroedvrouwen in Nederland tot 1865', *Focaal. Tijdschrift voor Antropologie* 14: 13–34.

Borg, H.A. (1992) *Vroedvrouwen: Beeld en Beroep. Ontwikkelingen in het Vroedvrouwschap in Leideun, Arnhem, 's-Hertogenbosch en Leewarden, 1650–1865*, Wageningen.

Dupuis, H.M. et al. (1987) *Een Kind Onder het Hart. Verloskunde, Volksgeloof, Gezin, Seksualiteit en Moraal Vroeger en Nu*, Amsterdam.

Frijhoff, W. (1983) 'Non satis dignitatis . . . Over de maatschappelijke status van geneeskundigen tijdens de Republiek', *Tijdschrift voor Geschiedenis* 96: 379–406.

—— (1985) 'Vrouw Schrader's beroepsjournal: overwegingen bij een publikatie over arbeidspraktijk in het verleden', *Tijdschrift voor de Geschiedenis der Geneeskunde, Natuurwetenschappen, Wiskunde en Techniek* 8: 27–38.

Hallema, A. (1955) 'Vroedvrouwen in stad en dorp in het westen van Noord-Brabant', *Nederlands Tijdschrift voor Geneeskunde* 99 (III): 2660–7.

Van Lieburg, M.J. (1982) 'Het verloskundig onderwijs te Rotterdam vóór 1828', in E. Scholte, M.J. van Lieburg and R.O. Aalbersberg, *Rijkskweekschool voor Vroedvrouwen te Rotterdam*, Leidschendam, 5–20.

—— (ed.) (1984) *C.G. Schrader's Memoryboeck van de Vrouwens. Het Notitieboek van een Friese Vroedvrouw 1693–1745* (with an obstetric commentary by G.J. Kloosterman), Amsterdam.

Van Lieburg, M.J. and Marland, H. (1989) 'Elisabeth en Neeltje van Putten: twee 18e-eeuwse grensgangers tussen de beroepsvelden van vroedvrouw en vroedmeester', *Tijdschrift voor de Geschiedenis der Geneeskunde, Natuurwetenschappen, Wiskunde en Techniek* 12: 181–97.

Marland, H. (1987) 'All well for mother and child. The notebook and practice of Vrouw Catharina Schrader, 1693–1745', *Nursing Times* 83 (7 Oct.): 49–51.

Marland, H., Van Lieburg, M.J. and Kloosterman, G.J. (1987) *'Mother and Child Were Saved'. The Memoirs (1693–1740) of the Frisian Midwife Catharina Schrader*, Amsterdam.

Post, C. R. (1985) 'De Amsterdamse vroedvrouw uit de 18de eeuw', *Bijdragen tot de Geschiedenis der Geneeskunde* 36: 1–8.

Van Reeuwijk, A.J. (1941) *Vroedkunde en Vroedvrouwen in de Nederlanden in de 17e en 18e Eeuw*, Amsterdam.

Ringoir, D.J.B. (1973) *Plattelandschirurgie in de 17de en 18de Eeuw. De Rekeningboeken van de 18de-Eeuwse Durgerdamse Chirurgijn Anthony Egberts*, Amsterdam.

Schilling, H. (1980) 'Religion und Gesellschaft in der calvinistischen Republik der Vereinigten Niederlande – "Öffentlichkeitskirche" und Säkularisation; Ehe und Hebammenwesen; Presbyterien und politische Partizipation', in F. Petri (ed.) *Kirche und gesellschaftlicher wandel in deutschen und niederländischen Städten der werdenden Neuzeit*, Köln, 197–250.

Spain

Cabré, M. (1988) 'Formes de cultura femenina a la Catalunya medieval', in M. Nash (ed.) *Mes enllà del silenci: Les dones a la història de Catalunya*, Barcelona, 31–5.

Conejo Ramilo, R. (1970) 'Los cirujanos y las matronas en Archidona durante la Edad Moderna', *Asclepio* 22: 125–9.

Cuadri Duque, M.J. (1985) 'La ciencia y el arte de partear. Antecedentes históricos de la enfermería maternal', *Revista Rol de Enfermería* 8 (84–5): 13–6.

García Herrero, M.C. (1989) 'Administrar del parto y recibir a la criatura'. Aportación al estudio de la obstetricia bajomedieval', in *Aragón en la Baja Edad Media. Homenaje al profesor Antonio Ubieto*, Zaragoza, vol. 8: 283–92.

Levine Melammed, R. (forthcoming) 'A sixteenth-century Castilian Midwife and her encounter with the Inquisition', in R.B. Waddington and A.H. Williamson (eds) *The Expulsion of the Jews: 1492 and After*, New York.

López Beltrán, M. (forthcoming) 'Espacio público y espacio privado: el trabajo extradoméstico en Málaga en el tránsito a la modernidad', in B. Villar (ed.) *Los espacios de las mujeres en el Antiguo Régimen. Inercias y cambios*, Málaga.

López-Cordón, M.V. (1982) 'La situación de la mujer a finales del Antiguo Régimen (1760–1860)', in R. Capel (ed.) *Mujer y sociedad en España. 1700–1975*, Madrid, 93–5.

Ortiz, T. (1992) 'Luisa Rosado, una matrona en la España de la Ilustración', *Dynamis* 12: 323–47.

Palacios Alcalde, M. (1987) 'Formas marginales de trabajo femenino en la Andalucía moderna', *VI Jornadas de Investigación Interdisciplinaria sobre la mujer. El trabajo de las mujeres: siglos XVI–XX*, Madrid, 83–92.

Riera, J. (1973) 'Dos parteras sevillanas', *IV Congreso Español de Historia de la Medicina, Granada, abril 1973*, vol. 1, Granada, 63–7.

Sánchez Arcas, R. (1970) 'La sustitución de las matronas por los cirujanos en Europa y España (S. XVII y sucesivos)', *Acta Obstétrica y Ginecológia Hispano-Lusitana* 18: 238–48.

—— (1971) 'Las comadronas españolas a través de los tiempos', *Surgere* 144: 2–19, and 'Conclusión', *Surgere* 145: 2–24.

Usandizaga, M. (1944) *Historia de la obstetricia y la ginecología en España*, Santander.

United States

Augur, H. (1930) *An American Jezebel: The Life of Anne Hutchinson*, New York.

Donegan, J.B. (1978) *Women and Men Midwives. Medicine, Morality, and Misogyny in Early America*, Westport, CT and London.

—— (1984) '"Safe delivered", but by whom? Midwives and men-midwives in early America', in J.W. Leavitt (ed.) *Women and Health in America*, Madison, WI, 302–17.

Dye, N.S. (1980) 'History of childbirth in America', *Signs: Journal of Women in Culture and Society* 6: 97–108.

Fox, C. E. (1966) 'Pregnancy, childbirth and early infancy in Anglo-American culture: 1675–1830', unpub. PhD diss., University of Pennsylvania.

Giardina Hess, A. (1994) 'Social aspects of local midwifery practice in latter seventeenth-century England and New England', unpub. PhD thesis, University of Cambridge.

Learned, M.D. and Bride, C. F. (eds) (n.d.) 'Susanna Müller, 1756–1815. An Old German Midwife's Record', n.p. (located at the Library of the College of Physicians of Philadelphia).

Leavitt, J.W. (1983) '"Science" enters the birthing room: obstetrics in America since the eighteenth century', *Journal of American History* 70: 281–304.

—— (ed.) (1984) *Women and Health in America*, Madison, WI.

—— (1986) *Brought to Bed. Childbearing in America 1750 to 1950*, New York and Oxford.

McGregor, D.K. (1989) '"Childbirth-travells" and "spiritual estates". Anne Hutchinson and colonial Boston, 1634–1638', *Caduceus* 5 (4): 1–33.

McMillan, S. (1990) *Motherhood in the Old South: Pregnancy, Childbirth, and Infant Rearing*, Baton Rouge, LA.

Nash, C. E. (1904) *The History of Augusta: First Settlements and Early Days as a Town Including the Diary of Mrs. Martha Moore Ballard*, Augusta, ME.

Rugg, W.K. (1930) *Unafraid: A Life of Anne Hutchinson*, Boston.

Scholten, C. M. (1977) '"On the importance of the obstetrick art": changing customs of childbirth in America, 1760–1825', *William and Mary Quarterly* 34: 426–45.

—— (1985) *Childbearing in American Society, 1650–1850*, ed. by L. Withey, New York and London.

Spruill, J.C. (1938) *Women's Life and Work in the Southern Colonies*, New York.

Thoms, H. (1933) *Chapters in American Obstetrics*, Springfield, IL.

Ulrich, L.T. (1989) '"The living mother of a living child": midwifery and mortality in post-revolutionary New England', *William and Mary Quarterly* 46: 27–48.

—— (1990) *A Midwife's Tale: The Life of Martha Ballard, Based on Her Diary, 1785–1812*, New York.

Wertz, R.W. and Wertz, D.C. (1979) *Lying-In. A History of Childbirth in America*, New York.

General and international

Achterberg, J. (1990) *Woman as Healer. A Panoramic Survey of the Healing Activities of Women from Prehistoric Times to the Present*, Boston.

Ackerknecht, E.H. (1974) 'Zur Geschichte der Hembammen', *Gesnerus* 31: 181–92.

—— (1976) 'Midwives as experts in court', *Bulletin New York Academy of Medicine* 52: 1224–8.

Ackerknecht, E.H. and Fischer-Homberger, E. (1977) 'Five made it, one not. The rise of medical craftsmen to academic status during the 19th century', *Clio Medica* 12: 255–67.

Bourdillon, H. (1988) *Women as Healers. A History of Women and Medicine*, Cambridge.

Carter, J. and Duriez, T. (1986) *With Child. Birth Through the Ages*, Edinburgh.

Cutter, I. and Viets, H. (1964) *A Short History of Midwifery*, Philadelphia.

Ehrenreich, B. and English, D. (1973) *Witches, Midwives, and Nurses: A History of Women Healers*, Old Westbury, NY.

Forbes, T.R. (1962) 'Midwifery and witchcraft', *Journal of the History of Medicine* 17: 264–83.

—— (1966) *The Midwife and the Witch*, New York.

Gélis, J. (1984) *L'Arbre et le Fruit. La naissance dans l'occident moderne (XVIe–XIXe siècle)*, Paris.

—— (1988) *La sage femme ou le médecin. Une nouvelle conception de la vie*, Paris.

—— (1991) *History of Childbirth. Fertility, Pregnancy and Birth in Early Modern Europe*, Cambridge.

Graham, H. (1950) *Eternal Eve. The Mysteries of Birth and the Customs that Surround It*, London.

Harley, D. (1990) 'Historians as demonologists: the myth of the midwife-witch', *Social History of Medicine* 3: 1–26.

Hurd-Mead, K.C. (1938) *A History of Women in Medicine*, London, repr. New York, 1977.

Laforge, H. (1985) *Histoire de la sage-femme dans la région de Québec*, Quebec.

Oakley, A. (1976) 'Wisewomen and medicine men: changes in the management of childbirth', in J. Mitchell and A. Oakley (eds) *The Rights and Wrongs of Women*, Harmondsworth, 17–58.

Radcliffe, W. (1967) *Milestones in Midwifery*, Bristol.

Shorter, E. (1982) *A History of Women's Bodies*, New York.

Snapper, I. (1963) 'Midwifery, past and present', *Bulletin New York Academy of Medicine* 39: 503–32.

Speert, H. (1958) *Obstetric and Gynecologic Milestones: Essays in Eponymy*, New York.

—— (1973) *Iconographia Gyniatrica. A Pictoral History of Gynaecology and Obstetrics*, Philadelphia.

Towler, J. and Bramall, J. (1986) *Midwives in History and Society*, London.

Witkowski, G.J. (1891) *Accoucheurs et sage-femmes célèbres*, Paris.

Medieval and Renaissance midwifery

Benedek, T.G. (1977) 'The changing relationship between midwives and physicians during the Renaissance', *Bulletin of the History of Medicine* 51: 550–64.

Benton, J.F. (1985) 'Trotula, women's problems, and the professionalization of medicine in the Middle Ages', *Bulletin of the History of Medicine* 59: 30–53.

Biller, P. (1986) 'Childbirth in the Middle Ages', *History Today* 36: 42–9.

Delva, A. (1983) *Vrouwengeneeskunde in Vlaanderen tijdens de late middeleeuwen*, Bruges (Genootschap voor Geschiedenis).

Diepgen, P. (1963) *Frau und Frauenheilkunde in de Kultur des Mittelalters*, Stuttgart.

Green, M.H. (1989) 'Women's medical practice and health care in Medieval Europe: review essay', *Signs: Journal of Women in Culture and Society* 14: 434–73.

—— (forthcoming) 'Problems of documenting medieval women's medical practice', in *Practical Medicine from Salerno to the Black Death*, Cambridge.

Greilsammer, M. (1984) 'The condition of women in Flanders and Brabant at the end of the Middle Ages', unpub. PhD diss., Hebrew University, Jerusalem.

—— (1991) 'The midwife, the priest, and the physician: the subjugation of midwives in the Low Countries at the end of the Middle Ages', *Journal of Medieval and Renaissance Studies* 21: 285–329.

Jacobsen, G. (1984) 'Pregnancy and childbirth in the medieval north: a topography of sources and a preliminary study', *Scandinavian Journal of History* 9: 91–111.

Laurent, S. (1989) *Naître au Moyen Age: de la conception à la naissance: la grossesse et l'accouchement (XIIe-XVe siècles)*, Paris.

Rowland, B. (1981) *The Medieval Woman's Guide to Health: The First English Gynaecological Handbook*, London.

Saunier, A. (1987) 'Le visiteur, les femmes et les "obstetrices" des paroisses de l'archidiaconé de Josas de 1458 à 1470', in *Santé, médecine et assistance au moyen âge*, Actes du 110e Congrès National de Sociétés Savantes, Montpellier, 1985, Paris, 43–62.

Sigal, P.A. (1987) 'La grossesse, l'accouchement et l'attitude envers l'enfant mortné à la fin du moyen âge d'après les récits de miracles', in *Santé, médecine et assistance au moyen âge*, Actes du 110e Congrès National de Sociétés Savantes, Montpellier, 1985, Paris, 23–41.

Stuard, S.M. (1975) 'Dame Trot', *Signs: Journal of Women in Culture and Society* 1: 537–42.

Index